The Politics of the Pandemic in Eastern Europe and Eurasia

This book provides a comprehensive overview of the political impact of the COVID-19 emergency in central and eastern Europe and Eurasia. Offering a theoretical framework linking the authoritarian, post-Soviet institutional legacy with patterns of political behavior, support and governments' policies, the expert contributors argue that domestic political regimes mediate and shape citizens' perceptions of public health crises, and the very regimes' political survival. The authors explore how the pandemic affected regime change, government stability, business groups and civil societies in more than 15 countries of the region from the discovery of the virus to the vaccination rollout. The studies rely on a broad range of empirical evidence from the region – survey, state statistics, ethnography and interviews.

Formulating, explaining and empirically testing the causal mechanisms that drive political accountability and support through a cross-country comparison and in-depth case studies of popular and electoral support attempting to highlight any patterns specific to the region, this book contributes to studies of governance and political accountability in low-trust countries with authoritarian legacies and proclivities. Drawing on an interdisciplinary approach that brings together area studies, history, sociology and political science, it will also be of value to those interested in systematic effect of political regimes on handling public health crises.

Margarita Zavadskaya is a senior research fellow at the Finnish Institute of International Affairs (FIIA) and researcher at the Aleksanteri Institute, University of Helsinki. She obtained her doctoral degree in social and political sciences from the European University Institute (EUI) in Florence, Italy.

Studies in Contemporary Russia
Series Editor: Markku Kivinen

Studies in Contemporary Russia is a series of cutting-edge, contemporary studies. These monographs, joint publications and edited volumes branch out into various disciplines, innovatively combining research methods and theories to approach the core questions of Russian modernisation; how do the dynamics of resources and rules affect the Russian economy and what are the prospects and needs of diversification? What is the impact of the changing state-society relationship? How does the emerging welfare regime work? What is the role of Russia in contemporary international relations? How should we understand the present Russian political system? What is the philosophical background of modernisation as a whole and its Russian version in particular?

The variety of opinions on these issues is vast. Some see increasingly less difference between contemporary Russia and the Soviet Union while, at the other extreme, prominent experts regard Russia as a 'more or less' normal European state. At the same time new variants of modernisation are espoused as a result of Russian membership of the global BRIC powers. Combining aspects of Western and Soviet modernisation with some anti-modern or traditional tendencies the Russian case is ideal for probing deeper into the evolving nature of modernisation. Which of the available courses Russia will follow remains an open question, but these trajectories provide the alternatives available for discussion in this ground-breaking and authoritative series.

The editor and the editorial board of the series represent the Finnish Centre of Excellence in Russian Studies: Choices of Russian Modernisation.

Stalin Era Intellectuals
Culture and Stalinism
Edited by Vesa Oittinen and Elina Viljanen

The Politics of the Pandemic in Eastern Europe and Eurasia
Blame Game and Governance
Edited by Margarita Zavadskaya

For more information about this series, please visit: www.routledge.com/series/ASHSER-1421

The Politics of the Pandemic in Eastern Europe and Eurasia

Blame Game and Governance

Edited by
Margarita Zavadskaya

Routledge
Taylor & Francis Group
LONDON AND NEW YORK

First published 2024
by Routledge
4 Park Square, Milton Park, Abingdon, Oxon OX14 4RN

and by Routledge
605 Third Avenue, New York, NY 10158

Routledge is an imprint of the Taylor & Francis Group, an informa business

British Library Cataloguing-in-Publication Data
A catalogue record for this book is available from the British Library

Library of Congress Cataloging-in-Publication Data
Names: Zavadskaya, Margarita, editor.
Title: The politics of the pandemic in Eastern Europe and Eurasia : blame game and governance / edited by Margarita Zavadskaya.
Description: Milton Park, Abingdon, Oxon ; New York, NY : Routledge, 2024. |
Series: Studies in contemporary Russia | Includes bibliographical references and index.
Identifiers: LCCN 2023015157 (print) | LCCN 2023015158 (ebook) | ISBN 9781032428772 (hardback) | ISBN 9781032429137 (paperback) | ISBN 9781003364870 (ebook)
Subjects: LCSH: COVID-19 Pandemic, 2020—Political aspects—Europe, Eastern. | COVID-19 Pandemic, 2020—Political aspects—Eurasia. | COVID-19 (Disease)—Government policy—Europe, Eastern. | COVID-19 (Disease)—Government policy—Eurasia.
Classification: LCC RA644.C67 P6515 2024 (print) | LCC RA644.C67 (ebook) | DDC 362.1962/41440094—dc23/eng/20230630
LC record available at https://lccn.loc.gov/2023015157
LC ebook record available at https://lccn.loc.gov/2023015158

ISBN: 978-1-032-42877-2 (hbk)
ISBN: 978-1-032-42913-7 (pbk)
ISBN: 978-1-003-36487-0 (ebk)

DOI: 10.4324/9781003364870

Typeset in Sabon
by codeMantra

Contents

Contributors

Alexandra Arkhipova is folklorist and a social anthropologist, and currently, she is a visiting research fellow at the Laboratory of Social Anthropology EHESS, Paris, France (for the year 2022–2023). She studies political jokes, rumors and legends; the concept of money in traditional society; and protest.

Valeria Caras is Junior Data Scientist at CSC – IT Center for Science in Finland. Valeria graduated as Master of Social Sciences from the University of Helsinki in 2021. She was an intern at the Aleksanteri Institute, University of Helsinki.

Vladimir Gel'man is Professor of Russian Politics at the Aleksanteri Institute, University of Helsinki. For many years, he has taught at the European University at St. Petersburg, Russia. He authored many books on politics and governance in post-Soviet Russia.

Mirzokhid Karshiev is a doctoral researcher in Political, Societal and Regional Change program at the University of Helsinki. His research interests include state-society relations and development patterns in Eurasia, particularly in Central Asia.

Shugyla Kilybayeva has worked as a postdoctoral researcher and senior lecturer at Al-Farabi Kazakh National University and KIMEP University, Kazakhstan. She is currently engaged in the EU-funded projects as a Marie Sklodowska-Curie visiting researcher at TalTech Law School, Tallinn University of Technology, Estonia.

Irina Kozlova is a folklorist and a social anthropologist, she holds a PhD in Russian Literature. In 2021, she completed an internship at the Nicolaus Copernicus University in Torun under the program of the Centre for Polish-Russian Dialogue and Understanding (in 2022, the Centre was transformed into Mieroszewski Centre).

Diana Kurtametova is a graduate of the HSE University and an independent researcher. She received a bachelor's degree in Political Science and a master's degree in Management and Analytics for Business. Her research interests include business environment and institutions.

Katalin Miklóssy is a political and legal historian and the head of Eastern European area studies. Her recent scholarship investigates how the evolution of the rule of law is conditioned by spatiality and what kind of consequences the historical threat perceptions had on choices of governance model and people-power relations.

Eemil Mitikka is a social scientist specializing in Russia and post-Soviet countries. He works as a doctoral researcher at the University of Helsinki and Aleksanteri Institute. His PhD research deals with the relationship between political participation and authoritarianism in Russia and ex-USSR.

Ryhor Nizhnikau is a senior research fellow at the Finnish Institute of International Affairs. He works on Russia's and EU's policies towards Ukraine, Moldova and Belarus. He received his PhD in Political Science from the Johan Skytte Institute of Political Studies, University of Tartu.

Boris Peigin is a legal anthropologist and a visiting scholar in the Department of Slavic and Eurasian Studies at the University of Texas at Austin.

Aleksandra Rumiantseva has been a researcher in the Department of Politics and Economics, Research Centre for East European Studies at the University of Bremen since spring 2022. She received a master's degree from the European University at Saint-Petersburg and the High School of Economics (SPB).

Kristiina Silvan is Postdoctoral Fellow in the Russia, EU's Eastern Neighbourhood and Eurasia research program at the Finnish Institute of International Affairs. Her research focuses on authoritarian governance and domestic and foreign policy issues in Russia, Belarus and Central Asia, as well as on Russia's changing role in the post-Soviet region.

Anna Tarasenko is a researcher at the Aleksanteri Institute, Helsinki University. Her research appeared in *Post-Soviet Affairs*, *East European Politics* and *Europe-Asia Studies*. She has proficiency in research on social policy and institutions, conducts qualitative and quantitative analysis and produces policy papers.

Margarita Zavadskaya is a senior research fellow at the Finnish Institute of International Affairs (FIIA) and researcher at the Aleksanteri Institute, University of Helsinki. She obtained her doctoral degree in social and political sciences from the European University Institute (EUI) in Florence, Italy.

Introduction

Facing the Global Pandemic: Regimes, Governance, and Post-communism

Margarita Zavadskaya[1]

In late February, early Spring 2020, when the COVID-19 pandemic hit Europe and the rest of the world, Poland's presidential elections were approaching. The incumbent Andrzej Duda, backed by the conservative Law and Justice party (*Prawo i sprawiedliwość or PiS*), faced off against the left-wing candidate and Mayor of Warsaw, Rafał Trzaskowski, supported by Civic Platform (*Platforma obywatelska*). The Polish government was faced with a tough dilemma: postpone the elections or hold them in the middle of a pandemic, thereby exposing voters to deadly health risks. Election day was scheduled for May 10, 2020. However, after extremely heated debates between the main competitors, elections were rescheduled for June 28. Initially, the government aimed to hold elections as planned, while other candidates as well as members of the Constitutional Court opposed it. The Law and Justice party also proposed to alter electoral legislation so that it would only allow mail-in voting. The latter triggered a new political conflict as some judges deemed it unconstitutional (Vashchanka 2020, Orzechowski et al. 2021). One way or another, Polish voters came to the polling stations in late June. None of the candidates received a majority of the vote, so the second round of elections took place in July. The incumbent, Andrzej Duda, won with a slim margin of 51.03%, compared to Rafał Trzaskowski's 48.97%. Electoral integrity was severely compromised due to unbalanced media coverage, attempts on behalf of the incumbent to jeopardise voters' private data, as well as changes to election rules for the benefit of PiS.[2] Out of all European Union (EU) states, Poland introduced some of the strictest restrictions during the pandemic. Despite this initial policy, the Polish government started to lift many restrictions comparatively early in order to hold the national vote in June (Orzechowski et al. 2021). Thus, the pandemic deepened political divides between parties as well as made the very backbone of democratic rule in Poland vulnerable.

Belarus shares a border with Poland as well as several historical and cultural similarities. Despite geographical proximity, the political system and the very nature of the political regime are nothing like Poland's. The Belarusian government scheduled presidential elections for August 9, 2020.

DOI: 10.4324/9781003364870-1

Compared to Poland, there was no public debate over the impact of the pandemic on voters as the incumbent, Aliaksandr Lukašenka, did not believe that COVID-19 was a deadly virus (Åslund 2020, Silvan and Kilybayeva this volume). Lukašenka is notoriously known for brutal repression of political opposition as well as civic dissent, allowing him to remain in power since 1994. Following the election, official results reported that Lukashenka won with a landslide victory of 81%, whereas the main opposition candidate Sviatlana Tsikhanouskaya, backed by a united opposition, allegedly only received 10% of the vote. The opposition claimed that she received at least 60% of the vote. This controversy led to large-scale peaceful protests as well as country-wide strikes including hundreds of thousands of Belarusians in Minsk and other large cities. From the outset, 'the long-term protest' seemed successful and gave hope that Lukashenka was finally losing his grip on power (Bedford 2021, Onuch and Sasse 2022). Quite soon, Lukashenka embarked on a massive deployment of brutal force with the help of the riot police and the military. At least ten persons perished during the protests and their aftermath, while hundreds of protesters as well as random citizens were detained and exposed to extremely cruel and inhumane treatment. The riot police used torture, beatings, rape, threats, and various forms of humiliation to punish the protesters for expressing their political stance (De Vogel 2022). The tragic events of August 2020 extended the rule of the longest lasting dictator in Europe, seemingly unaffected by the worldwide pandemic. Against the backdrop of political tension and civil resistance, the fight against COVID-19 turned out to be a minor issue.

Two referendums – in Armenia and Russia – were planned to take place during the pandemic. An Armenian constitutional referendum on the president's tenure and terms of constitutional judges were postponed from April until an undetermined date due to the pandemic. In the absence of a referendum, the parliament instead voted for the constitutional amendment directly, which also brought about additional political tensions.[3] Nevertheless, it did not seem to threaten the regime's stability or legitimacy in any significant way.

In the case of Russia, it was a popular vote for the constitutional amendments that aimed to extend Vladimir Putin's presidential terms. The constitutional vote was initially scheduled for April 2020, but due to the pandemic, it was postponed until July 1. Technically speaking, 'this type of change to the constitution did not qualify for the use of a referendum as outlined in the existing federal law on referendums' as its initiation did not conform with the federal law on referendums (Teague 2020, Kersting et al. 2023). On the other hand, it effectively extended Putin's presidential term until 2036, in case he wishes to run for another term. Voting on constitutional amendments is loaded with symbolic value for the Russian regime's stability. All this comes in a single package with extravagant textual novelties such as support for the 'traditional family', so as to shift attention and reinforce support for Putin in conservative and unsophisticated electorates. It is noteworthy that social distancing and other restrictive measures were not implemented in Russia until the last week of March because the authorities wanted to carry on with the constitutional plebiscite until the very last moment. On March 25, the president signed a decree postponing the constitutional referendum. Amendments passed with 78.56% in favour and 21.44% against. Observers noted multiple violations and fraud. The opposition boycotted the vote because of the illegality of the referendum (Krivonosova 2020).

These vignettes demonstrate how the nature of a political regime affects the imposition of COVID-19 constraints and related policies. The Polish and Armenian governments introduced the state of emergency right away and subsequently postponed voting, while Russian authorities never declared a state of emergency and mostly pursued a relaxed *laissez-faire* policy approach to COVID-19. The Belarusian government took the most radical stance and simply ignored the pandemic and consigned thousands of people to their fate. Authoritarian governments in many cases succeeded in capitalising on the pandemic, effectively shifting the blame for inefficient policies to other actors and in some cases, like Hungary or Russia, strengthening their rule even further. On the other hand, democratic governments handled the pandemic challenge with varying degrees of efficiency and effectiveness, leading to either a short-term 'rallying around' effect or a loss of political support like in Belarus and Poland. The initial stages of the pandemic set the dynamics that changed over time with every new wave of COVID-19, its mutation, and the vaccination campaign.

At first glance, these states have nothing in common, although it is not entirely true that all these states and societies share a legacy of communist rule as well as contentious post-communist transition. These legacies manifest themselves in a variety of forms – inherited institutional deficiencies, informal practices and shared knowledge, remnants of communist governments, as well as patterns of political participation and non-participation. Weak civil society structures and amorphous political parties coupled with low impersonal trust (Howard 2002) are known as the most prominent traces of communist rule. A low quality of governance, prone to corruption and clientelism (Grzymała-Busse 2008, Hooghe and Quintelier 2014), is also endemic to the region and is often attributed to the legacy of communist or authoritarian rule. Overall cynicism, lack of trust, and sceptical attitudes towards democracy are also believed to be traces of long exposure to communism and authoritarianism (Pop-Eleches and Tucker 2017).

Despite these problematic prerequisites, Poland, together with most Central and Eastern European states, made a fairly successful transition to electoral democracy under the influence of the EU conditionality and *acquis communautaire* (Vachudova and Hooghe 2009). Russia, however, became stuck in transition and slid back to a new authoritarian rule as soon as 2007. Belarus never democratised and fell victim to a corrupt personalist rule, purported by consolidated authoritarianism in Russia. Democracy does not spawn good governance *per se*, but it serves as a necessary condition to create it (Schmitter and Karl 1991). Good governance under autocracies is only possible in forms of 'pockets of effectiveness' that tend to be short-lived and highly susceptible to political patronage (Gel'man 2021). From this perspective, one may assume that democratic post-communist regimes are expected to handle public health crises more efficiently than autocracies.

Legacies differ across these societies and states. The impact of various aspects of communist and transitional legacies varies dramatically across former communist states. Shared pasts often reflect themselves in perplexing ways. For instance, through political parties that operate as successors of banished communist parties in Bulgaria, Romania, or Russia, nostalgia for the communist rule and grievance towards the EU are expressed (Bozóki and Ishiyama 2020). In all three states, communists are closely intertwined with the Orthodox church and during the pandemic, attempted to capitalise on COVID-19 scepticism. Remarkably, as of January 2022, Bulgaria had the largest share of COVID-19 sceptics and percentage of the population that is determined not to get vaccinated. Approximately 45% of the population in each of these three countries believe that COVID-19 resulted from a planned operation by hidden forces in an attempt to control the population (Hajdu 2021). The share of COVID-19 sceptics in Russia amounts to one-third of the population (Sokolov and Zavadskaya 2021). In the 1990s, the communist successor parties voiced the collective grievances of those who perceived themselves as 'losers of the economic transition' (Tucker et al. 2002). Three decades later, communists represent those alienated from the state and nostalgic for the past, all while denying any credibility to vaccination policies.

An interesting conundrum arose when these legacies quirkily manifest themselves during the COVID-19 pandemic. How did states that three decades ago shook off communist rule handle the global pandemic? Do these legacies of communist rule and transitions affect the way governments dealt with the pandemic? All in all, an overarching question of the volume is as follows: ***what kind of tangible political consequences did the global COVID-19 pandemic bring about in Central and Eastern Europe as well as Central Asia?*** More specifically, why did some states handle the pandemic efficiently, maximising their healthcare capacity and minimising the death toll, while others lost thousands? How did the nature of a political regime and state capacity mediate the ability to decrease human losses and strengthen systemic and performance legitimacy? Why did some governments capitalise on the exogenous shock while others lost their political credibility?

COVID-19 as an exogenous shock, though, differs from other natural disasters in terms of timing, visibility, and perceptions. The virus as an immediate threat is not directly visible. People were not exposed to the virus at the same time and in the same location. Rather, it spreads in waves and with varying paces. Finally, the most dangerous phase of the pandemic lasted for more than two years, which made governments and populations adapt to new realities and adjusted their political expectations, i.e., the pandemic ceased to be a shock after all.

We differentiate between the following types of political consequences: (1) the dynamics of political regimes, (2) political support and legitimacy, quality of government policies, and (3) the state of civil society. A political regime is the most fundamental characteristic of a polity. It defines how the 'rules of the game' for all political actors are set and followed. Political regimes – even if one sticks to a blunt dichotomy of differentiating between democracies and autocracies – to a great extent defined how timely and effectively governments managed the perfect storm of COVID-19. Some observers claim that autocracies perform better during emergencies as they rely less on mass support (Lo 2020). However, we do not find empirical support for the 'authoritarian advantage' thesis (Cheibub et al. 2020). From this perspective, autocracies are better equipped to manage emergencies as they are relatively free from popular pressure. That said, one would expect stronger rallying effects, even in the cases of policy failures autocrats usually enjoy a monopoly over mass media and can effectively shift blame for poor governance elsewhere. On the other hand, COVID-19 as an emergency created opportunities for vote-rigging, pressuring the opposition under the pretext of preventing the disease and hiding behind securitisation narratives. The example of China demonstrates that repressive and enforcement capacities of the state can be considered a rather efficient tool for handling COVID-19.

Elections served as a political focal point that allowed key political actors to coordinate on several hot policy issues. Sometimes, not just metaphorically but literally – on polling stations and while protesting (e.g., Israeli protesters maintained a two-metre distance between themselves; it was not an actual requirement, but just a bottom-up rule). During the pandemic, in the majority of countries all over the world, gatherings were banned, and social distancing was required. Not surprisingly, most autocracies from our sample immediately introduced restrictions or bans on all sorts of gatherings and events, including Russia. Meanwhile, other measures came with a delay and most autocracies covered in this volume never introduced full lockdowns or states of emergency.

For instance, during the COVID-19 crisis, electoral campaigns in all regimes were impacted in several ways. Firstly, the pandemic caused the postponement of elections worldwide, especially at the crisis' onset. The highest proportion of postponed elections was observed in March–April 2020. Countries gradually returned to the usual routine of electoral campaigns, especially in the autumn. Both autocracies and democracies rescheduled national elections, but in democratic systems, campaigns were twice as likely to be postponed than in autocracies. Democratic regimes tended to schedule the date of new elections while non-democratic regimes proposed a new date less often. In hybrid regimes, defined by IDEA Global State of Democracy Indices, campaigns are most likely to be postponed without a new date (Asplund and James 2020).

Earlier studies show that autocracies handle public health crises somewhat worse than democracies. The reason is not simply the lack of structural capacity and expertise, but, quite often, the sheer lack of accountability and, respectively, the lower value of human life in the eyes of the state (Gel'man 2021). Breaches in freedom of speech and state control over mass media allowed for effective blame-shifting in case of major failures (Maestas et al. 2008). The latter facilitates blame avoidance for poor policies by blaming external actors for malicious intentions, corrupt and incompetent officials who implement anti-COVID-19 measures haphazardly, or even the citizens themselves for irresponsible behaviour and failure to adhere to pandemic restrictions. Russian authorities took the lead in the blame game by accusing barbecue lovers and tourists for spreading the virus (Busygina and Filippov 2021, Chaisty et al. 2022).

According to International IDEA, since 2017, 'the number of countries moving toward authoritarianism are more than double those that are moving toward democracy. Of the 104 democracies included in the study, 52 are considered to be eroding, up from 12 a decade ago. Among non-democratic countries such as Afghanistan and Belarus, nearly half are becoming more repressive'.[4] The pandemic made a dramatic contribution to democratic backsliding, although as some analysts argue, *it did not cause it*. As Saikkonen and Rapeli put it, 'repercussions of the pandemic can aggravate the situation in countries that are already experiencing democratic erosion. However, the long-term economic effects of the pandemic may be more detrimental to non-democratic governance' (2020). Authoritarian leaders largely rely on politically induced distribution of benefits and tax exemptions and the provision of public goods to specific constituencies and segments of the electorate (Rapeli and Saikkonen 2020). The massive public health crisis undermined authoritarian regimes' ability to deliver goods and services as well as the size of these regimes' coffers.

At the same time, for established democracies, the pandemic did not seem to pose any significant threat to democratic sustainability. Rather, short-term increase in trust in current governments, also known as 'rallying around the flag' (Altiparmakis et al. 2021), was observed. Strong institutions, existing procedural constraints, and accountability prevented extensive abuses of human rights and political repression. Even in the case of denial of COVID-19 as a deadly threat, established democracies weathered the crisis. The US unequivocally exemplified this tendency under Donald Trump's government, which openly denied the dangers of COVID-19 and compromised the fight against the pandemic in 2020 (Kapucu and Moynihan 2021). However, the presence of several 'veto actors' prevented the US from spiralling downward into an abyss. Many Western European governments rode the short-lived wave of 'rallying' in 2020 that existed due to pre-existing stocks of institutional trust in these countries.

For relatively new democratic states where democratic institutions seem less stable as well as in states with recent authoritarian pasts, COVID-19 was a grave danger. In some states such as Spain,[5] there was a dramatic rise in trust for expert-led governance, i.e., technocratic, and non-representative government, which goes against the fundamental principles of democratic representation (Amat et al. 2020). In the face of deadly peril, citizens were ready to give up their rights and freedoms. Similar challenges arose for Central and Eastern European states, especially the *Visegrád Group* including Hungary, Poland, Czechia, and Slovakia. Hungary had already been downgraded to 'electoral autocracy' by the reputable V-Dem project (Maerz et al. 2020) by the time COVID-19 broke out. Poland had been experiencing a controversial constitutional crisis since 2015, accompanied by several attempts by the conservative PiS party to establish political control over the judiciary and freedom of speech (Miklóssy this volume). Czechia and Slovakia were under the rule of new populist leaders Andrej Babiš and Igor Matovič, respectively (Buštíková and Baboš 2020).

From the early days of the COVID-19 emergency, experts raised concerns regarding how the state of emergency and an unprecedented degree of danger may jeopardise democratic institutions through executive aggrandisement, official disinformation campaigns, restrictions on freedom of speech, absence of time limits on emergency measures, and outright discriminatory measures based on gender, age, race, or social origin (Edgell et al. 2021). Hungary and Serbia were listed in a group of countries at elevated risk of democratic backsliding in the Summer of 2020. Armenia, Azerbaijan, Belarus, Bulgaria, Kazakhstan, Kyrgyzstan, Russia, Tajikistan, Turkmenistan, and Ukraine appeared among the countries with milder risks of autocratisation (Edgell et al. 2021). At least two autocracies spiralled downward even further – Russia and Belarus. During the pandemic, Russia's government massively deployed anti-COVID-19 restrictions to oppress the freedom of gathering and freedom of speech, while Belarusian and Turkmen leaderships engaged in consciously misinforming the population without implementing any COVID-19-related policies. Ukraine and Georgia performed in line with the rest of the EU by imposing strict lockdowns and making COVID-19 testing, and later vaccinations, available (Buckley et al. 2020). Tragically, three of these countries are currently at war after Russia launched a full-scale invasion of Ukraine on February 24, 2022 (Belarus being a country that supports the aggressor). It would not be an exaggeration to argue that the pandemic contributed its fair share to the further alienation of the Russian leadership and corruption of decision-making processes in Moscow as well as social and elite feedback mechanisms (Sokhey 2020, Chaisty et al. 2022). Vladimir Putin's increased isolation and detachment from more critically minded elites led him to make the pernicious decision to again invading Ukraine. Once again, the pandemic *did not cause* the war, but it made it more likely.

The global public health crisis put both systemic and specific political support to a harsh test. At the pandemic's onset, democracies were slower to introduce restrictive measures, which can be explained by the more significant trade-off between healthcare necessities and respect for liberal rights in democracies compared to autocracies (Cheibub et al. 2020). However, the severity of the crisis pushed democratic leaders to eventually adopt similar restrictions to those adopted by authoritarian governments. While Western Europe at large experienced a short-term 'rallying' at the initial stage, Eastern Europe, with the prominent exception of Hungary, demonstrated more governmental instability and loss of political credentials by the ruling coalitions. This phenomenon is sometimes referred to as 'hyper-accountability', which has been seen in the Eastern Europe context before in relation to other natural disasters (Jastramskis et al. 2021).

In half of the CEE countries, governments changed – Lithuania, Czechia, Romania, Bulgaria, and Slovakia. There are instances of limited 'rallying', such as in Slovakia, where the government successfully handled COVID-19 with one of the lowest mortality rates in the EU in the early stages of the pandemic. However, when vaccination campaigns began, a full-blown scandal erupted over the purchase of Russian Sputnik vaccines, which were unapproved by the European Medicines Agency (EMA) (Guasti and Bílek 2022). The regional champions of autocratisation – Poland and Hungary – did not experience any dramatic shifts in their governments. The political leadership of Latvia, Estonia, Slovenia, and Croatia even capitalised on the pandemic. Poor handling of COVID-19, such as a lack of timely policy measures and policy coordination as well as shortages of medical facilities and trainings impacted voters' behaviours, causing major crises in Romania and Bulgaria.

In Montenegro, a significant shift of power happened after parliamentary elections held in August 2020. This took place against the background of a shrinking economy and a huge drop in gross domestic product (GDP), mainly due to the impact of the pandemic on the country's tourism sector (12–14% drop in GDP). The Democratic Party of Socialists (DPS), led by President Milo Đukanović since 1991, passed power to a coalition government formed by For the Future of Montenegro. The electoral defeat was preceded by protests in 2019, which demanded President Đukanović and the government's resignation over widespread corruption. Although elections were organised competitively, the OSCE election observation mission noted that the ruling party attempted to monopolise press coverage and state resources to influence the campaign's results (Caras 2021).

Finally, the global pandemic severely affected civil society groups, opposition, and social movements. Authoritarian governments used leverage to restrict undesirable political activities using quarantine measures as a legitimate pretext. Repertoires of political resistance shrank dramatically during the pandemic in democratic countries as well. Although social movement groups became creative and, in many instances, found ways to voice their claims without violating COVID-19 restrictions, long-term restrictive measures caused over 25 significant protests worldwide.[6] In some cases, protests were attended by a relatively modest number of COVID-19 dissidents, as seen in Bulgaria, the Netherlands, Spain, and Slovakia. In other cases, protests acted as a conduit to express dissatisfaction with the economy, corruption, and elections. For instance, in Argentina, people protested corruption, judicial reform, as well as stringent lockdown measures. In Bolivia, the public criticised a second delay in general elections due to the pandemic. In Serbia, the opposition contested the results of the parliamentary elections and blamed the incumbent president, Aleksandar Vučić, for using lockdowns to his party's advantage (Caras 2021).

The bottom line is that when deciding upon strategies to address COVID-19, states must take several aspects into account. Political leaders do care about citizens' support regardless of political regime, and whenever national elections are at stake, their response to the COVID-19 outbreak might be affected by it. There are some patterns in how various regimes prioritise public health: in more accountable regimes restrictions proved to be tougher, while less accountable regimes attempted to balance between a crumbling economy and silencing the opposition that could potentially dwell on COVID-19-related issues. This volume addresses questions of how the global COVID-19 pandemic altered political landscapes in Central-Eastern Europe as well as Eurasia. The following chapters also address how and why the pandemic boosted political legitimacy and mass support, or vice versa, brought down governments. Finally, the contributions found in this volume address how the pandemic changed patterns of street politics and social movements and how the pandemic affected various political actors such as political parties, governments, business groups, and opposition forces.

Each chapter addresses either regime changes in relation to policy implementation or the impact on citizens' political participation and activism. The geographical scope of the volume intentionally goes beyond Europe and includes Central Asia – Kazakhstan and Uzbekistan. These chapters deploy a variety of analytical tools and approaches to answer more specific research questions related to the political effects of the COVID-19 pandemic. The first part addresses Central and Eastern Europe and the dynamics of political support based on mass surveys. These contributions explore the effects of political attitudes, especially the role of COVID-19 scepticism and beliefs in conspiracy theories. Conspiracy thinking thrives on more generic distrust. Therefore, as part of a post-communist legacy, conspiracy thinking exercises an enormous impact on the effectiveness of pandemic restrictions, vaccination rates, as well as political blame attribution. Zavadskaya and Caras in their chapter argue that COVID-19 scepticism correlates with the lack of political punishment in some states and blurred the mechanisms of blame attribution. Miklossy demonstrates how Hungarian and Polish authorities capitalised on the COVID-19 emergency and tweaked existing political rules, especially constitutional regulations, to their advantage. She refers to this as 'the COVID-19 rule of law' indicating the pathways of how political institutions deteriorated under external pressure. COVID-19 gave the opportunity to finetune discursive strategies so that governments could effectively channel citizens' attention away from one crisis to another. For example, away from the rule of law mechanism endangering the countries' budgetary interests in EU funds to COVID-19. Nizhnikau's chapter brings us to pre-war Ukraine and the implementation of EU governance reforms, which included the overhaul of the healthcare sector. The latter posed a double challenge to Volodymyr Zelensky's institutional building. Silvan and Kilybayeva draw parallels between two post-Soviet authoritarian states: Belarus and Kazakhstan, showing how the political leadership in both countries sought to legitimise its rule by portraying the state as 'socially oriented' (in Belarus) or 'listening' and pro-business (in Kazakhstan). The state's inability to deliver welfare at a moment of crisis exacerbated popular resentment, thus changing the political opportunity structure of each state. The chapter explains how the pandemic affected the outbursts of violence during political protests.

The second part of the volume mostly focuses on Russian political developments in light of the global pandemic. As Gel'man puts it, although it is too early to provide a comprehensive account of the response to the COVID-19 pandemic and its consequences across the globe, even preliminary and incomplete data tell us that Russia has coped with the pandemic much worse than most developed and developing countries. Russia demonstrated one of the highest excess mortality rates given the well-grounded suspicions of systematically underreporting the number of patients and deaths due to COVID-19. He attributes the blame to 'bad governance' that drives major policy decisions by Russia's authorities, which can be characterised as 'muddling through at any cost, including the cost in lives and health of Russian citizens'. Kurtametova and Tarasenko focus on how small businesses survived the pandemic through various adaptations to new circumstances as well as eternally changing and inconsistent regulatory policies. According to their estimates, unemployment and the average age of a population accounts for a large share of SMEs per capita in addition to factors such as the cost of innovation and votes for the incumbent in presidential elections in 2018. Mitikka, by analysing patterns of administrative and criminal law enforcement, shows how the pandemic restrictions were deployed to repress the political opposition in Russia during the pandemic. Rumiantseva and her co-authors lay out explanations for the massive number of anti-vaxxers and COVID-19 sceptics in Russia who took to the streets, echoing the findings of Zavadskaya and Caras from Eastern Europe. Drawing on quantitative and qualitative data, they explain why the Russian vaccination policy failed and show how Russians struggled against vaccine mandates. The main reasons for this policy failure were the campaign's inconsistency, citizens' lack of trust in the government, and the vaccine initiative's obligatoriness, which influenced the perceptions of even the most loyal citizens of the regime. Looking at Russian domestic politics during the pandemic provides a complex picture of how the regime sought to keep its legitimacy, manoeuvring between fighting COVID-19, vaccination campaigns, political distribution of benefits and tax exemptions or reliefs, and appeasement of protest groups. These chapters offer a gruesome depiction of one of the most notorious autocracies that soon after the pandemic crisis, launched a full-scale invasion of its neighbour Ukraine. Finally, Karshiev and Silvan's chapter tells the story of fighting COVID-19 in another Central Asian autocracy – Uzbekistan, caught in the middle of political liberalisation and administrative reforms through the lens of performance legitimacy.

The novel COVID-19 virus has left deep traces in Central and Eastern Europe, including Russia, in terms of economic development, healthcare, and overall political support. COVID-19 as an exogenous shock reshaped political opportunity structures to the advantage of some political actors and the disadvantaging of others: in the incumbent's favour in Hungary and Russia or against the government in Belarus. All economies worldwide were hit hard by the COVID-19 crisis, which caused a dramatic slowdown in domestic business activities, border closures, a rise in unemployment, and pressure on national welfare systems, which extended governments' discretionary powers. On the other hand, the pandemic has exacerbated the challenges of government efficiency, transparency, and accountability (namely, 'good governance'). The pandemic and subsequent states of emergency made citizens more vulnerable and dependent on their governments, opening up possibilities for political and administrative abuse and manipulations, all of which may ultimately undermine the rule of law. The latter especially holds true for states with authoritarian legacies and a legacy of politically motivated redistribution, i.e., the old communist rule, an oversized state apparatus, and politicised bureaucracies.

In this book, it is hypothesised that COVID-19 as an exogenous shock shifts access to political, media, economic, and administrative resources towards the state, politicised welfare spending, and thereby fostered authoritarian tendencies in the region. Moreover, previous research has shown that external crises tend to force citizens 'to rally around' their governments and leaders, acknowledging no blame, expressing solidarity, and appreciating the operation of public services. In this context, CEE societies, including Russia, are known for their extremely low institutional and interpersonal trust due to a lack of efficiency and breaches in public governance. Numerous rumours and conspiracy theories accompanied the COVID-19 pandemic. This trend is primarily attributed to the lack of information about the disease and the inevitable inconsistency of the scientific data. In the CEE region, conspiracy thinking thrives on distrust. Coupled with the recent conservative and populist turn, it brings about long-term consequences for political accountability and governance.

At the same time, conspiracy theories pose a significant threat to public welfare. Politicians and officials who do not believe in the existence of the virus or underestimate its danger can impede the timely introduction of measures to combat the disease or promote inadequate options to face the challenge. COVID-19 sceptics, in turn, are less inclined to observe basic precautions, such as wearing masks or social distancing. They are more likely to oppose vaccinations and thereby endanger their own and other people's health.

These obstacles facilitate the so-called 'blame game', where incumbents then enjoy more opportunities for shifting the responsibility for COVID-related policy failures to other actors – subnational and local authorities, businesses, other countries, and 'unfriendly' international community or fellow citizens. Countries with populist governments obtained more opportunities to consolidate their support as seen in Hungary and Poland. States with authoritarian rule slide further into repressive and autarchic forms of governance, as seen in Russia and Belarus. The outcomes for other states are yet to be explored.

We seek to formulate, explain, and empirically test the causal mechanisms that drive political accountability and support in 'the hard times' of the COVID-19 pandemic in countries of Central and Eastern Europe. With cross-country comparisons and in-depth case studies of popular and electoral support, this volume attempts to highlight patterns specific to the region. This book contributes to the studies of governance and political accountability in low-trust countries with authoritarian legacies and proclivities.

I would like to express my deepest gratitude to the University of Helsinki and their three-year grant programme that made the publication of this volume possible as well as the research team of the ElMaRB project – Elena Gorbacheva, Valeria Caras, and Viktor Lambin. We are indebted to Aleksei Gilev, Monika Hajdu, Bradley Reynolds, Boris Sokolov, and Jonáš Syrovátka for commenting the chapters, providing access to the data, and assisting with preparation of this volume. On behalf of the contributors, we would like to thank the Aleksanteri Institute at the University of Helsinki and its Director Markku Kangaspuro for encouraging us to proceed with this project and providing an inspiring environment for us.

Notes

1 Margarita Zavadskaya is a senior research fellow at the Finnish Institute of International Affairs and researcher at the Aleksanteri Institute, University of Helsinki.
2 See OSCE Republic of Poland, Presidential Election June 28–July 12, 2020, Final report. https://bip.brpo.gov.pl/sites/default/files/Poland%20Presidential%20Election%202020%20%20final%20report.pdf.
3 Harout Manougian. 2022. "Armenia's Constitutional Journey Continues." January 31, 2022. https://constitutionnet.org/news/armenias-constitutional-journey-continues.
4 Karl, Vick. 2020. "The COVID-19 Pandemic Is Weakening Democracy Around the World, Report Finds." October 2, 2020. https://time.com/5895315/covid-19-pandemic-democracy/
5 As a post-Communist state, Spain experienced a long-term authoritarian rule under Francisco Franco up until 1975.
6 Carothers, Thomas and Wong David. 2020. "The Coronavirus Pandemic is Reshaping Global Protests." May 4, 2020. https://carnegieendowment.org/2020/05/04/coronavirus-pandemic-is-reshaping-global-protests-pub-81629

References

Altiparmakis, Argyrios, Abel Bojar, Sylvain Brouard, Martial Foucault, Hanspeter Kriesi, and Richard Nadeau. 2021. "Pandemic politics: Policy evaluations of government responses to COVID-19." *West European Politics* 44, no. 5–6: 1159–1179.

Amat, Francesc, Arenas Andreu, Falcó-Gimeno Albert, and Muñoz Jordi. 2020. "Pandemics meet democracy. Experimental evidence from the COVID-19 crisis in Spain." *SocArXiv*, April 6, 2020. https://doi.org/10.31235/osf.io/dkusw.

Åslund, Anders. 2020. "Responses to the COVID-19 crisis in Russia, Ukraine, and Belarus." *Eurasian Geography and Economics* 61, nos. 4–5: 532–545.

Asplund, Erik, and James Toby. 2020. "Elections and Covid-19: Making democracy work in uncertain times." *Democratic Audit Blog*. https://eprints.lse.ac.uk/107847/1/dit_com_2020_03_30_elections_and_covid_19_making_democracy_work_in.pdf.

Bedford, Sofie. 2021. "The 2020 presidential election in Belarus: Erosion of authoritarian stability and re-politicization of society." *Nationalities Papers* 49, no. 5: 808–819.

Bozóki, András, and John T. Ishiyama. 2020. *The communist successor parties of Central and Eastern Europe*. London: Routledge.

Buckley, Cynthia J., Ralph S. Clem, and Erik S. Herron. 2020. "The COVID-19 pandemic and state healthcare capacity: Government responses and citizen assessments in Estonia, Georgia, and Ukraine." *Problems of Post-Communism* 69, no. 1: 14–25.

Buštíková, Lenka, and Baboš Pavel. 2020. "Best in Covid: Populists in the time of pandemic." *Politics and Governance* 8, no. 4: 496–508.

Busygina, Irina, and Filippov Mikhail. 2021. "COVID and federal relations in Russia." *Russian Politics* 6, no. 3: 279–300.

Caras, Valeria. 2021. "COVID-19 impact on electoral support worldwide: An overview." *Electoral Malpractice, Cybersecurity and its Political Consequences in Russia and Beyond (ElMaRB) Blog*, May 3, 2021. https://blogs.helsinki.fi/elmarb-project/2021/05/03/covid-19-impact-on-electoral-support-worldwide-an-overview/.

Chaisty, Paul, Christopher J. Gerry, and Stephen Whitefield. 2022. "The buck stops elsewhere: Authoritarian resilience and the politics of responsibility for COVID-19 in Russia." *Post-Soviet Affairs* 38, no. 5: 366–385.

Cheibub, Jose A., Ji Yeon J. Hong, and Adam Przeworski. 2020. "Rights and deaths: Government reactions to the pandemic." *SocArXiv*, July 9, 2020. doi:10.31235/osf.io/fte84.

De Vogel, Sasha. 2022. "Anti-opposition crackdowns and protest: The case of Belarus, 2000–2019." *Post-Soviet Affairs* 38, nos. 1–2: 9–25.

Edgell, Amanda B., Jean Lachapelle, Anna Lührmann, and Seraphine F. Maerz. 2021. "Pandemic backsliding: Violations of democratic standards during Covid-19." *Social Science & Medicine* 285: 114244.114244.

Gel'man, Vladimir. 2021. "Exceptions and rules: Success stories and bad governance in Russia." *Europe-Asia Studies* 73, no. 6: 1080–1101.

Grzymała-Busse, Anna. 2008. "Beyond clientelism: Incumbent state capture and state formation." *Comparative Political Studies* 41, nos. 4–5: 638–673.

Guasti, Petra, and Bílek Jaroslav. 2022. "The demand side of vaccine politics and pandemic illiberalism." *East European Politics* 38, no. 4: 594–616.

Hajdu, Dominika, Klingova Katarina, Milo Daniel, and Sawiris Miroslava. 2021. "GLOBSEC Trends 2021: Central and Eastern Europe one year into the pandemic." *GLOBSEC Bratislava*. June 3, 2021. https://www.globsec.org/what-we-do/press-releases/globsec-trends-2021-key-highlights.

Hooghe, Marc, and Quintelier Ellen. 2014. "Political participation in European countries: The effect of authoritarian rule, corruption, lack of good governance and economic downturn." *Comparative European Politics* 12: 209–232.

Howard, Marc M. 2002. "The weakness of postcommunist civil society." *Journal of Democracy* 13, no. 1: 157–169.
Jastramskis, Mažvydas, Vytautas Kuokštis, and Matas Baltrukevičius. 2021. "Retrospective voting in Central and Eastern Europe: Hyper-accountability, corruption or socio-economic inequality?" *Party Politics* 27, no. 4: 667–679.
Kapucu, Naim, and Moynihan Donald. 2021. "Trump's (mis) management of the COVID-19 pandemic in the US." *Policy Studies* 42, nos. 5–6: 592–610.
Kersting, Norbert, Zavadskaya Margarita, and Magne Tiphaine. 2023. "Direct democracy integrity in modern authoritarian systems-The constitutional referendum in Turkey 2017 and Russian plebiscite in 2020." Unpublished manuscript.
Krivonosova, Iuliia. 2020. "Electoral events in Russia during the COVID-19 pandemic: Remote electronic voting, outdoor voting and other innovations." *International IDEA Case Study*, 6.
Lo, Bobo. 2020. "Global order in the shadow of the coronavirus: China, Russia, and the West." Report by Lowy Institute, 29.
Maerz, Seraphine F., Lührmann Anna, Lachapelle Jean, and Amanda B. Edgell. 2020. "Worth the sacrifice? Illiberal and authoritarian practices during Covid-19. Illiberal and Authoritarian Practices during Covid-19" (September 2020). *V-Dem Working Paper*, 110.
Maestas, Cherie D., Lonna Rae Atkeson, Thomas Croom, and Lisa A. Bryant. 2008. "Shifting the blame: Federalism, media, and public assignment of blame following Hurricane Katrina." *Publius: The Journal of Federalism* 38, no. 4: 609–632.
Miklossy, Katalin. forthcoming. "Legislative advantages of multiple crises in the Europe in-between." In *Politics of the Pandemic: Blame Game and Governance in Russian and Central-Eastern Europe*, edited by M. Zavadskaya. Routledge.
Onuch, Olga, and Sasse Gwendolyn. 2022. "The Belarus crisis: People, protest, and political dispositions." *Post-Soviet Affairs* 38, nos. 1–2: 1–8.
Orzechowski, Marcin, Schochow Maximilian, and Steger Florian. 2021. "Balancing public health and civil liberties in times of pandemic." *Journal of Public Health Policy* 42, no. 1: 145–153.
Pop-Eleches, Grigore, and Joshua A. Tucker. 2017. *Communism's shadow: Historical legacies and contemporary political attitudes*. Vol. 3. Princeton: Princeton University Press.
Rapeli, Lauri, and Saikkonen Inga. 2020. "How will the COVID-19 pandemic affect democracy?" *Democratic Theory* 7, no. 2: 25–32.
Schmitter, Philippe C., and Terry L. Karl. 1991. "What democracy is... and is not." *Journal of Democracy* 2, no. 3: 75–88.
Silvan, Kristiina, and Shugyla Kilybayeva. forthcoming. "The state failing people's expectations: Resentment at the pandemic policy in Belarus and Kazakhstan." In *Politics of the Pandemic: Blame Game and Governance in Russian and Central-Eastern Europe* edited by. M. Zavadskaya. London: Routledge.
Sokhey, Sarah W. 2020. "What does Putin promise Russians? Russia's authoritarian social policy." *Orbis* 64, no. 3: 390–402.
Sokolov, Boris O., and Margarita A. Zavadskaya. 2021. "Socio-demographic profiles, personality traits, values, and Covid-skeptics in Russia." *Monitoring Obshchestvennogo Mneniya: Ekonomicheskie i Sotsial'nye Peremeny*, 410–435.
Teague, Elizabeth. 2020. "Russia's constitutional reforms of 2020." *Russian Politics* 5, no. 3: 301–328.

Tucker, Joshua A., Alexander C. Pacek, and Adam J. Berinsky. 2002. "Transitional winners and losers: Attitudes toward EU membership in post-communist countries." *American Journal of Political Science* 46, no. 3: 557–571.

Vachudova, Milada A., and Hooghe Liesbet. 2009. "Postcommunist politics in a magnetic field: How transition and EU accession structure party competition on European integration." *Comparative European Politics* 7: 179–212.

Vashchanka, Vasil. 2020. "Political manoeuvres and legal conundrums amid the COVID-19 pandemic: The 2020 presidential election in Poland." *International Institute for Democracy and Electoral Assistance.* https://www.idea.int/sites/default/files/political-manoeuvres-and-legal-conundrums-2020-presidential-election-poland.pdf.

1 (No) Blame for the Crisis

COVID-19 Sceptics and Political Support in Central-Eastern Europe during COVID-19

Margarita Zavadskaya and Valeria Caras

Introduction

In the spring of 2021, Slovak prime minister Igor Matovič proudly declared his government as being 'best in COVID'. Indeed, Slovakia's death toll due to the pandemic proved to be remarkably low, one of the lowest in the EU (Buštíková and Baboš 2020). At the same time, vaccination campaigns kicked off quickly and without encountering dramatic resistance from COVID-19 dissidents and sceptics. However, the Matovič government was dissolved in April 2021 ending a scandal over importing the Russian Sputnik V vaccine, which was not approved by the EU. Matovič bet on Sputnik V to boost his declining popularity, by 'importing it behind the back of his coalition partners' (Guasti and Bílek 2022: 595). In May 2021, only 24% of Slovaks supported the government, indicating the clear end of any 'rallying' in the country (Hajdu et al. 2021).

The Hungarian government, to the contrary, was poorly equipped to mitigate the crisis: the healthcare sector was underfinanced, doctors and nurses were leaving the country for better jobs elsewhere in the EU, and long-serving Prime Minister Viktor Orbán replaced leading civil servants with his partisan allies. By the start of the pandemic, only one of the previously existing seven laboratories in Hungary licensed to carry out PCR testing remained in operation (Batory 2022: 6–7; Miklóssy Forthcoming). Nevertheless, the first wave of COVID-19 ended with a comparatively low number of fatalities. However, the next wave resulted in a healthcare disaster. According to official records, Hungary had one of the highest mortality rates in the winter of 2021 – 144 deaths per 100,000 (Batory 2022). At the same time, Fidesz had one of the most relaxed pandemic regulations despite the imminent danger to the public health of thousands of Hungarians. The government's political support remained fairly high, maintaining a 54% approval rating in May 2021. One of the reasons was that Orbán capitalised on 'vaccine diplomacy' by importing both Russian and Chinese vaccines, thereby bypassing the lack of the European Medicines Agency (EMA) authorisation. Although this trick 'killed' the reputation of the Slovak prime minister, it kept the Hungarian

DOI: 10.4324/9781003364870-2

leader politically afloat for the 2022 fall elections (Kazharski and Makarychev 2021; Palócz 2022).

Why did some governments successfully handle the crisis, but were dismissed when they tried to speed up vaccination campaigns? And, vice versa, why did inefficient pandemic policies that resulted in excess mortality fail to bring about any punishment? In the CEE region, conspiracy thinking thrives on the soil of distrust. Coupled with the recent conservative and populist turn, it brings about long-term consequences for political accountability and governance. At the same time, conspiracy theories pose a significant threat to public welfare. Politicians and officials who do not believe in the existence of the virus or underestimate its danger can impede the timely introduction of measures to combat the disease or promote inadequate options to face the challenge. COVID-19 sceptics among ordinary citizens, in turn, are less inclined to observe basic precautions, such as wearing masks or social distancing. They are more likely to oppose vaccinations and thereby endanger their own and other people's health. These obstacles facilitate the so-called 'blame game' when the incumbents enjoy more opportunities for shifting the responsibility for COVID-19-related policy failures to other actors – subnational and local authorities, businesses, other countries, 'unfriendly' international community, or even fellow citizens. Countries with populist governments obtained more opportunities to consolidate their support as seen in Hungary and Poland (Miklóssy this volume). States with authoritarian rule slid further into more repressive and autarkic forms of governance, as seen in Russia and Belarus (Gel'man this volume, Silvan and Kilybayeva this volume). The outcomes for other states are yet to be explored. This chapter provides an overview of case studies as well as a comparative analysis of nine EU countries that share communist pasts.

Our main research question asks: why did some governments in Central and Eastern Europe capitalise on the COVID-19 pandemic while others failed to do so? Why was there rallying in some countries and not in others? On the other hand, why did some governments avoid blame for inefficient policies despite high mortality rates and sluggish paces of vaccination campaigns? We argue that scepticism as part of attitudinal and institutional legacies facilitated blame avoidance in the region and is likely to have played down 'the rallying' effect.

We rely on two surveys – a cross-country survey conducted by the Global Security think tank in the late spring of 2021. This survey contains a battery of questions on COVID-19 denialism and scepticism. We also utilise a cross-country survey conducted by Eurobarometer, carried out at the same time, which contains a comprehensive set of economy-related questions. We estimate a series of country-specific OLS regression models to test the correlation between support for the government or the government's coalition. Altogether, these data cover nine countries – Bulgaria, Czechia, Slovakia, Hungary, Poland, Estonia, Lithuania, Latvia, and Romania. Looking at spring 2021 allows us to capture data from a period when COVID-19 was still a high priority on political agendas, most restrictions were still in place, and when the vaccination campaigns were just beginning. Our data do not allow us to observe rallying effects as they did not vary over time, but we rely on electoral statistics as well as earlier survey data to evaluate the presence of noticeable spikes in public support.

We start with the theoretical framework of blame attribution and blame avoidance that has been widely used to study European politics. We then attempt to apply it to the CEE region while adjusting the theoretical frame to the disproportionate spread of conspiracy thinking to consider mistrust as one of the most prominent parts of post-communist and authoritarian legacies. Then, we proceed with hypotheses and operationalisation: a descriptive analysis of each country in the sample by means of regression analysis. Finally, we conclude this chapter with interpretations of the results obtained and a discussion.

COVID-19 as an Exogenous Shock

The pandemic is often viewed as an example of a perfect storm that appears out of the blue and creates a calamity in economic and political developments. It is an established fact that different exogenous shocks affect electoral behaviour: terrorist attacks (Abramson et al. 2007), natural disasters (Healy and Malhotra 2009), and epidemics (Beall et al. 2016; Baccini et al. 2021) tend to foster a 'rallying around the flag' effect that manifests itself in a short-term surge in political support. On the other hand, back in 2009, the H1N1 epidemic brought about a significantly lower turnout and a lower proportion of votes for the incumbent party in Mexico (Gutiérrez, Meriläinen, and Rubli 2020). The Ebola outbreak negatively affected support for the incumbent party in Liberia (Maffioli 2021) and spurred a conservative shift in the context of the disasters and high risks in the US (Beall et al. 2016; Campante et al. 2020). Earlier studies on COVID-19 show evidence of rallying effects in Western Europe (Bol et al. 2021; Esaiasson et al. 2021; Johansson et al. 2021; Schraff 2021). Although in America, voters punished the Trump administration for incompetent actions (Baccini et al. 2021), COVID-19-instigated 'rallying' proved to be a strategy for citizens to cope with anxiety that in turn resulted from high uncertainty (Renström and Bäck 2021) and it was not an identity-driven emotion.

As opposed to natural disasters and wars, pandemics tend to result in a broader variety of politically relevant reactions. Pandemics do not typically have a single trigger that is simultaneously observed by a large number of people (Zavadskaya and Sokolov 2020). There is no unambiguously delineated location that would be understood as a dangerous place. Finally, the pandemic turned out to be a long-term phenomenon that several governments and societies adapted to. We rather observe an overall fatigue of pandemic-related agendas. Thus, the pandemic kept its features of 'a perfect storm' for only the first few months.

Accountability and Blame Attribution during Crisis

What accounts for changes in political support during crises? Classic theories of 'economic voting' predict punishment for poor economic and social policies and, vice versa, positive appraisal due to economic growth (Powell and Whitten 1993). Voters may be driven by either 'pocketbook' voting or by 'sociotropic' motives. One way or another, negative economic experiences such as loss of employment, decreased income, or bankruptcy tend to spill over into negative evaluations of a government's performance. Short-term 'rallying' makes incumbents exempt from political accountability as they did not cause trouble. However, voters assess how a government handles the crisis and after an initial upsurge in 'patriotism' still hold their politicians accountable. Thus, economic performance does not automatically translate into adequate evaluations (Hobolt and Tilley 2014). Similarly, evaluations and opinions do not automatically translate into voting decisions (Iyengar 1996).

Previous studies provide abundant evidence that blame attribution encounters obstacles even in peaceful times. There is usually a lack of clarity regarding who is supposed to be held responsible, especially in the case of coalition governments. Citizens selectively evaluate political actors by disproportionately punishing political opponents and ignoring the policy failures of their chosen parties (Hobolt and Tilley 2014). Partisanship forms 'a perceptual screen' through which individuals filter their evaluations. Selective assessment and punishment are known to affect political support in Western Europe during the financial crisis (Tilley and Hobolt 2011). Finally, mass media mediates the intensity of political punishment (Mutz 2001).

Countries of Central and Eastern Europe tend to have weaker partisan ties and less stable political affiliations. Some governments tend to utilise media to skew the political agenda, especially in Hungary and Poland (Pirro and Stanley 2022). The latter subsequently facilitates *blame avoidance* by the incumbent governments. Traditional media such as print, radio, and television are less trusted, while 'new' online media has gained more leverage in influencing individuals' opinions (Trujillo and Motta 2021). A lack of trust in media coupled with a growing menu of online outlets eased the spread of unreliable and unchecked information on the pandemic. This is known as 'the online accessibility hypothesis' that grasps the impact of internet media on the spread of vaccine hesitancy, conspiracy theories, and outright denial of COVID-19 as a deadly virus (Trujillo and Motta 2021; Rumiantseva et al. this volume; Zarocostas 2020).

Social media plays an essential role in spreading COVID-19 denial. The uncontrolled spread of inaccurate information about the COVID-19 pandemic was called 'infodemic' (Zarocostas 2020). Both the poor quality of information and a considerable amount of its quantity impacted the spread of COVID-19 denialism (Wang and Kim 2021). Conspiracy theories, in general, are successfully disseminated through various channels, both informally by means of private communication or via social networks and officially by means of traditional media. The typical presentation format, which presupposes emotionality and appeals to a sense of danger or group identity, facilitates conspiracy theories circulation (Törnberg 2018; Valenzuela et al. 2019). Social network publications are usually not verified and fact-checked (Cinelli et al. 2020). Research conducted with US online survey samples gathered in April 2020 demonstrated that conspiracy believers reported higher trust in social media and information coming from Trump about COVID-19 (Earnshaw et al. 2020). As such, beliefs in a COVID-19 conspiracy are connected with distrust in scientists, trust in populist governments, and trust in information coming from Facebook rather than from institutional websites such as WHO and national healthcare institutions.

There are multiple mechanisms through which perceptions translate into accountability. Assessment of public services in the heat of the emergency adds more credits to the executive (Bechtel and Hainmueller 2011), while attempts to accommodate uncertainty and anxiety often result in increased political support (Renström and Bäck 2021; Schraff 2021). Pre-COVID-19 levels of political trust provided governments with a stock of support, while excessive polarisation prevented any 'rallying' (Altiparmakis et al. 2021). Overall levels of institutional trust in CEE countries are somewhat lower, while the overall performance of public services is on average more modest. Put together, these factors are likely to prevent governments from capitalising on the pandemic. On the other hand, as we mentioned earlier, weaker institutional checks and authoritarian ambitions of some political leaders in the region facilitate establishing control over mass media and give a disproportionate advantage to one political party. This is how the 'blame game' jumps in and helps explain the lack of punishment in cases of outright policy failure during the pandemic.

First, blame-avoidance strategies dwell on shifting the blame to political opponents, subordinates (e.g., regional actors or municipal authorities), medical experts, or even malicious external forces. Some of these narratives are easily enforced by state-controlled media outlets. Hungary and Russia serve as paradigmatic illustrations of these strategies. Second, blame avoidance may occur whenever the threat is downplayed or even ignored by the media, experts, and political actors. Belarus is an example of pandemic denialism by the state. Third, when government policies face intentional sabotage on behalf of COVID-19 sceptics and vaccine-hesitant groups. The issue of handling COVID-19 looms larger if these grievances are spelled out by certain political parties. Bulgaria and Romania have the highest percentages of COVID-19 sceptics in the region – 17% and 30%, respectively (Hajdu et al., 2021). In both cases, scepticism and hesitancy to get a jab creates fertile ground for marginal political actors to expand their support base.

COVID-19 Denialism and Conspiracy Thinking

There are several types of COVID-19-related conspiracy theories. Van Mulukom et al. (2022) distinguish between three types. The first type combines the so-called hoax theories that underestimate the danger of a virus and a pandemic. This type denies the very existence of the virus, or claim that COVID-19 does not present more risk than an ordinary flu. The second type is made up of dogmas that imply the purposeful invention and spread of the virus to obtain material or political benefit. Examples include beliefs that COVID-19 is a secret biological weapon, a military development, the result of a big pharma conspiracy, or an instrument to establish a new world order. Finally, the third type consists of ideas that place the pandemic in the context of initially unrelated conspiracy theories (e.g., the negative consequences of the proliferation of 5G networks, the Bill Gates conspiracy, etc.).

The phenomenon of COVID-19 scepticism might have various shades and degrees. Its most radical form is broadcasted by the so-called 'COVID deniers' or 'COVID dissidents' who question the virus' very existence.[1] We further define 'COVID sceptics' as individuals who generally recognise the virus' presence but do not consider it dangerous enough or disagree with the measures taken by national governments to combat the pandemic, deeming them excessive. COVID-19 scepticism is closely related to conspiracy thinking (Douglas et al. 2019), a type of compensatory mechanism allowing illusionary control of reality in conditions of low levels of social trust and high levels of uncertainty (Imhoff and Lamberty 2020). COVID-19 scepticism can be analysed within the framework of the more general phenomenon of medical denialism: the totality of theories and practices of denying medical science's authority and expressions of distrust in health institutions (Diethelm and McKee 2009). The most striking example here is HIV dissidence, which denies the disease's presence or the danger of its consequences (Heller 2015; Rykov, Meylakhs, and Sinyavskaya 2017). In general, the denial of medical expertise is associated with both (1) the problems of national healthcare systems and their low level of efficiency and (2) an individual predisposition to conspiracy theories (Barkun 2003).

The vast majority of conspiracy studies have been published in the last five years, focusing extensively on the US and Europe (Goreis and Voracek 2019). However, the COVID-19 pandemic has been explicitly studied worldwide, including in the Central and Eastern European region (Nowak et al. 2020; Kohút, Kohútová, and Halama 2021). Such research predominantly uses survey data where respondents are recruited via online platforms or, in some cases, are interviewed by phone. In most cases, study designs are cross-sectional.

Conspiracy Thinking as Part of Post-Communist Legacy

Conspiracy thinking dwells on the deficit of institutional trust. The latter is believed to constitute part of the communist legacies and traumas of economic transition in the 1990s that CEE states share (Offe 1994). Legacies manifest themselves in a variety of forms: attitudes, institutions, and policies. Beissinger and Kotkin define legacies as an 'endurable causal relationship between past institutions and policies on subsequent practices or believes, long beyond the life of the regimes, institutions, and policies that gave birth to them' (Beissinger and Kotkin 2014: 7). It is helpful to differentiate between communist legacies and legacies of transition as they may affect subsequent political developments differently.

Communist legacies translate into a set of attitudes and predispositions that individuals internalised during their early and/or professional socialisation in communist times (Pop-Eleches and Tucker 2017). Exposure to communist rule happened in schools and universities, political organisations (youth organisations or political parties), as well as the army, trade unions, and workplaces. According to earlier accounts, communist socialisation made individuals more perceptive of economic inequalities, left-wing ideologies, paternalistic views of the state, as well as participation habits in top-down organised political events (Lankina et al. 2016). The left-right party dimension operates differently in the Eastern European context. For instance, far-right political views are associated with less popular conspiracy beliefs in Romania where traditionally right-of-centre voters are more pro-European, less religious, less nationalistic compared to left-of-centre voters (Stoica and Umbreş 2021). Among left-wing voters, a lower level of education is more widespread, as is an attachment to tradition and authority. Transitional legacies often transmit into collective memories of traumatic transitions to market economies, new statehood, and democracy. These changes in certain cases caused disillusionment and ressentiment (Vogt 2004; Libman and Rochlitz 2019).

Going back to the major attitudinal legacies, which also have a clear institutional dimension, are the systematic shortages of institutional trust, interpersonal trust, and omnipresent cynicism (Rozenas and Zhukov 2019). We do believe that these stem from any authoritarian regime, regardless of its ideological leanings where human rights are severely compromised (Nunn and Wantchekon 2011). Researchers who study the formation of trust in different institutions prove that facing a novel virus personally determines people's attitudes. For example, a study based on a panel survey conducted in Spain in late March 2020 among 1,600 citizens revealed the negative relationship between personal exposure to COVID-19 and trust in the Spanish government, the EU, and democracy in general (Amat et al. 2020). Respondents who were personally exposed to COVID-19 were more willing to sacrifice a certain amount of civil liberties to combat the pandemic. They also shared preferences for authoritarian rule during a state of emergency. It should be noted that the survey was conducted in Spain during the strict lockdown, and the country witnessed one of the fastest escalations in the number of COVID-19 cases and deaths in Europe. Slightly opposing results come from another study conducted on a similar sample of 1,600 respondents in the same period of March 2020 but in the Dutch context (Schraff 2021). The author concluded that the rise of COVID-19 infections is related to higher political trust.

State capture by crony groups or so-called *oligarchs,* coupled with widespread corruption and clientelism, reinforced citizens' distrust and paved the way for the anomalous popularity of conspiracy thinking. Marinov and Popova (2022: 222) explicitly draw the link between witnessing state capture and COVID-19 scepticism:

> 'Eastern European democracies' original sin of state capture has been exacerbated by the rise of conspiracy theories, whose stock has only increased with the addition of COVID misinformation.
>
> (2022: 222)

The tragic congruence between a lack of trust and state capture by vested economic interests results in an odd denial of COVID-19 and the absence of effective blame attribution in the region. States that were less economically stable and possessed a strong record of corruption, such as Romania and Bulgaria, exhibit this pattern to the greatest degree. At the same time, both the Romanian and Bulgarian governments lost power because of the pandemic, meaning that some form of punishment took place regardless of COVID-19 denialism. Previous studies showed that there is a strong correlation between political support and COVID-19 scepticism (Sokolov et al. 2022). Those who believe that the pandemic was a hoax and any governmental measures are overreactions systematically correlate with lower levels of government support.

For instance, an early study, based on a Romanian survey in May 2020, revealed that higher education levels, as well as older age, are connected with a belief in conspiracy theories (Stoica and Umbreș 2021). People with higher levels of education may overestimate their policy evaluation abilities and trust the government in Romania less. The authors connect these findings with the local Romanian context and a post-communist legacy of a lower trust in institutions. Moreover, at the outbreak of the pandemic, local politicians, experts, and media tended to underestimate the threat of COVID-19, which provided a solid base for conspiracies to flourish. The results also indicated a strong association between pro-Russian political views, anti-Western views (meaning anti-EU, anti-NATO, and anti-US), and predisposition to conspiracy thinking and simultaneous neglection for health measures (Achimescu, Sultănescu, and Sultănescu 2021). Pro-Russian political opinions on the edge of the pandemic possibly act as alternative explanations for EU citizens who tend to distrust national authorities and supranational institutions. Left-wing and religious citizens are more likely to become COVID-19 deniers (Achimescu, Sultănescu, and Sultănescu 2021). The research conducted in Slovakia shows that behavioural and emotional responses to the pandemic have decreased, meaning that people have developed adaption mechanisms (Kohút et al. 2021).

Studies also illustrate that trust in government, health institutions, and expert knowledge are significant predictors of compliance with restriction measures and quarantine (Nestik 2021). A compelling interaction has been found between conservatively minded individuals, low levels of trust in other persons, and high knowledge, which all together endorse conspiracy beliefs (Miller, Saunders, and Farhart 2016). Research based on a representative survey in Slovakia supports the positive correlation between the perceived lack of control, low trust in institutions, feelings of anxiety and conspiracy, and pseudoscientific beliefs (Šrol et al. 2021).

How are conspiracy theories, legacies, and blame attribution strategies connected? The first mechanism implies that the very denial of COVID-19 is a tangible threat; therefore, governments are punished for attempts to compartmentalise the pandemic through restrictions. Paradoxically, political leaders may be punished for technically well-meaning policies (Bulgaria and Romania). The presence of communist parties may partially hijack an agenda sceptical of COVID-19, thereby shifting the blame. However, most governments quickly realised electorate priorities and despite the threats to public health, lifted pandemic constraints. The latter kickstarted the second mechanism of blame avoidance (Hungary). In higher trust countries such as the Baltic states, which have a relatively small share of sceptics and a long-standing tradition of coalition governments, rallying is stronger and blame attribution operates similar to other EU states.

Drawing on these considerations, we articulate the following hypotheses:

1 COVID-19 sceptics and vaccine-hesitant individuals demonstrate systematically lower degrees of political support for the government (conspiracy thinking);
2 Those who support the incumbent government would estimate its COVID-19-related policies as more efficient (political partisanship effect);
3 Those who trust 'new' media (social networks, internet outlets) possess lower levels of political support for the government (information availability hypothesis);
4 Those who perceive the economy as declining possess lower levels of political support for the government (economic punishment).

We also include socio-demographic controls, such as gender, age, and education. It is expected that the elderly and females would perceive risks more acutely as the former belonged to a major risk group, while the latter tends to care about underage and elderly members of households. Educated respondents should have more adequate evaluations of the country's government's policies.

Analysis

We take individual attitudes as the starting point for our empirical analysis. We rely on two surveys that were carried out in late that spring and summer of 2021, i.e., after the second wave of the pandemic and after the start of vaccination campaigns. It is likely that we do not grasp the initial rallying that analysts observed in the spring of 2020, but it makes the whole set-up closed to regular economic punishment models, rather than a reaction to an emergency. The first survey is a standard Eurobarometer 95.3 requested and coordinated by the European Commission, a poll whose main topic was attitudes towards COVID-19 vaccinations, COVID-19 in general, and economic perceptions. The survey draws on national representative samples from 27 EU states. The second survey is carried out by the think tank Global Security and is specifically tailored to explore various forms of COVID-19 scepticism: outright denialism, COVID-19 as a result of clandestine conspiring, and vaccine hesitancy. Survey fieldwork took place in March 2021. The latter covers eight CEE countries and includes variables on political support. Taking advantage of two surveys provides additional cross-validation for the analysis.

We used simple OLS regression as a preliminary way of estimating correlations between COVID-19 scepticism and political support, while also controlling for other variables. The major caveat is that such an empirical strategy does not allow one to make any causal claims and rather aims at exploring the existing links. We run regression country by country as the number of cases is not sufficient for more sophisticated hierarchical modelling. On the other hand, such an approach permits having a more nuanced gaze into each case. The main dependent variable is trust in government, which is operationalised as a four-item Likert scale, where one stands for the lowest degree of trust and four for the highest.

In Figure 1.1, we present the country percentages of the main variables of interest: political support of the government (striped bars), beliefs that COVID-19 is fake (dark grey bars), and beliefs that COVID-19 is planned (light grey bars). The highest share of those who trust their government is observed in the Baltic states and Hungary. In Estonia, the grand coalition of the Reform Party and the Centre Party enjoyed the highest support with 62.3%. The Hungarian Fidesz government scored second in the sample with 53.3% of public support. Romania's centre-right coalition of the National Liberal Party (PNL), USR PLUS, and the Democratic Alliance of Hungarians (UDMR/RMDSZ) with Florin Cîțu as prime minister had the lowest support of just 31.8%. Romanian politics went through turbulent times in the spring of 2021, which resulted in a full-blown crisis in the fall of 2021 (Stan and Zaharia 2022).

Czechia also reveals a low share of those who supported the government – just 32.7%. Prime Minister Andrej Babiš and his populist ANO party were losing their grip on power. Support for the Bulgarian government was 34%, and this number reflects the 2021–2023 Bulgarian political crisis. The country held five elections over two years, demonstrating an abnormal degree of governmental instability. At the time of the survey, Bulgaria faced large-scale protests against the long-standing prime minister and

GERB leader Boyko Borissov. Legislative elections were scheduled for April 2021. According to several accounts, the government followed an inconsistent pattern of anti-COVID-19 policies that resulted in a slow vaccination rollout and high mortality (Spirova 2022). Political support, or lack thereof, translates into electoral choices. Incumbents lost in half of the CEE countries in question: Lithuania, Czechia, Slovakia, Bulgaria, and Romania. Polish and Hungarian governments passed the COVID-19 test quite successfully in terms of electoral performance.

Two of those countries with the lowest levels of trust in the government have the largest share of COVID-19 sceptics – Romania and Bulgaria. More than one-third of Romanians believe that COVID-19 is fake and almost 20% of Bulgarians share the same opinion. Almost 56% of Bulgarians deem COVID-19 as planned by hidden political forces, while in Romania, this share is also remarkable – 45% of respondents. All in all, conspiracy thinking seems to be widespread in the region – around 30% of respondents in Poland, Hungary, and Lithuania think the same. Czechia on the other hand has the smallest share of outright COVID-19 deniers – 5.7% and 6.6%, respectively.

Looking at the vaccination rollout, Latvia, Lithuania, and Hungary demonstrated the fastest speed with more than 60% of the population receiving at least one dose of the vaccine until Summer 2021. Hungary's engagement with vaccine diplomacy and import of Sinovac and Sputnik V boosted vaccination rates. In all these countries, the share of COVID-19 scepticism is below 10% (Johns Hopkins Coronavirus Resource Center 2021). Romania and Bulgaria lagged behind other CEE states with less than 50% of those who received the first dose and extremely large numbers of COVID-19 sceptics.

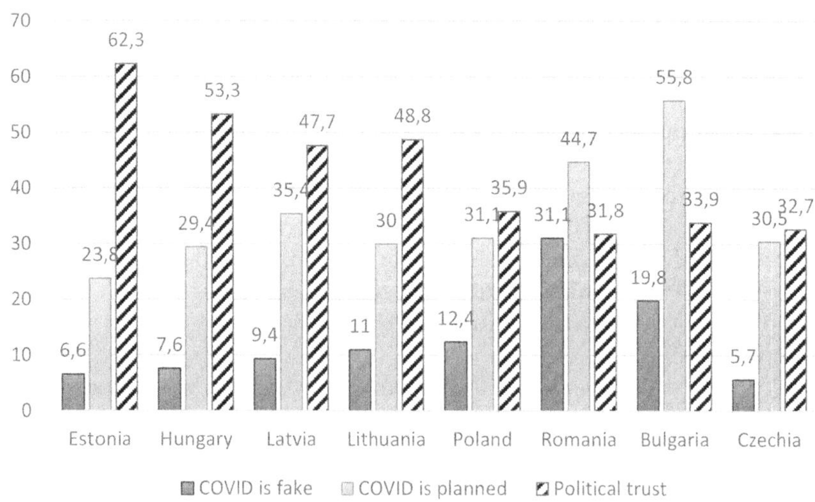

Figure 1.1 Political support and COVID-19 scepticism in CEE countries.
Source: Haidu et al. (2021)

Table 1.1 summarises political outcomes, the overall situation with COVID-19 in the spring of 2021, and strategies for blame avoidance. The latter includes more general breaches in democracy that permit tweaking the rule of law (e.g., abusing state of emergency legislation), repressing political opposition under the guise of the pandemic, and exercising media control. Attempts to import Russian and Chinese vaccines, bypassing EU regulations, demonstrate the electorate's political independence of leadership and its alleged efficiency (vaccine diplomacy). Provisions for additional vaccines aimed at creating an image of governments that care about public health and who dare to act independently from EU authorities. Finally, 'the blame game' stands for systematic attempts to spotlight 'scapegoats' who allegedly undermine the government's policies to handle COVID-19. Hungary is the only country whose government enjoyed a proper 'authoritarian advantage' at the onset of the pandemic and successfully deployed a full array of policies (Miklossy this volume). Viktor Orbán actively blamed his opponents from the Social Democratic party for sabotaging the vaccination campaign (Batory 2022), while importing Sputnik V and Sinovac to gain a populist advantage in the eyes of the population. Hungarian media has been under the government's and Orbán's affiliates' control for the last decade (Magyar 2016), thereby facilitating the spread of narratives favouring the government. Orbán's government pushed all the buttons that allowed Fidesz to triumphantly sidestep potential political ramifications of the COVID-19 emergency. Polish PiS enjoyed similar advantages except for one: it could not engage in vaccine diplomacy and boost the vaccination rate, since pro-Russian or pro-Chinese sentiments are extremely unpopular. Polish parties adamantly blame each other for the poor handling of the pandemic as well as for endangering citizens' health and lives (Lipiński 2021). Bulgarian and Romanian political actors deployed the pandemic as an additional reason to shift the blame to the opponent. The major underlying reasons for both political crises were of economic nature. Slovak and Czech populist leaders attempted to follow the Hungarian government's lead and import non-EU vaccines but largely failed. Slovenia, Estonia, Latvia, and Lithuania did not show any evidence of abusing the existing rules and avoided blame. To a great extent, these countries managed the COVID-19 emergency quite successfully, so there was no need to resort to any dubious strategies.

Thus, there are two main scenarios that distorted blame attribution: (1) the weakness of the state and large numbers of COVID-19 sceptics and (2) authoritarian options. While in other cases, blame attribution followed the logic of economic punishment or appraisal. Bulgarian and Romanian governments suffered for economic reasons, lack of efficient governance and corruption. Hungary and Poland engaged in strategies that undermine democratic rule. although Poland to a much lesser degree than Hungary.

In Tables 1.2 and 1.3, we present the estimate of how various variables are associated with trust in government. Regression estimates in Table 1.3 provide similar models for eight CEE countries based on Eurobarometer

Table 1.1 COVID-19 and Strategies of Blame Avoidance

Country	*Incumbent lost?*[a]	*Vaccination rate, at least 1 dose, %*[b]	*% of COVID-19 sceptics*[c]	*State of democracy: tweaking the rule of law and oppressing opposition*[d]	*Media control*[d]	*Vaccine diplomacy*	*Blame game*
Hungary	No	67,7	7	Poor	Yes	Yes	Yes
Poland	No	59,6	12	Poor	Yes	No	Yes
Lithuania	Yes	69,7	10	Okay	No	No	No
Latvia	No	70,7	9	Okay	No	No	No
Estonia	No	64,6	6	Okay	No	No	No
The Czech Republic	Yes	65	6	Okay	No	Yes	No
Romania	Yes	42,3	30	Okay	No	No	Yes
Bulgaria	Yes	NA	17	Okay	No	No	Yes
Slovenia	No	60,2	NA	Okay	No	No	No
Slovakia	Yes	51,7	11	Okay	No	Yes	No

a IDEA, International Institute for Democracy and Electoral Assistance. Databases. https://www.idea.int/data-tools.
b Johns Hopkins Coronavirus Resource Center (2021).
c Globsec (2021), Hajdu et al. (2021).
d V-Dem Project. https://www.v-dem.net/publications/democracy-reports/.

data that include (1) economic variables, (2) attitudes towards the EU and their own country, (3) COVID-19 scepticism, and (4) demographic controls. Unfortunately, this survey does not cover preferences for certain political parties; therefore, we cannot estimate the effect of political leanings in these models. All in all, economic perceptions play a crucial role in individuals' support of a government.

We used multiple tools to tease out respondents' economic perceptions: perceptions of one's financial situation, perceptions of the national economy, employment prospects in general and respondent's situation, and overall assessment of whether a country develops in the right direction. All variables vary from one to four, Likert scale. More positive assessments systematically increase political support: perceptions of employment make the strongest covariate of political support; a one-unit increase is associated with a 0.01-unit increase in support that varies from one to four (see Table 1.2). More positive perceptions of the national economy tend to increase political support by 0.5–0.1 points. Although the estimates are not statistically significant for all countries, employment perceptions fail to reach conventional thresholds of statistical significance in Czechia. Egocentric perceptions are significant only in Estonia and Czechia. Individual perceptions of employment prospects significantly correlate with political support only in Bulgaria. Regardless of operationalisation, more economic perceptions – sociotropic or egocentric – are likely to boost trust in a government.

The effects of COVID-19 scepticism were less consistent across CEE countries. We include respondents' perceptions of pandemic restrictions and their willingness to follow them, also known as vaccine hesitancy. The Eurobarometer survey does not include direct questions about COVID-19 denialism and conspiracy thinking, but these variables approximate general attitudes towards COVID-19 and the risks it bears. In all CEE countries except Bulgaria, a one-unit increase in positive COVID-19 restrictions is associated with approximately a 0.1 increase in political support. This is in line with our idea that a large number of COVID-19 sceptics and an absence of efficient government responses made the pandemic resemble a more traditional economic crisis. In Bulgaria, respondents held their government accountable for economic outcomes, rather than public health issues. Against our expectations, 'anti-vaxxer' attitudes systematically decrease political support only in Estonia and Lithuania. In other countries, there is no clear-cut correlation between vaccine hesitancy and support.

To track the proclivities of respondents to endorse the import of Sputnik V and Sinovac, we add attachment to the EU and respondents' country into the equation. A stronger pro-EU stance is expected to negatively correlate with political support for the Hungarian government, which indulged in 'vaccine diplomacy' and, perhaps, in Czechia and Slovakia where some political groups supported the use of Sputnik V. Stronger identification with one's own country is expected to boost government support in any case, but stronger in more nationalistic and less pro-EU governments. Indeed, a stronger attachment to

Table 1.2 Correlates of Political Support in CEE, May 2021

	BU		*CZ*		*HU*		*PL*		*EST*		*LA*		*LT*		*RO*	
Predictors	*Coef.*	*P-value*	*Coef.*	*p-value*	*Coef.*	*p-value*	*Coef.*	*p-value*	*Coef.*	*p-value*	*Coef.*	*p-value*	*Coef.*	*p-value*	*Coef.*	*p-value*
Gender	−0.1	0.219	0.07	0.297	0.08	0.283	0.05	0.432	−0.1	0.142	0.11	0.085	0.11	0.192	0	0.943
Age	0	0.207	0	0.288	0	0.809	0	0.439	0	0.912	0	0.288	0	0.629	0	0.466
Education (ranks)	−0.08	**0.044**	−0.03	0.388	−0.05	0.145	−0.05	0.208	0.07	0.187	−0.06	0.203	0.05	0.461	0.04	0.375
Do not want vaccination	0.08	0.086	0.09	**0.007**	0.03	0.38	0.01	0.798	0.07	0.06	0.04	0.28	0.14	**0.001**	0.02	0.547
COVID is a fake	0.03	0.555	−0.09	0.103	−0.08	0.159	−0.11	**0.016**	0.03	0.616	−0.02	0.749	−0.06	0.343	−0.03	0.478
No trust in vaccination firms	−0.08	0.174	−0.04	0.268	−0.04	0.291	−0.05	0.157	−0.16	**<0.001**	−0.14	**0.002**	−0.07	0.207	−0.11	**0.006**
COVID-19 was planned	−0.15	**0.005**	−0.06	0.157	−0.05	0.19	−0.01	0.758	−0.15	**0.003**	−0.1	**0.01**	0.02	0.788	0.03	0.489
Preference for a strong leader	0.08	0.072	0.05	0.171	0.03	0.285	0.08	**0.002**	−0.08	**0.006**	−0.06	0.051	−0.13	**0.001**	0.01	0.681
Democracy is good for my country	0.19	**0.001**	0	0.966	0.13	**0.01**	0.06	0.153	0.21	**<0.001**	0.04	0.458	0.13	**0.035**	0.14	**0.002**
Media need more restrictions	0.02	0.668	0.05	0.164	0.11	**<0.001**	0.13	**<0.001**	0.04	0.259	0.12	**<0.001**	0.03	0.49	0.01	0.712
Non-voter	−0.22	0.082	0.21	**0.009**	0.51	**<0.001**	0.44	**<0.001**	−0.21	0.08	−0.3	**0.002**	−0.27	**0.047**	−0.13	0.146
Winner			1.11	**<0.001**	1.79	**<0.001**	1.46	**<0.001**	0.33	**<0.001**	0.41	**<0.001**	0.5	**<0.001**	0.4	**<0.001**
Partisan (no voting rights)									0.25	**0.034**	0.03	0.839				
Observations	404		529		446		531		443		449		306		623	
R^2/R^2 adjusted	0.140/0.116		0.338/0.322		0.626/0.616		0.537/0.526		0.364/0.345		0.366/0.347		0.409/0.385		0.156/0.139	

Source: Standard Eurobarometer 95 – Wave EB95.3 – Kantar Public.

the home country boosts political support for the government in Hungary and Czechia. Meanwhile, in Slovakia and Romania, more patriotic respondents tend to demonstrate more sceptical views of the governments. Stronger pro-EU leanings positively and significantly correlate with political support everywhere except for in Hungary, Poland, and Czechia. In Poland, the correlation is even the opposite: more pro-EU respondents assess their government's performance more critically and it perfectly reflects attitudes towards EU sceptic isolationist policies by PiS.

In Table 1.3, we present the OLS regression estimate for the Global Security survey that covers various aspects of COVID-19 scepticism, though it does not include question items on the state of the economy. Four variables account for COVID-19 scepticism: hesitancy towards vaccination, belief that COVID-19 is fake, a lack of trust in vaccination firms, and belief that COVID-19 was planned by hidden political forces. Effects of partisanship are operationalised through whether a respondent supports the incumbent or goes to national elections. We expect to observe 'a winner-loser gap' in respondents' perceptions of their government's performance. We also include the variable indicating whether a respondent consistently abstains from participation in national elections. The latter is likely to indicate a lack of trust in the very political institutions in the country. Finally, the Global Security survey contains questions on support for authoritarian rule (preference for a stronger political leader) and support for democracy (whether democracy is good for one's country).

Those who do not want to get a jab tend to assess their governments more negatively. Especially, in Czechia and Lithuania, regardless of if the association is statistically significant. A belief that COVID-19 is fake also negatively correlates with political support, but turns out to be significant only for Poland. Lower trust in companies that produced the vaccine tends to systematically decrease support in Romania, Latvia, and Estonia. Finally, beliefs that COVID-19 was planned by clandestine political forces drove political support down in Bulgaria, Estonia, and Latvia.

Authoritarian leanings prove to be more visible in Poland, Estonia, and Latvia. Apparently, in Poland, a one-unit increase in preference for a strong political leader increases political support by 0.3 points (political support varies from one to four). In Estonia and Lithuania, the correlation is the opposite: a stronger preference for authoritarian rule tends to decrease political support for the government. A preference for democratic rule, and vice versa, increases political support in most of the countries: a one-unit increase in democratic preferences (a Likert scale from one to four) is positively associated with 0.1–0.2 points increases in political support. What is telling is that the respondents in Poland, Hungary, and Latvia, who are more supportive of media restrictions, support their governments more strongly. In the case of Poland and Hungary, these are likely to be conservative respondents, while in Latvia this trend is likely connected with Russian-language media, which is widespread in the country. Quite predictably, those who voted for the incumbent tend to support the government more. This is the most consistent and strong correlation across all CEE countries,[2] boarding on tautology.

It is interesting that non-voters tend to support the government in Czechia, Hungary, and Poland: non-voting brought an additional 0.2–0.5 points to political support. While in Latvia and Lithuania, non-voters share more sceptical attitudes towards the government. Respondents with no voting rights – most likely Russian-speaking minority groups – share a more positive stance towards their respective governments, although the regression coefficient is significant only for Estonia. The bottom line is that partisanship is the most decisive factor that accounts for variance in political support.

Demographic controls remain largely insignificant. More elderly respondents in Poland and Czechia share more positive attitudes towards the government. Women in Czechia express, on average, somewhat lower support for the Babiš' government (see Table 1.3). More educated respondents tend to dislike the government more in Bulgaria (see Table 1.3).

Bringing empirical evidence from regression analysis together, economic variables, and broadly understood partisanship (adherence to a certain political party, support for the EU or one's own country) explains domestic variance in political support. Meanwhile, COVID-19 scepticism, manifested in various forms, proves to operate differently from country to country. Denialism, conspiracy thinking, and vaccine hesitancy do not necessarily translate into political support or lack thereof. At the same time, it may interfere with economic attitudes and identity-related variables.

To trace the effects of communist legacies is far from a straightforward task, but the regression estimates provide no evidence that support for communist parties or age anyhow affect political support. EU scepticism in some contexts can be congruent with a pro-Russian stance, as is the case in Bulgaria or Hungary. However, it does not necessarily stem from communist or even transitional legacies. We rely on the concept of legacies to theorise the role of conspiracy thinking, but we do not test its effects empirically in this chapter. Nevertheless, we hypothesise that the effects on the level of individual attitudes are weaker than one would expect and play out in a combination with other factors.

Conclusion

How did some governments avoid blame for inefficient policies despite high mortality rates and the sluggish pace of vaccination campaigns? Why did some governments in Central and Eastern Europe capitalise on the pandemic, while others did not? The results of our exploratory analysis offer a framework of political blame attribution and strategies of blame avoidance that were available in the region due to its shared post-communist and transitional legacy. We argue that a systematic deficit of institutional and interpersonal trust that is endemic in many post-authoritarian societies created fertile ground for conspiracy thinking, COVID-19 denialism, and vaccine

Table 1.3 Correlates of Political Support in CEE, March 2021

	BU		*CZ*		*EE*		*HU*		*LT*		*LV*		*PL*		*SK*		*RO*	
Predictors	*Coef.*[a]	*p-value*	*Coef.*	*p-value*	*Coef.*	*p-value*	*Coef.*	*p-value*	*Coef.*	*p-value*	*Coef.*	*p-value*	*Coef.*	*p-value*	*Coef.*	*p-value*	*Coef.*	*p-value*
Female	−0.01	0.86	−0.06	**0.041**	0.03	0.315	0.04	0.234	−0.04	0.198	0.03	0.249	0.02	0.641	0.01	0.674	0.07	0.064
Age	0	0.935	0.04	**0.007**	0.01	0.632	0	0.957	−0.01	0.444	0.02	0.254	0.09	**<0.001**	0.03	0.099	0.01	0.541
Financial situation	−0.02	0.683	−0.09	**0.001**	0.07	**0.022**	0.04	0.209	0.01	0.691	−0.04	0.092	0.08	**0.014**	−0.01	0.862	0.02	0.568
National economy last year	0.12	**<0.001**	−0.01	0.556	0.08	**<0.001**	0.07	**<0.001**	0.09	**<0.001**	0.1	**<0.001**	0.05	**0.025**	0.02	0.368	0.04	0.051
Employment prospects	0.12	**<0.001**	0.01	0.717	0.1	**<0.001**	0.18	**<0.001**	0.06	**0.006**	0.11	**<0.001**	0.11	**<0.001**	0.13	**<0.001**	0.12	**<0.001**
Job situation	−0.09	**0.042**	0.03	0.19	0.05	0.056	0.01	0.849	0.04	0.173	0.04	0.128	0.03	0.36	0.04	0.2	0.04	0.124
Life goes in the right direction	0.14	**0.01**	0.11	**0.016**	0.06	0.214	0.14	**0.002**	0.05	0.184	0.09	**0.012**	0.02	0.595	0.11	**0.009**	−0.03	0.41
Good to follow COVID-19 restrictions	0.03	0.238	0.03	0.053	0.02	0.277	0	0.895	0	0.813	0.02	0.089	0.04	**0.018**	0.01	0.429	0.03	0.093
COVID-19 restrictions are just	−0.02	0.515	0.18	**<0.001**	0.06	**0.005**	0.12	**<0.001**	0.13	**<0.001**	0.11	**<0.001**	0.07	**0.003**	0.12	**<0.001**	0.1	**<0.001**
Do not want to get vaccinated	0.02	0.669	0.03	0.446	−0.13	**0.007**	−0.15	**0.001**	−0.11	**0.005**	−0.03	0.269	−0.01	0.863	0.01	0.817	0.03	0.6
Attached to one's own country	0.02	0.454	0.08	**<0.001**	0.03	0.252	0.07	**0.014**	0.03	0.139	0.03	0.126	0.05	0.097	−0.08	**0.001**	−0.06	**0.024**
Attached to the EU	0.09	**<0.001**	−0.02	0.218	0.13	**<0.001**	−0.03	0.172	0.11	**<0.001**	0.04	0.007	−0.09	**<0.001**	0.06	**0.004**	0.08	**0.002**
Other (gender)			−0.15	0.543	0	0.993			−0.48	0.256								
Observations	472		873		1010		703		992		902		672		626		646	
R^2/R^2 adjusted	0.204/0.183		0.202/0.190		0.235/0.225		0.318/0.306		0.291/0.281		0.269/0.259		0.212/0.198		0.281/0.267		0.143/0.127	

Source: Hajdu et al. (2021).

a Table entries are non-standardised b-coefficients.

hesitancy. We hypothesised that the latter affected blame attribution in such a way that some governments succeeded in escaping punishment for poor policies. For instance, in post-Soviet states, especially Russia, COVID-19 deniers altered public perceptions of policy efficiency (Gel'man forthcoming). However, it turned out that a significant share of COVID-19 sceptics did not facilitate blame avoidance, but rather exacerbated economic problems, overloaded public health capacities, and, in the end, caused dramatic excess mortality. Voters did punish the governments harshly but not primarily for poor handling of COVID-19.

The best governments in avoiding political blame turned out to be Hungary and Poland, whose incumbents took advantage of the 'blame game', mass media domination, and EU sceptic stances. However, the portion of COVID-19 sceptics in both countries is relatively small compared to other countries in the region. No political force capitalised on COVID-19 denialism, although there was more speculation over possible economic conspiracies behind vaccination campaigns. Breaches in the rule of law coupled with aggressive media campaigns kept governments afloat. Finally, other countries handled the public health crisis well with relatively low death tolls, making blame-avoidance strategies both unavailable and unnecessary. Attempts to engage in vaccine diplomacy failed to work out in Czechia and Slovakia as they did in Hungary. That said, COVID-19 scepticism and low trust tend to cause governmental destabilisation, but abusive political institutions play a more decisive role in avoiding political accountability. Pro-authoritarian leanings and EU scepticism produce more leeway for incumbents to prop up their support.

To summarise the findings from the hypotheses, we find confirmation that sceptics and vaccine-hesitant respondents demonstrate a systematically lower degree of political support for the government. Although various aspects of COVID-19 scepticism seem to play differently across the CEE region. We found no uniform pattern: outright denialism is more widespread only in Bulgaria and Romania, while pro-conspiracy attitudes tend to be more widespread. Some countries, despite a shared post-communist past, enjoyed a high degree of political trust, primarily Baltic countries, thereby resembling trends in the Nordic countries rather than Southern Europe. Partisanship played a major role in the selective evaluation and blame attribution in all instances presented here, regardless of other factors. From this perspective, CEE voters are no different from any other. Unfortunately, our data do not allow for any systematic estimate of how media shaped respondents' perceptions, although we find out that support for media restrictions tends to correlate with more loyal political behaviour and a preference for strong political leadership. Not surprisingly, these tendencies were strongest in Poland and Hungary and were part of the pre-pandemic democratic decline. Finally, the logic of retrospective economic punishment remains a reliable correlate of political support. Thus, the region resembles other electoral democratic regimes around the world.

Our analysis has important limitations such as a non-experimental design that is based on non-dynamic cross-country data. Due to this, causal interpretations are not possible. We do not estimate more complex relations between the independent variables or interaction effects that may be in operation. To do that, more elaborated theoretical mechanisms are to be developed. Future research may draw more attention to the interplay between COVID-19 scepticism and partisan support in a more dynamic format, i.e., relying on panel data. The effects of political institutions and the peculiarities of national healthcare systems on political support are to be considered. Since we do not explore the immediate impact of post-communist or transitional legacies, this offers another pathway for future study. Last, but not least, a broader cross-country comparison would be a better way to systematically estimate the role of COVID-19 in blame attribution and political support.

Notes

1 This term is generally vaguer, but to avoid unnecessary terminological confusion, in this work, it is used as a synonym for 'COVID deniers'. Both concepts are special cases of the more general phenomenon of COVID-19 scepticism.
2 There is no estimate for Bulgaria as there was a non-partisan caretaker government at the time of the survey.

References

Abramson, Paul R., John H. Aldrich, Jill Rickershauser, and David W. Rohde. 2007. "Fear in the voting booth: The 2004 presidential election." *Political Behavior* 29: 197–220.

Achimescu, Vlad, Dan Sultănescu, and Dana C. Sultănescu. 2021. "The path from distrusting Western actors to conspiracy beliefs and noncompliance with public health guidance during the COVID-19 crisis." *Journal of Elections, Public Opinion and Parties* 31, no. sup1: 299–310.

Altiparmakis, Argyrios, Abel Bojar, Sylvain Brouard, Martial Foucault, Hanspeter Kriesi, and Richard Nadeau. 2021. "Pandemic politics: Policy evaluations of government responses to COVID-19." *West European Politics* 44, no. 5–6: 1159–1179.

Amat, Francesc, Albert Falcó-Gimeno, Andreu Arenas, Jordi Muñoz. 2020. "Pandemics meet democracy. Experimental evidence from the COVID-19 crisis in Spain." *SocArXiv*. 10.31235/osf.io/dkusw.

Baccini, Leonardo, and Abel Brodeur. 2021. "Explaining governors' response to the COVID-19 pandemic in the United States." *American Politics Research* 49, no. 2: 215–220.

Barkun, Michael. 2003. *A Culture of Conspiracy. Apocalyptic Visions in Contemporary America*. Berkeley: University of California Press.

Batory, Agnes. 2022. "More power, less support: The Fidesz government and the coronavirus pandemic in Hungary." *Government and Opposition*: 1–17. doi:10.1017/gov.2022.3

Beall, Alec T., Marlise K. Hofer, and Mark Schaller. 2016 "Infections and elections: Did an Ebola outbreak influence the 2014 US federal elections (and if so, how)?" *Psychological Science* 27, no. 5: 595–605.

Bechtel, Michael M., and Jens Hainmueller. 2011. "How lasting is voter gratitude? An analysis of the short- and long-term electoral returns to beneficial policy." *American Journal of Political Science* 55, no. 4: 852–868.

Beissinger, Mark, and Stephen Kotkin. 2014. Eds. *Historical Legacies of Communism in Russia and Eastern Europe*. Cambridge: Cambridge University Press.

Bol, Damien, Marco Giani, André Blais, and Peter John Loewen. 2021. "The effect of COVID-19 lockdowns on political support: Some good news for democracy?" *European Journal of Political Research* 60, no. 2: 497–505.

Buštíková, Lenka, and Pavol Baboš. 2020. "Best in Covid: Populists in the time of pandemic." *Politics and Governance* 8, no. 4: 496–508.

Campante, Filipe R., Emilio Depetris-Chauvin, and Ruben Durante. 2020. *The Virus of Fear: The Political Impact of Ebola in the US*. No. w26897. National Bureau of Economic Research. https://econpapers.repec.org/paper/nbrnberwo/26897.htm.

Cinelli, Matteo, Walter Quattrociocchi, Alessandro Galeazzi, Carlo Michele Valensise, Emanuele Brugnoli, Ana Lucia Schmidt, Paola Zola, Fabiana Zollo, and Antonio Scala. 2020. "The COVID-19 social media infodemic." *Scientific Reports* 10, no. 1: 1–10.

Diethelm, Pascal, and Martin McKee. 2009. "Denialism: What is it and how should scientists respond?" *The European Journal of Public Health* 19, no. 1: 2–4.

Douglas, Karen M., Joseph E. Uscinski, Robbie M. Sutton, Aleksandra Cichocka, Turkay Nefes, Chee Siang Ang, and Farzin Deravi. 2019. "Understanding conspiracy theories." *Political Psychology* 40: 3–35.

Earnshaw, Valerie A., Lisa A. Eaton, Seth C. Kalichman, Natalie M. Brousseau, E. Carly Hill, and Annie B. Fox. 2020. "COVID-19 conspiracy beliefs, health behaviors, and policy support." *Translational Behavioral Medicine* 10, no. 4: 850–856.

Enders, Adam, Christina Farhart, Joanne Miller, Joseph Uscinski, Kyle Saunders, and Hugo Drochon. 2022. "Are republicans and conservatives more likely to believe conspiracy theories?" *Political Behavior*: 1–24. https://link.springer.com/article/10.1007/s11109-022-09812-3.

Esaiasson, Peter, Jacob Sohlberg, Marina Ghersetti, and Bengt Johansson. 2021. "How the coronavirus crisis affects citizen trust in institutions and in unknown others: Evidence from 'the Swedish experiment'." *European Journal of Political* Research 60, no. 3: 748–760.

Gel'man, Vladimir. (forthcoming). "Bad governance in times of exogenous shocks: The case of the pandemic in Russia." In *Politics of the Pandemic: Blame Game and Governance in Russian and Central-Eastern Europe*, edited by M. Zavadskaya. London: Routledge.

Goreis, Andreas, and Voracek Martin. 2019. "A systematic review and meta-analysis of psychological research on conspiracy beliefs: Field characteristics, measurement instruments, and associations with personality traits." *Frontiers in Psychology* 10: 205.

Guasti, Petra, and Jaroslav Bílek. 2022. "The demand side of vaccine politics and pandemic illiberalism." *East European Politics* 38, no. 4: 594–616.

Guasti, Petra, and Lenka Buštíková. 2020. "A marriage of convenience: Responsive populists and responsible experts." *Politics and Governance* 8, no. 4: 468–472.

Gutiérrez, Emilio, Jaakko Meriläinen, and Adrian Rubli. 2022. "Electoral repercussions of a pandemic: Evidence from the 2009 H1N1 outbreak." *The Journal of Politics* 84, no. 4: 1899–1912.

Hajdu, Dominika, Katarína Klingová, Daniel Milo, and Miroslava Sawiris. 2021. *GLOBSEC Trends 2021: Central and Eastern Europe one year into the pandemic*. Bratislava: GLOBSEC. https://www.globsec.org/what-we-do/publications/globsec-trends-2021-central-and-eastern-europe-one-year-pandemic.

Healy, Andrew, and Neil Malhotra. 2009. "Myopic voters and natural disaster policy." *American Political Science Review* 103, no. 3: 387–406.

Heller, Jacob. 2015. "Rumors and realities: Making sense of HIV/AIDS conspiracy narratives and contemporary legends." *American Journal of Public Health* 105, no. 1: 43–50.

Hobolt, Sara B., and Tilley James. 2014. *Blaming Europe?: Responsibility without accountability in the European Union*. Oxford: Oxford University Press.

Imhoff, Roland, and Pia Lamberty. 2020. "Conspiracy beliefs as psycho-political reactions to perceived power." In *Routledge Handbook of Conspiracy Theories*, edited by Michael Butter, Peter Knight, 192–205. London: Routledge.

Iyengar, Shanto. 1996. "Framing responsibility for political issues." *The Annals of the American Academy of Political and Social Science* 546, no. 1: 59–70.

Johansson, Bengt, Jacob Sohlberg, Peter Esaiasson, and Marina Ghersetti. 2021. "Why swedes don't wear face masks during the pandemic-a consequence of blindly trusting the government." *Journal of International Crisis and Risk Communication Research* 4, no. 2: 335–358.

Kazharski, Aliaksei, and Makarychev Andrey. 2021. "Belarus, Russia, and the escape from geopolitics." *Political Geography* 89. https://doi.org/10.1016/j.polgeo.2021.10237.

Kohút, Michal, Veronika Kohútová, and Peter Halama. 2021. "Big Five predictors of pandemic-related behavior and emotions in the first and second COVID-19 pandemic wave in Slovakia." *Personality and Individual Differences* 180: 110934.

Lankina, Tomila V., Alexander Libman, and Anastassia Obydenkova. 2016. "Appropriation and subversion: Precommunist literacy, communist party saturation, and postcommunist democratic outcomes." *World Politics* 68, no. 2: 229–274.

Libman, Alexander, and Rochlitz Michael. 2019. *Federalism in China and Russia*. Northampton, MA: Edward Elgar Publishing.

Lipiński, Artur. 2021. "Poland: 'If we don't elect the President, the country will plunge into chaos'." *Populism and the Politicization of the COVID-19 Crisis in Europe*, edited by Giuliano Bobba, Nicolas Hubé, 115–129. Camden: Palgrave Macmillan.

Lunz Trujillo, K., and Motta Matthew. 2021. "How internet access drives global vaccine skepticism." *International Journal of Public Opinion Research* 33, no. 3: 551–570.

Maffioli, Elisa M. 2021. "The political economy of health epidemics: Evidence from the Ebola outbreak." *Journal of Development Economics* 151.

Magyar, Bálint. 2016. *Post-Communist Mafia State. The Case of Hungary*. Central European University Press.

Marinov, Nikolay, and Maria Popova. 2022. "Will the real conspiracy please stand up: Sources of post-communist democratic failure." *Perspectives on Politics* 20, no. 1: 222–236.

Miklossy, Katalin. forthcoming. "Legislative advantages of multiple crises in the Europe in-between." In *Politics of the Pandemic: Blame Game and Governance in Russian and Central-Eastern Europe*, edited by M. Zavadskaya. London: Routledge.

Miller, Joanne M., Kyle L. Saunders, and Christina E. Farhart. 2016. "Conspiracy endorsement as motivated reasoning: The moderating roles of political knowledge and trust." *American Journal of Political Science* 60, no. 4: 824–844.

Mutz, Diana C. 2001. "Facilitating communication across lines of political difference: The role of mass media." *American Political Science Review* 95, no. 1: 97–114.

Nestik, Timothy. 2021. "Socio-psychological predictors and types of personal long-term orientation." *Psikhologicheskii zhurnal* 42, no. 4: 28–39.

Nowak, Bartłomiej, Paweł Brzóska, Jarosław Piotrowski, Constantine Sedikides, Magdalena Żemojtel-Piotrowska, and Peter K. Jonason. 2020. "Adaptive and maladaptive behavior during the COVID-19 pandemic: The roles of Dark Triad traits, collective narcissism, and health beliefs." *Personality and Individual Differences* 167: 110232.

Nunn, Nathan, and Leonard Wantchekon. 2011. "The slave trade and the origins of mistrust in Africa." *American Economic Review* 101, no. 7: 3221–3252.

Offe, Claus. 1994. "Capitalism by democratic design? Democratic theory facing the triple transition in Central and Eastern Europe." *The Political Economy of Transformation*, edited by Hans-Jürgen Wagener, 25–43. Berlin: Springer – Verlag Berlin.

Palócz, Márk. 2022. "COVID-19: Democratic Backsliding and Vaccine Diplomacy–The Hungarian Case." https://ruj.uj.edu.pl/xmlui/handle/item/293841.

Pirro, Andrea L.P., and Ben Stanley. 2022. "Forging, bending, and breaking: Enacting the "illiberal playbook" in Hungary and Poland." *Perspectives on Politics* 20, no. 1: 86–101.

Powell Jr, G. Bingham, and Guy D. Whitten. 1993. "A cross-national analysis of economic voting: Taking account of the political context." *American Journal of Political Science*: 391–414.

Renström, Emma A., and Hanna Bäck. 2021. "Emotions during the Covid-19 pandemic: Fear, anxiety, and anger as mediators between threats and policy support and political actions." *Journal of Applied Social Psychology* 51, no. 8: 861–877.

Rozenas, Arturas, and Yuri M. Zhukov. 2019. "Mass repression and political loyalty: Evidence from Stalin's 'terror by hunger'." *American Political Science Review* 113, no. 2: 569–583.

Rumiantseva, Aleksandra, Arkhipova Alexandra, Kozlova Irina, and Peigin Boris. forthcoming. "Protest as an appeal: How and why Russians struggled with vaccinations in 2021." In *Politics of the Pandemic: Blame Game and Governance in Russian and Central-Eastern Europe*, edited by M. Zavadskaya. London: Routledge.

Rykov, Yuri G., Peter A. Meylakhs, and Yadviga E. Sinyavskaya. 2017. "Network structure of an AIDS-denialist online community: Identifying core members and the risk group." *American Behavioral Scientist* 61, no. 7: 688–706.

Schraff, Dominik. 2021. "Political trust during the Covid-19 pandemic: Rally around the flag or lockdown effects?" *European Journal of Political Research* 60, no. 4: 1007–1017.

Silvan, Kristiina, and Kilybayeva Shugyla. forthcoming. "The state failing people's expectations: Resentment at the pandemic policy in Belarus and Kazakhstan." In *Politics of the Pandemic: Blame Game and Governance in Russian and Central-Eastern Europe*, edited by M. Zavadskaya. Routledge.

Sokolov, Boris O., Margarita A. Zavadskaya, and K. Sh. Chmel. 2022. "Dinamika individualnoi politicheskoi poddershki v Rossii v khode pandemii COVID-19: Analiz dannykh oprosa 'Tsennosti v krizise'" (The dynamics of political support in

Russia during the COVID-19 pandemic: An analysis of the survey data 'Values in Crisis'). *Politicheskaia nauka* 2: 122–143.

Spirova, Maria. 2022. "Bulgaria: Political developments and data in 2021: The year of the three parliaments." *European Journal of Political Research Political Data Yearbook* 61, no. 1: 47–70.

Šrol, Jakub, Eva Ballová Mikušková, and Vladimíra Čavojová. 2021. "When we are worried, what are we thinking? Anxiety, lack of control, and conspiracy beliefs amidst the COVID-19 pandemic." *Applied Cognitive Psychology* 35, no. 3: 720–729.

Stan, Lavinia, and Razvan Zaharia. 2022. "Romania: Political developments and data in 2021: Covid crisis and unexpected political changes in the absence of elections." *European Journal of Political Research Political Data Yearbook* 61, no. 1: 385–397.

Stoica, Cătălin A., and Radu Umbreş. 2021. "Suspicious minds in times of crisis: Determinants of Romanians' beliefs in COVID-19 conspiracy theories." *European Societies* 23(sup1): 246–261.

Tilley, James, and Sara B. Hobolt. 2011. "Is the government to blame? An experimental test of how partisanship shapes perceptions of performance and responsibility." *The Journal of Politics* 73, no. 2: 316–330.

Törnberg, Petter. 2018. "Echo chambers and viral misinformation: Modeling fake news as complex contagion." *PLoS One* 13(9): e0203958. https://doi.org/10.1371/journal.pone.0203958.

Pop-Eleches, Grigore, and Joshua A. Tucker. 2017. *Communism's shadow: Historical legacies and contemporary political attitudes*. Princeton, NJ: Princeton University Press.

Valenzuela, Sebastián, Daniel Halpern, James E. Katz, and Juan Pablo Miranda. 2019. "The paradox of participation versus misinformation: Social media, political engagement, and the spread of misinformation." *Digital Journalism* 7, no. 6: 802–823.

Van Mulukom, Valerie, Lotte J. Pummerer, Sinan Alper, Hui Bai, Vladimíra Čavojová, Jessica Farias, Cameron S. Kay, Ljiljana B. Lazarevic, Emilio J.C. Lobato, Gaëlle Marinthe, Irena Pavela Banai, Jakub Šrol, Iris Žeželj. 2022. "Antecedents and consequences of COVID-19 conspiracy beliefs: A systematic review." *Social Science & Medicine* 301: 114912. https://www.sciencedirect.com/science/article/pii/S0277953622002180.

Vogt, Henri. 2004. *Between Utopia and Disillusionment: A Narrative of the Political Transformation in Eastern Europe*. New York: Berghahn Books.

Wang, Jaesun, and Kim Seoyong. 2021. "The paradox of conspiracy theory: The positive impact of beliefs in conspiracy theories on preventive actions and vaccination intentions during the COVID-19 pandemic." *International Journal of Environmental Research and Public Health* 18(22): 11825. doi: 10.3390/ijerph182211825.

Zarocostas, John. 2020. "How to fight an infodemic." *The Lancet* 395(10225). https://www.thelancet.com/journals/lancet/article/PIIS0140-6736(20)30461-X/fulltext.

Zavadskaya, Margarita, and Sokolov Boris. 2020. "Linkages between experiencing COVID-19 and levels of political support in Russia." PONARS Policy Memo No. 677. https://www.ponarseurasia.org/linkages-between-experiencing-covid-19-and-levels-of-political-support-in-russia/.

2 Legislative Advantages of Multiple Crises in the Europe In-between

Katalin Miklóssy

Introduction

The COVID-19 pandemic introduced limitations on civil rights around the world, offering extraordinary powers to governments – regardless of the underlying political system. Even in liberal democracies, people supported strong leadership and obeyed without protest when their civic freedom, livelihood, and constitutional rights were restricted. Borders around and within countries became sealed, justified in the name of national emergencies. COVID-19 allowed state actors to implement new strategies, which challenged established perceptions of democracy. Nevertheless, stable democracies have been protected also in such extraordinary times by checks and balances, regulating people–power relationships, embedded in traditionally strong institutions.

This is where temporal factors are of significance. The underlying historical conventions, frequency, and length of the practice of the rule of law bear grave consequences on the prospects of the supposedly short-term outreach of power in times of crisis. Whereas Western liberal democracies are more resilient to authoritarian backsliding, in the Eastern members of the European Union (EU), democratic institutions are younger. In other words, they had less time to ingrain the practice of the rule of law and are thus more fragile to undemocratic flashbacks. These authoritarian memories of strong centralised power, which are based on century-old experiences, are also resilient.

According to the typology presented by Ollson and his colleagues, the resilience of a political system can be perceived conceptually either as an '*ability to cope with stress and bounce back*' or '*bounce back and transform*' (Olsson et al. 2015). From the perspective of liberal democracies, their solidity makes them sustainable because it endows them with the capacity to absorb disturbances and resist major changes within their core values (Walker et al. 2006; Boese et al. 2021, 885–907). There is however another type of resilience where 'bouncing back', i.e., safeguarding the main structures and values of the system, is dependent on the transformative capacity (Folke et al. 2010; Obrist, Pfeiffer, and Henley 2010, 283–293). The difference between these two types is that the latter offers more leeway because

DOI: 10.4324/9781003364870-3

it relies on a richer palette of policy tools to choose from and is therefore characteristically unpredictable. Whereas in the case of liberal democracies, the storehouse of means is more limited, and their usages are transparent and well circumscribed. In comparison, the continuous need for flexibility makes the non-democratic regimes more innovative and fluid than the solid framework of liberal democracies allows or even necessitates.

This chapter analyses why and how liberal democracies, enacting a *solid type of resilience,* offered a new chance and ammunition for the flawed democracies to strengthen their own path of development by a *fluid type of resilience*. The cases of Hungary and Poland are selected for analysis. After two decades of EU membership, the '*former star performers of democratic transition*' (Lugosi and Thorlakson 2014) are the main objects of EU criticism of turning away from liberal democratic values (Cabada 2017, 75–87). According to various reports and indexes, it became obvious that EU membership in fact weakened democratic evolution in the Eastern members. Between 2010 and 2022, the decline of democracy was noticeable in all Visegrád countries but particularly in Hungary and Poland (e.g., Freedom House 2019, World Justice Project 2021, Global Economy 2022, The World Bank 2022).

The main argument presented here is that the moments of overlapping multiple crises provide illiberal regimes an invaluable leverage to consolidate their institutions and core values. This study focuses on how COVID-19 became a 'godsend' opportunity to accelerate authoritarian evolution, conducted in parallel to and behind the scenes of COVID-crisis management. By analysing legal sources, official state documents, public and parliamentary debates, and media references, crisis legislation and its consequences are investigated. The main objective is to understand the step-by-step process of how the disease was instrumentalised over the two years' time of the pandemic. Methodologically, the applied qualitative content analysis relies on identifying three types of crisis management, which also reveal the purpose of the legislative processes, such as (a) power-boosting efforts, (b) atmosphere-tuning goals, and (c) constituency-building outreach. These underlying goals behind the implemented COVID-19 policies were targeted in multiple areas simultaneously but with different intensity, depending always on the estimation of what kind of response the *ad hoc* pandemic situation would require.

Multiple-Crises Moment: Time and Leverage

The pandemic hit and spread around the world with a devastating number of casualties, extraordinary pressure on healthcare services, and fast slope to economic recession in 2020 (The World Bank 2022). The global nature of the pandemic with similar signs of the emerging disaster concealed the fact that the crisis had divergent effects on different regimes. There is a fast-growing literature on the idea of 'autocratisation by decree' (Lührmann and Rooney 2020), analysing the types of threats on democracy by emergency measures during the COVID-19 pandemic (e.g., Diamond 2020; Hale et al.

2020; Maerz et al. 2020; Petrov 2020). These studies concentrate on the crisis as a sudden change to 'normalcy' that brings attention to the various governmental responses, liberal and illiberal ones. This chapter, in contrast, emphasises the long-standing experience and endurance of crises in Eastern Europe. To get a better understanding why the COVID-19, from the long chain of crises in the past 30 years, became *the* chance for illiberal regimes to take advantage of, we need to explore the nature of crises.

Obviously not any crisis carries a *crossroad moment* that opens a new horizon of possibilities. While one could say that crises come and go – yet every now and then, there appears a temporal juncture point when the overlap of multiple crises emerges on multiple levels. The cross section of time and space is important only if the actors are aware of the potential of the moment. It can be argued that the skill evaluating the emerging opportunities is rooted in the constant urge to mitigate long-term exogenous pressure. This ability can develop over time and by continuous practice in areas located in-between oppositional powers. The geographical position *in between* two ideologically, politically, or economically divergent great entities (akin to the well-known oppositions of East vs. West, democracy vs. authoritarianism) affects a state's policy perspectives.

East Central Europe represents a complex 'in-between-ness', situated at spatial crossroads where Eastern (mostly Russian) and Western (mostly German) influences have mixed, and great power interests clashed over centuries (Mackinder 1904, 421–437; 1919/1981). In-between-ness also refers to *buffer zone* entities indicating that they carry a particular weight (military security, political or economic value). A 'buffer' is a space in between two antagonist poles, where one of outside forces considers that area to be of primary importance for its interests. The purpose is to deepen an area's buffer potential by accommodating its values, political system, and social and economic structures with the power that exercises it. In-between-ness produces a consciousness of double options the juxta-positioned poles' competition offers. The poles' competition does not require or push the countries necessarily to choose between them but opens a possibility to skilfully play with two sets of cards (Miklóssy and Smith 2019, 250–266).

In-between-ness gets activated in *crossroad moments,* which the pandemic represents – enabling the Hungarian and Polish power elite to reinvent itself. It creates a suitable 'state of exception' (Schmitt 1922/2004; 1926/1988; Agamben 2005, 32–40, 74–88; Agamben 2021, 26–30, 82–85) overturning traditional hierarchical relation between causes and effects: it is a moment when illegitimate legislative practices become legitimate, enabling the power to overstep its institutional boundaries. In our case, the intensity of the crossroad moment, originally launched by the pandemic, grew in significance from the point of view of Hungary and Poland. The global pandemic intersected with the European-level rule of law crisis. The increasing Western criticism of illiberal tendencies created a gradually growing exogenous stress on these administrations. The domestic political opposition mirrored the EU discontent; thus, exogenous pressure was intensified by endogenous tension over the rule of law. The simultaneous COVID-19 pandemic was also originally an exogenous effect on every country, yet it converted into a domestic stress everywhere because it required primarily national crisis strategies that relied on the quality of healthcare services and public management. The significance of the Hungarian and Polish political elite's ability to neutralise both endogenous and exogenous pressures grew because parliamentary elections were coming up in April 2022 in Hungary and in November 2023 in Poland.

This chapter argues that simultaneous crises on multiple levels provide, ironically, an extraordinary leverage to mitigate crises on all levels. The aim is to investigate the legislative and political impact of the COVID-19 pandemic, yet in the time of writing, the ongoing war in Ukraine offers an interesting addition to the discussion on resilience, space of manoeuvre within the pretext of crisis management.

The Historical Legacy of Crisis Management

Timing is important, especially when overlapping exogenous pressures appear. The sudden COVID-19 hit simultaneously with a new wave of EU policies regarding the Hungarian and Polish cases. The long-lasting and fruitless dispute over the rule of law led to the introduction of a novel instrument. The rule of law mechanism was to cause serious financial damage to the Hungarian and Polish elite by withholding the EU funds – these regimes have been relying on (EU Regulation 2020/2092). While officially the new mechanism was issued on December 22, 2020, nevertheless, the warning signs of the mounting Europe-wide frustration were clearly articulated for several years before the EU legislation (Miklóssy 2023).

Since the new crisis, created by the COVID-19, was shared by all EU countries, the situation offered embedded opportunities. The crisis management strategies in Hungary and Poland evolved gradually due to the unexpected duration and consecutive waves of the pandemic. It can be argued that concentration of power by the assistance of extraordinary measures was not in essence a new *modus operandi* that these regimes have not already implemented previously. What was strikingly different was that the Western pandemic strategies offered an argumentative frame for moving onto a new phase of accelerating the concentration of power. Argumentatively, actions aiming further centralisation of power could be reasoned as a necessary but temporary solution during the pandemic. This type of keen monitoring of every possibility and sensitive reaction to take advantage of the moment relied on a long practice. History provides us an understanding of the role of traditions in adaptive resilience. These regimes look back to a common and lengthy period of the Eastern Bloc where they had to balance between continuous exogenous pressure from the Soviet centre and national interest. The Hungarian Kádárist regime was exemplary of *tight-rope dancing* strategy, and similarly, the consecutive Polish administrations managed to avoid direct Soviet army involvement even in revolutionary periods of social unrest.

Historical strategies became relevant again in the contemporary crises, especially the *rhetorical* and *institutional* instruments, by which these countries had learned to constantly calibrate their abilities to circumvent mounting hardship inflicted from the outside. The practice of doublespeak was one of the well-functioning means that was designed to turn the limelight away from real intentions. This discursive strategy was invented in the 1950s, with the purpose to show ideological obedience to the Kremlin, by which they protected national interests that were articulated in a down-to-earth language that the domestic audience could understand. This well-tested practice was transplanted later into the EU context (Török 2012). The countries sought leverage *vis-a-vis* the EU by accommodating to the rhetorical conventions of the EU, on the one hand, but ensured domestic popularity by national interpretations of the EU intentions, on the other hand. This discursive tool has been constantly finetuned to meet the changes in the inflicted exogenous pressure; hence, it secured a fluid *semantic elbowroom*. This meant that central concepts were used frequently with a different connotation, without making the diverging content transparent. This technique creates a fuzzy and complex web of misunderstandings where the opponent, coming from a different political culture, does not realise the rule of the game (Turtiainen 2019, Miklóssy 2023).

The institutional toolkit relies on the same idea as the semantic elbowroom and was also invented during the communist era – when both means, the rhetoric and institutions, were carefully and transparently regulated. Thus, the clearly defined boundaries of the major institutions, i.e., the Warsaw Pact, the Comecon or the Friendship, Cooperation and Mutual Assistance Treaty network, provided the framework of formal cooperation and destined the modus operandi of the Eastern Bloc countries. The challenge was to develop a veiled practice on how to take advantage of these institutions and expand the manoeuvring space – and as it happened a comprehensive systemic crisis opened the opportunity. Because of the economic dead end of the Stalinist development model,[1] the deteriorating standard of living led to protests, strikes, and uprisings in the Eastern Bloc. In this systemic disaster, a thorough revision of the governance model was necessary to maintain the system at all. The request for restructuring of the economic management and rethinking societal development offered a new leverage for the Bloc members. Reform communism introduced socialist market economy and a more liberal atmosphere that did not meet the Soviet expectations, but since the communists maintained power maintained, the Kremlin. 'Reform communism introduced socialist market economy and a more liberal atmosphere that did not met the Soviet expectations but since the communists maintained power, the Kremlin did not intervene first, and than it was too late to revise the process.' Expanding the elbowroom for national decision-making by the disguise of reform communism was a typical in-between endeavour that relied on blending Western elements with the Eastern system, including entrepreneurship, small scale private property, and consumption-led industry (Miklóssy 2010, 150–170; Kansikas 2011, 193–209).

The communist experience taught an invaluable lesson that exogenous crisis moments can be utilised for national purposes. The struggle against the COVID-19 also forced Western liberal democratic states to take on extraordinary measures that were incompatible with their basic liberal democratic values, restricting civil rights (Lührmann et al. 2020). Transparency of decision-making processes became fuzzy, but people accepted it because they were reassured that crisis demanded quick solutions and mandatory policies. To understand the significance of overlapping crisis, the attention is always on how the powerholders evaluate the volume of parallelly occurring crises in comparison. From the Hungarian and Polish regimes' points of view, the major threat was undoubtedly posed by the EU. While these regimes wanted to maintain integrity of decision-making, their visions of development path and core values, the COVID-19 was comparably a lesser threat.

Empowered by Pandemic

Hungary and Poland carried out resembling crisis management, in every respect. There are similarities in the starting situation, i.e., in the phase of the erosion of the rule of law – but significant differences in the extent of power. The Hungarian Fidesz party has been able to secure supermajority in four consecutive elections since 2010, foreseeably will stay in power until 2026. Supermajority, i.e., two third of parliamentary seats, gives completely free hands in all legislative fields, including the Constitution. This also means that the executive power overshadows the role of the Parliament. The Polish Law and Justice (PiS) party has never acquired a similar supermajority, and hence, it had to rely on coalitions to form a government. The different power balances translated into different spaces of manoeuvre in Hungary and Poland, irrespective of the fact that they have been pursuing a similar governance model and have been strong allies on the EU arena ever since 2015. The differences in power position were also reflected in the toolkit, which was developed to tackle the pandemic, but at the same time, it would help to achieve also various goals related to consolidating power.

The focal point in the Hungarian crisis management became known as the 'Enabling Act' (2020. évi XII. Törvény), issued at the end of March 2020. The law was meant to be in force as long as the 'crisis and its consequences' would demand it, depending on how the government assessed the pandemic situation, without any predeclared time boundaries. The Hungarian administration got free hands to govern by statutes, and to deal with the pandemic, it established a special Task Force (1012/2020. Korm.határozat). In comparison, Poland did not introduce the 'state of emergency' as Hungary and many other countries did around Europe. The Polish authorities launched restrictive lockdowns in 2020, but it was not unusual even by Western standards. The decision-makers issued instead the 'Anti-Crisis Shield', which constituted a chain of new laws and various amendments to existing laws (Journal of Laws 2020, sections 374, 568, 695, 1086). It became a broad legal toolkit enabling the government to go beyond the pandemic management – and thus, it greatly resembled with the Hungarian 'Enabling Act'.

In both countries, the new legislation was not inevitable. The Enabling Act was not necessary because crisis legislation had already existed in the Constitution and codes the Hungarian legal system (Szitás 2020). In addition, at the time the virus arrived in early March, the Hungarian administration in fact did not need the extra COVID-19 assistance to acquire new constraints on the residual space of democracy. The governing Fidesz party had it all: with its two-thirds parliamentary majority, it could pass a new Constitution any time by itself, without any democratic constraints on its overwhelming power. And yet, the Fidesz could not help leaping at the chance. Similarly, in Poland, the government had existing legal instruments available designed for these types of crises. The Constitution provides the possibility to declare the State of Emergency or the *State of Natural Disaster* (Constitution, Ch.XI 1997). This law, however, was too effective for the political purpose of upcoming elections because it banned all gatherings for 90 days. Presidential elections were scheduled in May 2020 and the PiS party was determent to maximise the chances of its candidate, Andrzej Duda, to be re-elected. The party feared that the assumable spread of the pandemic and its dead tolls could bear high political costs for the government. So, time was an essence to cement the position of the party, and after a heated domestic debate, the election was announced to be organised between June 28 and July 12 (TVN24: Wybory prezydenckie 2020) – and the PiS-incumbent president was able to renew his mandate. Since the president has the power to veto laws, having a loyal man in office gave the PiS party an extra confidence to its overall parliamentary majority to continue its old practice of power.

Some scholars, like Makowski and Waszak (2021), assessed the purpose of the Anti-Crisis Shield laws as 'closing the gaps'. This notion refers to the alleged process by the PiS-dominated government's intention to gradually build control over society, ever since the Law and Justice party came to power in 2015. Now, the endeavour of the new laws was to finalise the centralisation of power, and many of them contained sections that had obviously nothing to do with the management of the pandemic. Hence, one example was to take over institutions that bore special importance from the point of view of power, such as the media. In addition, the president of the Office of Electronic Communication was removed, and the election criteria for the position was changed so that the Senate, leaning on an opposition-majority, would not be able to influence it. Pandemic empowerment was to serve a wide range of purposes, and therefore, creating the 'right kind of atmosphere' in society, optimal to carry out covered goals, was inevitable.

Calibrating the Atmosphere

Crisis rhetoric is always a powerful political instrument by which politicians appeal to people's insecurities and acquire exceptional entitlements for their mandates, as Barry Buzan, Ole Weaver, and Jaap de Wilde (1998) defined the key concept of 'securitization', applicable here. To introduce new ways of 'crisis management' in Hungary and Poland, the people had to be prepared to accept extraordinary measures. Global crisis was easy to instrumentalise: mediatising death tolls in other countries made people increasingly sensitive to centrally rationed information. Public awareness was directed to the fact that the disease was *dragged in* from abroad, by foreigners – as if the people were threatened from the outside. As it happened, the first registered patients in Hungary were Iranian exchange students, a detail that became handy for the administration's more durable anti-migration politics. Thus, the government emphasised that it was right to block immigration from the Middle East and Africa since these people were obviously *virus-centrifuges,* aiming to stir up anti-migrant sentiments and draw attention away from crisis management. The government decided accordingly to also abolish the transit zones, i.e., channels of entrance for refugees, which was a constant target of EU criticism against Hungary (Zubor 2020).

Besides the official securitisation discourse, there were also other means to create fear by COVID-related regulations. All critical voices were to be silenced by a simple redefinition of the public space. The Enabling Act, mentioned above, forbade all public gatherings, but the government went further and made amendments to the Criminal Code to also restrict the freedom of speech. Rumours and disinformation about the pandemic situation or the way the authorities handled the pandemic would be punished by up to five years of imprisonment. This was an effective way to bring back communist-time self-censorship and not only for the journalists. By mid-May 2020, it became obvious that this was an excellent means to strike against civil society, ordinary citizens active in social media, and independent local governments. In addition, to take full control over information, the hospitals were ordered to be led by military commanders who took over the management of the hospitals, and the healthcare professionals were warned not to communicate with the media about the conditions in the hospitals (Hung. Gov. Koronavirusinformation 2020; Szabó and Writh 2021).

Poland chose a similar strategy, but its arrowhead was directed against the media. The aim was to minimise the damage that the mismanagement of the pandemic would have caused for the government. Thus, the flow of information of the first months' chaotic situation in the hospitals had to be hindered. Granting access to public information, normally a constitutional right (Constitution 1997, Art. 61, Par. 1–4), was now fast suspended and all requests for information could be ignored by the first Shield law (Journal of Laws 2020, Section 374, Art. 15zzr, Par. 1). The restrictions on information did not regard only the pandemic affair but all decision-making procedures during the pandemic, like, for instance, enabling the government to cover also budgetary overspending.

The Hungarian administration, in comparison, did not need to worry about the media since it controlled over 85% of the media landscape. The massive concentration of over 400 media enterprises into a media holding, Central European Media Foundation, was carried out already in 2018, establishing hence the Fidesz-run media empire. The Foundation was declared to belong to the sphere of *national strategic importance* and thus not subject of EU competition legislation (229/2018. (XII.5.) Korm). The Commissioner for Values and Transparency, Vera Jourova, admitted in May 2021 that there was nothing the EU could do about it (Zsiros 2021).

Yet, from the Polish perspectives, after the third wave of the pandemic and rising death tolls, it became important to appeal rather openly to the national sentiment and make people realise how well actually the administration's prompt actions, and especially the Anti-Crisis Shield laws, protected the nation. In July 2021, PM Morawiecki (2021) underlined that the 'Poles could count on the state that got actively involved in helping all those in need'. The prime minister trying to turn attention from disastrous healthcare services was proud to announce of his country's excellent economic performance records – the third best in Europe – as a proof of the government's ability to cope with disastrous pandemic impact (ibid.).

Motivating Constituents' Compliancy through Economic Assets

The pandemic hit hard the economic sphere everywhere, and all states around the world tried to mitigate the damage for economic actors, with a keen eye on the overall national economic performance. These measures were designed to keep economy running and invest to post-pandemic restoration. In Poland, the *Financial Shield* under the Anti-Crisis Shield legislative umbrella, issued already on June 23, 2020, was marketed as an efficient tool to avoid the drastic economic setback, experienced in other European countries. The new law addressed not only companies and entrepreneurs but also jobs, local governments, and consumers. The new shield was to distribute over 100 billion zlotys (i.e., about 22 billion euros). One of the articulated goals was to protect Polish companies, facing COVID-related difficulties and value-depreciation, from being taken over by outsiders. Since the EU law would forbid this kind of discrimination of European actors, the Financial Shield mentions as an excuse that the 'anti-takeover laws' are following the German, French, and Italian models and targeting only investors coming from the 'outside of Europe and the OECD'. The companies that were under protection were defined as working in key areas ensuring public safety, such as energy and health sectors, water and food supply, transport, army, and police, etc. (Shield 4.0, 2000). Yet the idea was not new. Already in 2018, a *Special Investment Zone* was established to provide public support to small- and medium-sized Polish businesses (Reg. Poz. 1162). This Council of Ministers' regulation was changed during the pandemic in December 2021 to help to channel state aid to certain Polish enterprises and grant them tax evasion (Reg. Poz. 2483). Extra funds were channelled to local governments.

These protective shields affected market dynamics under the pretence of pandemic strategy even though there was a questionable link between the COVID damage and the action taken, as, for instance, was the case of *Shield Three* that amended the Telecommunication law. The new bill changed the rules of competition for frequencies and construction of 5G Internet networks (Journal of Laws 2020, Section 695) which was a lucrative business in a relatively big country like Poland. The central government's influence was maximised with another law that would enable the administration to rule out any parties from the competition by referring to national security (Bill on the Amendment of the Law on National Cybersecurity).

In July 2021, PM Morawiecki warned that times of historical disaster require a new approach (Morawiecki 2021). The 'Polish Deal' (Pol. *Polski Ład*), announced already in May, was not only targeting the economic recovery after the pandemic but was to 'set a new path of development' altogether. The new programme was basically a tax reform, which advocated for social justice and was deemed as a solidarity project. It raised the minimum income tax threshold, gave tax exemption for the elderly, and distributed money to young families – all of them were the core social layers of the traditional constituency of the PiS party (PWC 2021). The idea besides the direct support of the electorate was boosting employment by investing in infrastructure and consumption. While the law package was called 'Polish Deal', nevertheless, a significant portion of the resources was expected from the EU's recovery funds. Initially, 58 billion euros were earmarked for Poland (National Recovery and Resilience Plan). The problem was that the EU was withholding the delivery of the money because of the serious reservations about the rule of law situation (EP Resolution March 10, 2022). While the Polish administration was well aware of the fact that the critical stand of the EU will influence the funds, still the government pushed ahead with the Polish Deal by which it prepared the public stage for the simplest of all blame games: the EU was against the post-pandemic recovery and development of Poland.

In Hungary, the economic support policy was affected by the changes in the domestic power balance. The local election in October 2019 brought an unexpected result for the Fidesz administration that won every election since 2010. The opposition now acquired several stronghold areas from the government party (Választási Iroda, Municipal Elections 2019). The power shifted in Budapest, 10 cities out of 23, and 50 towns out of 100. Some political scientists argue that local elections would predict a forthcoming transformation of authoritarian regimes because these can be challenged only from the grass-roots level (Lucardi 2016; Carothers 2018). A few months after the Hungarian local elections, the COVID-19 pandemic broke out.

The pandemic economic measures were directed against the opposition-led municipalities with the aim to drain resources from local self-governments by taking away their core income. The government established in April 2020 a *Fund for Protecting the Economy* (Hung. *Gazdaságvédelmi Alap*) that was justified by the urgency to minimise the damage caused by the pandemic for the economy and its actors (Government Decree 92/2020). This new decree gave free hands for the government to redirect key tax areas from the municipalities to the central budget. For example, losing taxation on motorcars hit hard both small villages, where this was the only income, and big cities, where the number of vehicles was significant. Similarly, parking in public areas became prescribed to be free of charge – to prevent people using public transport (Pandemic communique 2020). Parking has been a considerable income for local administrations, and this intervention was particularly targeted against Budapest, led by non-Fidesz Mayor and controlled predominantly by opposition forces. An equally drastic decision was simply refusing to transfer the already budgeted resources for regional development in Budapest. The money, as argued, was spent for fighting the disease, and the local administrations should just make sacrifices (Undersecretary Pogácsás 2020). The most drastic decision decreasing immensely the income of the municipalities was restricting the right to revenues of local enterprises, which made up about 32% of their budget and 90% of the municipalities had access to this type of taxation (Németh 2020). A similarly vivid example was the introduction of 'special economic belts'. By the pretext of the pandemic, lucrative economic areas were cut off from the opposition-run local governance and centralised, with the purpose of taking over the revenues. The first such a region was Göd where a huge Samsung factory was sited. After Göd, the government established two other similar territories where profitable economic assets could be found (Government Decrees 136/2020, 44/2021, and 362/2021). The gradual opening of Hungary after COVID-19 in the summer of 2021 did not cure the economic situation of oppositional local administration but accelerated their distress. The government started to compensate the budgetary losses of politically loyal municipalities and left others unattended.

Accelerating property transfer to loyal supporters was another key function in this process. The continuous 'emergency situation', prolonged the temporal window of opportunities to seize new economic assets. The emergency law encompassed companies that were considered *vital for the crisis management* (Government Decree 128/2020). The fight against the epidemic necessitated a special attention to *strategically important enterprises*, some of which, like an unlikely suspect, a carton factory, were simply taken over by the state (Domány 2020). There were over 100 businesses on the same list to be nationalised (Hungary Today 17.4.2020). These production areas, including, for example, information technology, construction industry, transport, logistics, food industry, agriculture, tourism, etc., are listed in a government statute in April 2021 (Government Decree 289/2020). Furthermore, the party loyal oligarchs were able to expand economic control over new enterprises. They possess the banking sector, insurance companies, agricultural lands, media firms, and energy enterprises (Szabó and Gyenis 2021). While the 'emergency situation' was to end officially in June 2022, nevertheless, the acquired economic assets would not be transferred back to their original owners. This was obviously a careful preparation to tackle the EU's new instrument, the rule of law mechanism, which was not designed to change the property ownership structure of a country on political grounds – and it would also run counter with the core EU values of liberal democracy and market economy.

War in Ukraine: A New Crossroad Moment

The war in Ukraine created yet another crossroad moment of overlapping crises. While the pandemic opportunity was fading away, the war now substituted it as a new pan-European crisis, and it was an important asset in the EU debate over the rule of law that was revived in the Spring 2022. The strategies developed during COVID were now reinvented. The utilisation of this crossroad moment, however, differed in Hungary and Poland because of their positioning towards Russia relied on different historical experiences and security perceptions (Miklóssy and Pierzynska 2019, 83–114).

The Russian invasion carried out in the near vicinity of Poland launched painful memories of Second World War traumas, underlying the loss of contemporary Western Ukraine to the aggressive then-Soviet power. The remembering of the profound fragility of territorial integrity triggered a strong sense of solidarity with Ukraine (Radio Poland May 26, 2022). The war also reactivated an existential fear that urged the Polish administration to create a strategy that would serve Poland's needs for the Western community providing shelter against the potentially dangerous Russia. So, the government was ready to bend and respond to EU requirements. Poland overwhelmingly welcomed numerous Ukrainian refugees, which was a new feature in comparison to the stubborn refusal of sharing the common burden of refugees since 2015. Furthermore, the Polish administration made some concessions regarding the rule of law and abolished the much-criticised judicial disciplinary chamber (AP June 14, 2022). As the war continued, it turned out that the EU equally needed Poland to support its sanction policies and military aid to Ukraine. This mutual understanding provided a crossroad opportunity to increase Poland's influence in forging European politics. Poland had a good reputation as being the main driver of European sanction politics ever since the Russian occupation of Crimea in 2014. The Polish political elite was united in advocating for stricter policies against Russia and supported extended military help since the war broke out in February 2022. By these EU compatible actions, Poland was able to acquire a more central role on the European scene (Cienski 2022; The Economist June 30, 2022). The new and stronger position was to help unlock post-pandemic recovery funds from the EU that were previously withheld due to the rule of law situation.

Hungary chose an entirely different approach to the war in Ukraine than Poland. The Hungarian ruling elites' understanding of security has been historically connected to economic development that guaranteed the people's standard of living – and in the end legitimacy for the powerholders.

Hungary's dependency on Russian energy supply grew over the years and thus the government succeeded to get exceptions from EU sanctions on energy (Rankin 2022). In addition, the administration has established close relations with the Putinist regime since 2011, which offered investments and lucrative trade deals and financed the construction of a nuclear power plant in Hungary (Miklóssy and Pierzynska 2019, 83–114). The Hungarian PM Viktor Orbán has been reluctant to take a clear stand against Putin, and the government-controlled media echoed the official Russian interpretation of the war. Hungary also refused to help the Ukrainians with weapons and forbade all arms transfer over Hungarian territory. This unveiled position stirred up controversial attitudes and great annoyance in the EU.

From the EU's point of view, the Ukrainian crisis seemingly overrode the significance of the rule of law debate. It can be argued that the new rule of law mechanism became a subject of bargaining in the game of compromise over the sanctions on Russia. The best example is how differently EU officials treated Poland than Hungary. In October 2021, Poland had to pay a considerable fine of one million euros per day due to the reform that undermined the freedom of judiciary (Euronews October 27, 2021), and in May 2022, the European Parliament still debated the situation of the rule of law of Hungary and Poland (European Parliament May 3, 2022). Nevertheless, on June 1, 2022, the Commission was ready to accept the Polish post-pandemic recovery plans for 35,4 billion euros (European Commission June 1, 2022), even though the European Court of Justice found that Poland failed to improve judiciary freedom (Orlando 2022). In contrast, while the Hungarian government was also ready to compromise by the summer of 2022 (Hungary Today June 17, 2022), the recovery plan of Hungary for 5.8 billion euros was finally approved on December 12, 2022 but only conditionally upon the fulfilment of reforms to strengthen the rule of law (European Council: NextGenerationEU). In other words, the long-warned rule of law mechanism may still be implemented against the Hungarian administration – whereas the European institutions were seemingly more lenient vis-à-vis Poland (Euronews April 27, 2022; European Parliament: Motion 2022).

It has been argued that the historical friendship and strong alliance between Hungary and Poland is soon coming to end because of their diverging positions on Russia. Sticking together under EU pressure strengthened the bond between them that relied on the exchange of knowledge between leaderships (Kovács 2020; Hungarian Government: *Justice Minister* 2021). There are also similar steps now being taken to reintroduce the 'state of emergency' in both countries that enables the governments to move on to decision-making by statutes, marginalising the Parliament. Now, after the pandemic, the war provides a suitable excuse for an extraordinary legal order.

In Hungary, before the pandemic, a state of emergency would have ended on June 1, 2022 (Miniszterelnökség – törvényjavastlat 23.11.2021). However, the government announced on May 24 the necessity of emergency, due to the war (2022/VI törvény). The new state of emergency was declared on

June 8, 2022, which practically continued the previous consecutive periods of emergency, started already in March 2020 (40/2020. Kormányrendelet). Now, in two days, the government issued a new tax regulation to gain extra income, as explained, 'to protect the Hungarians against the negative impact of the war' (Magyarország Kormánya, Kormányinfó, May 26, 2022). To keep ordinary households' energy and food prices at bay, the government introduced an 'extra profit tax' on companies that got too rich during the pandemic. The new tax targeted particularly international companies, seen as a response to the EU's rule of law procedure withholding the recovery fund. In addition, even though that the pandemic was mostly over by October 2022, the government refused to give any information of the previous two years of COVID-related decisions and the use of public money. While some journalist turned to the judiciary claiming the right to public information and the Court of Budapest also decided to demand access to COVID documents, the government, using its extra-powers endowed by the state of emergency, came up with a new decree prohibiting all information to be sealed from the public for ten years (HVG 2022).

Poland also brought a new Act on 'Defence of the Homeland' that was to concentrate crisis management in case of war (Journal of Laws 2022/655). While the purpose of the Polish defence bill was to modernise the army in times of acute crisis, the new regulation introduced extraordinary powers to the government over the local authorities and businesses. The state of emergency would be operated without the control of the Sejm or the president and could be introduced by the declaration of the minister of internal affairs or the prime minister. During that time, the government could gain direct control over local governments and change their personnel, with embedded threats especially to opposition-run municipalities (Podolski 2022).

The COVID-19 offered a chance to learn what kind of crisis strategies work to navigate profound national interest and neutralise increasing warning signs from the EU that threatened the core of the system in Hungary and Poland. The war gave a new opportunity to recycle the lessons learned during COVID-19 and develop an effective strategy. The two cases, the pandemic and the war, indicate that any new global or European crisis will likely produce a similar type of modus operandi.

Concluding Remarks: The Advantage of Overlapping Crises

This chapter discussed how the overlapping crises can offer new leverage for power elites to deal with pressures arising in parallel. The Hungarian and the Polish cases revealed the significance of timing in the sequencing of decisions. Since the pandemic has been a universal phenomenon, the spatial and cultural factors are often underestimated. The power of spatiality was in fact embedded in the temporal context. The sudden appearance of the COVID-19 crisis overlapped with an underlying, more durable crisis. That being the prolonged conflict between the EU, on the one hand, and Hungary and Poland on the other hand, over the erosion of the rule of law. A gradually growing EU pressure has been targeting Hungary since 2011 and Poland since 2016, yet without mentionable results because the effectiveness of EU threats is inhibited due to their long-lasting nature. Warning rhetoric and constant delays in taking serious actions on EU complaints offered time to the Polish and Hungarian administrations to adjust and reinvent their strategies in tackling the intended measures. Similarly, the COVID-19 crisis also continued for over two years, and it created more time and opportunities for Poland and Hungary to further adjust to EU 'challenges'. The Hungarian and Polish governments not only learned to deal with the pandemic but also saw their chance to further their national interests, as well as mitigate the underlying more durable crisis. Thus, while articulating the necessary fight against the disease and seemingly following Western practices, the Hungarian and Polish administrations were able to tighten their grip over society and further erode the remaining traces of the rule of law. The core question has been, which was a more serious crisis from the perspectives of each regime's resilience.

COVID-19 gave the opportunity to finetune discursive strategy with a purpose to channel attention away from one crisis to another, i.e., from the rule of law mechanism endangering the countries' budgetary interests in EU funds to COVID-19. New waves and new mutations of the virus were capitalised on by magnifying the *ad hoc* crisis at hand, and the pandemic character that required extreme measures also in the West. What became evident over the two years of pandemic was that both countries earned the dubious position of extraordinarily high death tolls in Europe and even in the world (Statista 2022). Yet, people did not punish the powerholders for their mismanagement and failures of dealing with the disease. In the parliamentary elections, on April 3, 2022, the Fidesz party was able to renew its strong mandate by acquiring a two-third supermajority. This will allow Fidesz to rewrite the Constitution if it so pleases (Nemzeti Választási Iroda 2022). The Polish parliamentary elections will be held in November 2023. The PiS party has never enjoyed such a strong majority position like the Fidesz in Hungary; hence, it most probably will be harder to renew its mandate. Yet, the prompt and well-articulated strategy dealing with the Polish existential crisis, due to the war in Ukraine, might offer a chance to successfully capitalise on.

Note

1 The Stalinist model relied on heavy industry, and extensive growth that is based on the increase of industrial production by the quantitative extension of input of raw materials, energy, and human workload.

References

AP. 2022. "Poland changes judiciary law; demands EU release COVID funds." 14 June 2022. Accessed June 17, 2022. https://apnews.com/article/COVID-health-poland-business-553e8aa610cd3c772f866a7a37634681.

"Bill on the Amendment of the Law on National Cybersecurity System and the Public Procurement Law." Accessed September 30, 2022. https://legislacja.rcl.gov.pl/projekt/12337950/katalog/12716608#12716608.

Boese, Vanessa A., Amanda B. Edgell, Sebastian Hellmeier, Seraphine F. Maerz, and Staffan I. Lindberg. 2021. "How democracies prevail: Democratic resilience as a two-stage process." *Democratization* 28, no. 5: 885–907.

Buzan, Barry, Ole Wæver, and Jaap de Wilde. 1998. *Security: A New Framework for Analysis*. Boulder: Lynne Rienner Publishers, 1998.

Cabada, Ladislav. 2017. "Democracy in East-Central Europe: Consolidated, semi-consolidated, hybrid, illiberal or other." *Politics in Central Europe* 13, no. 2/3: 75–87.

Carothers, Christopher. 2018. "The surprising instability of competitive authoritarianism." *Journal of Democracy* 29, no. 4: 129–135.

Cienski, Jan. 2022. "Poland goes from zero to hero in EU thanks to Ukraine effort." *Politico*, March 3, 2022. https://www.politico.eu/article/poland-goes-from-zero-to-hero-in-eu-thanks-to-ukraine-effort/.

Crowcroft, Orlando. 2022. "Poland judicial reforms are in breach of European law, court rules." *Euronews*, June 15, 2022. https://www.euronews.com/my-europe/2021/07/15/poland-judicial-reforms-are-in-breach-of-european-law-court-rules.

Diamond, Larry. 2020. "America's COVID-19 disaster is a setback for democracy." *The Atlantic*, April 16, 2020. https://www.theatlantic.com/ideas/archive/2020/04/americas-COVID-19-disaster-setback-democracy/610102/.

Domány, András. 2020. "Azonnali hatállyal állami felügyelet alá vonták a Kartonpackot." *HVG*, April 17, 2020. https://hvg.hu/gazdasag/20200417_Azonnali_hatallyal_allami_felugyelet_ala_vontak_a_Kartonpackot?fbclid=IwAR0ZLXAAsv9qfkpT7TIvA6fNfeyJ4AQGG68GtQUL6hYina5VWw4z8GHhFZY.

"Dunaújváros Government Decree 362/2021 (VI. 28)." Magyar Közlöny June 28, 2021, pp. 5620.

EUR-LEX. 2020. "Regulation (EU, Euratom) 2020/2092 of the European Parliament and of the Council of 16 December 2020 on a general regime of conditionality for the protection of the Union budget" *The EU website*. Accessed June 5, 2022. https://eur-lex.europa.eu/legal-content/EN/TXT/?uri=CELEX:32020R2092.

Euronews. 2021. "Poland must pay €1 million daily over judiciary reform, ECJ rules." October 27, 2021. Accessed June 13, 2022. https://www.euronews.com/my-europe/2021/10/27/poland-must-pay-daily-fines-of-1-million-over-its-controversial-judiciary-reforms-ecj-rule.

Euronews. 2020. "Brussels triggers rule of law mechanism for very first time against Hungary." April 27, 2022. Accessed June 13, 2022. https://www.euronews.com/2022/04/27/brussels-triggers-rule-of-law-mechanism-for-very-first-time-against-hungary.

European Commission. 2022. "NextGenerationEU: European Commission endorses Poland's €35.4 billion recovery and resilience plan." June 1, 2022. Accessed June 13, 2022. https://ec.europa.eu/commission/presscorner/detail/en/ip_22_3375.

European Council of the EU. 2022. "NextGenerationEU: Member states approve national plan of Hungary." December 12, 2022. Accessed December 19, 2022. https://www.consilium.europa.eu/en/press/press-releases/2022/12/12/nextgenerationeu-member-states-approve-national-plan-of-hungary/.

European Parliament. 2022. "European Parliament resolution of 10 March 2022 on the rule of law and the consequences of the ECJ ruling." Accessed June 14, 2022. https://www.europarl.europa.eu/doceo/document/TA-9-2022-0074_EN.html.

European Parliament. 2022. "Motion for a Resolution." May 3, 2022. Accessed June 13, 2022. https://www.europarl.europa.eu/doceo/document/B-9-2022-0264_EN.pdf.

European Parliament. 2022. "News: Rule of law in Hungary and Poland: Plenary debate and resolution." May 3, 2022. Accessed June 13, 2022. https://www.europarl.europa.eu/news/en/agenda/briefing/2022-05-02/6/rule-of-law-in-hungary-and-poland-plenary-debate-and-resolution.

Folke, Carl, Stephen R. Carpenter, Brian Walker, Marten Scheffer, Terry Chapin, and Johan Rockström. 2010. "Resilience thinking: Integrating resilience, adaptability and transformability." *Ecology and Society* 15, no. 4. https://www.jstor.org/stable/26268226?seq=1#metadata_info_tab_contents.

Freedom House. 2019. "Democracy in Retreat: Freedom in the World 2019." https://freedomhouse.org/report/freedom-world/freedom-world-2019/democracy-in-retreat.

Giorgio Agamben. 2005. *State of Exception.* Chicago: Chicago University Press. 32–40, 74–88.

Giorgio Agamben. 2021. *Where Are We Now? The Epidemic as Politics.* Eris. 26–30, 82–85.

"Government Decree 92/2020 (IV.6)." Magyar Közlöny, April 6, 2020, 1814–1819.

Hale, Thomas, Noam Angrist, Beatriz Kira, Anna Petherick, Toby Phillips, and Samuel Webster. 2020. "Variation in government responses to COVID-19." Blavatnik School of Government Working Paper.

Hungarian Government. 2021. "Justice Minister: Hungary and Poland Represent Common Sense in the EU." August 25, 2021. Accessed June 16, 2022. https://abouthungary.hu/news-in-brief/justice-minister-hungary-and-poland-represent-common-sense-in-the-eu.

Hungarian Government Koronavirusinformation. 2020. "Hétfôtôl kórházparancsnokok segítik a kórházak mûködését és az egészségügyi készlet védelmét." March 28, 2020. https://koronavirus.gov.hu/cikkek/hetfotol-korhazparancsnokok-segitik-korhazak-mukodeset-es-az-egeszsegugyi-keszlet-vedelmet.

Hungarian National Assembly. 2020. "Undersecretary Tibor Pogácsás' Speech in the Parliament." May 18, 2020. Accessed August 2, 2021. https://www.parlament.hu/web/guest/aktiv-kepviseloi-nevsor?p_p_id=hu_parlament_cms_pair_portlet_PairProxy_INSTANCE_9xd2Wc9jP4z8&p_p_lifecycle=1&p_p_state=normal&p_p_mode=view&p_auth=2YdkryMy&_hu_parlament_cms_pair_portlet_PairProxy_INSTANCE_9xd2Wc9jP4z8_pairAction=%2Finternet%2Fcplsql%2Fogy_naplo.naplo_fadat%3Fp_ckl%3D41%26p_uln%3D129%26p_felsz%3D113%26p_szoveg%3D%26p_felszig%3D113.

Hungary Today (HT). 2020. "Coronavirus: Military Taskforces to Oversee More Strategic Companies." April 17, 2020. https://hungarytoday.hu/coronavirus-hungary-companies-military-taskforces/.

Hungary Today (HT). 2022. "Minister Navracsics: Hungary Ready to Make Compromises with Brussels to Unblock Recover Funds." June 17, 2022. Accessed June 13, 2022. https://hungarytoday.hu/minister-navracsics-hungary-ready-to-make-compromises-with-brussels-to-unblock-recovery-funds/.

HVG. 2022. "HVG bírósági perének közepén írta át a kormány a szabályokat, hogy eltitkolhassa, mirôl szóltak az operatív törzs ülései." HVG.HU. September 20, 2022. https://hvg.hu/itthon/20220920_Operativ_torzs_birosagi_per_kormany_szabalyvaltoztatas_titkolozas.

Journal of Laws 2020, Section 568 (31 March 2020), Amending the Act on special arrangements for the prevention, counteracting and combating of COVID19, other infectious diseases and the crisis situations caused by them.

Journal of Laws 2020, Section 695 (16 April 2020), Law on Specific Support Instruments in Connection with the Spreading SARS-CoV-2 Virus.

Journals of Laws 2020, Section 374 (2 March 2020), Law on Specific Measures to prevent, Counteract and Combat COVID-19 and Other Contagious Diseases and associated Crisis Situations and certain Other Laws.

Journal of Laws 2020, Section 1086 (19 June 2020), Law on Subsidised Interest on Bank Loans Extended to Enterprises affected by COVID-19 and Simplified Process of Composition approval in Connection with the Incidence of COVID-19.

Kansikas, Suvi. 2011. "Room to manouvre? National interests and coalition building in the CMEA, 1969–1974." In *Reassessing Cold War Europe*, edited by Sari Autio-Sarasmo and Katalin Miklóssy, 193–209. London and New York: Routledge.

Kovács, Zoltán. 2020. "PM Orbán: This debate is not about money." Hungarian government, About Hungary, Blog. November 26, 2020. Accessed June 16, 2022. https://abouthungary.hu/blog/pm-orban-this-debate-is-not-about-money.

Lucardi, Adrián. 2016. "Building support from below? Subnational elections, diffusion effects, and the growth of the opposition in Mexico, 1984-2000." *Comparative Political Studies* 49, no. 14: 1855–1895.

Lugosi, Nicole and Lori Thorlakson. 2014. "Theorizing democratic development after EU accession: Bringing comparative politics back in." ECPR: European Consortium for Political Research. Accessed July 6, 2021. https://ecpr.eu/Events/Event/PaperDetails/16351.

Lührmann, Anna and Bryan Rooney. 2020. "Autocratization by Decree: States of Emergency and Democratic Decline. 2020." *V-Dem Working Paper* 85.

Lührmann, Anna, Seraphine F. Maerz, Sandra Grahn, Nazifa Alizada, Lisa Gastaldi, Sebastian Hellmeier, Garry Hindle, and Staffan I. Lindberg. 2020. "Autocratization Surges, Resistance Grows." University of Gothenburg, V-Dem Institute.

Mackinder, Harold. 1919/1981. *Democratic Ideals and Reality: A Study in the Politics of Reconstruction.* Westport, CT: Greenwood Press.

Mackinder, Harold. 1904. "The Geographical Pivot of History." *Geographical Journal* 13, no. 3: 421–437.

Maerz, Seraphine F., Anna Lührmann, Jean Lachapelle, and Amanda B. Edgell. 2020. "Worth the sacrifice? Illiberal and authoritarian practices during Covid-19." *Illiberal and Authoritarian Practices during Covid-19 (September 2020).* V-Dem Working Paper 110.

Magyarország Kormánya, Kormányinfó. 2022. "A kormány az ország biztonságát és a gazdaságot is megvédi." May 26, 2022. Accessed June 17, 2022. https://kormany.hu/hirek/a-kormany-az-orszag-biztonsagat-es-a-gazdasagot-is-megvedi.

Makowski, Grzegorz and Marcin Waszak. 2021. "Polish Legislation during the Pandemic vs. Corruption Anti-crisis Shields: Completing the Law and Justice State Project?" *IdeaForum.* Warsaw: Stefan Batory Foundation.

Miklóssy, Katalin and Hanna Smith. 2019. "Concluding remarks: In between-ness and strategic culture." In *Strategic Culture in Russia's Neighborhood*, edited by Miklóssy Katalin and Smith Hanna, 259–266. Lexington: Lexington Books.

Miklóssy, Katalin and Justyna Pierzynska. 2019. "Regional strategic culture in the Visegrad countries: Poland and Hungary." In *Strategic Culture in Russia's*

Neighborhood: Change and Continuity in an In-between Space, edited by Miklóssy Katalin and Smith Hanna, 83–114. 1 ed. Lexington: Lexington Books.

Miklóssy, Katalin. 2010. "Khrushchevism after Khrushchev: The rise of National interest in the Eastern bloc." In *Khrushchev in the Kremlin: Policy and Government in the Soviet Union, 1953–1964*, edited by Jeremy Smith and Melanie Ilic, 150–170. London and New York: Routledge.

Miklóssy, Katalin. forthcoming in 2023."Tackling EU-conditionality with the Hungarian legal manoeuvres." In *The Rule of Law's Anatomy in the EU: Foundations and Protections*, edited by Allan Rosas, Juha Raitio and Pekka Pohjankoski. Oxford: Hart Publishing

Miniszterelnökség. 2021. "Törvényjavaslat, 23.11.2021." https://www.parlament.hu/irom41/17671/17671.pdf.

Morawiecki, Mateusz. 2021."New Deal." Website of the Republic of Poland, July 10, 2021. Accessed June 5, 2022. https://www.gov.pl/web/denmark/new-deal---the-article-of-the-pm-m-morawiecki.

"National Recovery and Resilience Plan." Website of the Republic of Poland, May 3, 2021. Accessed June 14, 2022. https://www.gov.pl/web/planodbudowy/kpo-wyslany-do-komisji-europejskiej.

Németh,Tamás.2020."Jelentősbevételtképeznek–mindentaziparűzésiadóról."Pénzügyi Szemle,August6,2020.AccessedAugust3,2021.https://www.penzugyiszemle.hu/tanulmanyok-eloadasok/jelentôs-bevetelt-kepeznek-mindent-az-iparuzesi-adorol.

Nemzeti Választási Iroda (National Election Office). 2019. "Local Municipal Elections 2019." October 13, 2019. Accessed July 14, 2021.https://www.valasztas.hu/helyi-onkormanyzati-valasztasok-2019.

Nemzeti Választási Iroda (National Election Office). 2022. "Parliamentary Elections 2022." April 3, 2022.Accessed June 5, 2022. https://vtr.valasztas.hu/ogy2022.

Obrist, Brigit, Constanze Pfeiffer, and Robert Henley. 2010. "Multi-layered social resilience: A new approach in mitigation research." *Progress in Development Studies* 10, no. 4: 283–293.

Olsson, Lennart, Anne Jerneck, Henrik Thoren, Johannes Persson, and David O'Byrne. 2015. "Why resilience is unappealing to social science: Theoretical and empirical investigations of the scientific use of resilience." *Science Advances* 1, no. 4: e1400217.

"Pandemic Communique of the Hungarian Government." The Hungarian Government website, April 6, 2020. https://koronavirus.gov.hu/cikkek/orszagos-tisztifoorvos-az-ingyenes-parkolas-jarvany-lassitasat-szolgalja.

Petrov, Jan. 2020. "The COVID-19 emergency in the age of executive aggrandizement: What role for legislative and judicial checks?" *The Theory and Practice of Legislation* 8: 1–22.

Podolski, Antoni. 2022. "PiS's new bill. Protection of the people or protection of the authorities?" Rule of Law website, March 28, 2022. https://ruleoflaw.pl/piss-new-bill-protection-of-the-people-or-protection-of-the-authorities/.

PWC. 2021. "The Polish Deal -10 changes important from the point of view of employers and individuals. Package of modifications to the tax laws." August 2, 2021. Accessed June 8, 2022. https://www.pwc.pl/en/articles/the-polish-deal-polski-lad-tax-changes-important-from-the-employers-and-individuals-perspective.html.

Radio Poland. 2022. "Poland stands in solidarity with Ukraine amid war, envoy tells US Helsinki Commission." May 26, 2022. Accessed June 13, 2022. https://www.

polskieradio.pl/395/9766/Artykul/2966307,Poland-stands-in-solidarity-with-Ukraine-amid-war-envoy-tells-US-Helsinki-Commission.
Rankin, Jennifer. 2022. "Hungary 'holding EU hostage' over sanctions on Russian oil." *The Guardian*, May 16, 2022. Accessed June 17, 2022. https://www.theguardian.com/world/2022/may/16/hungary-sanctions-russian-oil-embargo-eu.
"Regulation of the Council of Ministers of 28 August 2018." Dziennik Ustaw Rzeczypospolitej Polskiej, Poz.1162. Accessed June 5, 2022. https://www.invest-ksse.com/files/?id_plik=3549.
"Regulation of the Council of Ministers of 28 December 2021." Dziennik Ustaw Rzeczypospolitej Polskiej, Poz. 2483. Accessed June 6, 2022. https://www.ksse.com.pl/files/?id_plik=6239.
Schmidt, Carl. 1922/2004. *Political Theology: Four Chapters on the Concept of Sovereignty*. Chicago: Chicago University Press.
Schmitt, Carl. 1926/1988. *The Crisis of Parliamentary Democracy*. Cambridge, MA: MIT Press.
Statista. 2022. "Number of Novel Coronavirus (COVID-19) Deaths Worldwide as of June 1, 2022, by Country." Accessed June 3, 2022. https://www.statista.com/statistics/1093256/novel-coronavirus-2019ncov-deaths-worldwide-by-country/.
Szabó, András and Zsuzsanna Writh. 2021. "Oltással akarta elkerülni Orbán a kórházi drámákat. Végül csak eltitkolni tudta azokat." *Direkt36*, August 23, 2021. https://telex.hu/direkt36/2021/08/23/orban-viktor-oltas-harmadik-hullam-korhazi-dramak.
Szabó, Yvette and Ágnes Gyenis. 2021 "A fülkeforradalom felfalja sajátjait: bevált receptek alapján viszik Fidesz-közeliek cégeit is." *HVG*, November 25, 2021. https://hvg.hu/360/20211125_fulkeforradalom_Fidesz_uzlet_felvasarlas_kleptokracia_Vitezy_Tamas_Meszaros_Lorinc_Garancsi_Istvan_Orban_Viktor.
Szitás, Katalin. 2020. "Nem jelenti a kritika hiányát." *Political Capital*, March 22, 2020. https://www.politicalcapital.hu/hirek.php?article_read=1&article_id=2510.
"The Constitution of the Republic of Poland of 2nd April 1997, Article 61, Paragraphs 1–4." The Polish Sejm Website. Accessed May 31, 2022. https://www.sejm.gov.pl/prawo/konst/angielski/kon1.htm.
"The Constitution of the Republic of Poland of 2nd April 1997, Chapter XI Extraordinary Measures." The Polish Sejm Website. Accessed May 29, 2022. https://www.sejm.gov.pl/prawo/konst/angielski/kon1.htm.
The Economist. 2016. "Illiberal Europe. Big, bad Visegrad." January 28, 2016. http://www.economist.com/news/europe/21689629-migration-crisis-has-given-unsettling-new direction-old-alliance-big-bad-visegrad.
The Economist. 2022. "Poland is being given an opportunity to matter in Europe." June 30, 2022. https://www.economist.com/europe/2022/06/30/poland-is-being-given-an-opportunity-to-matter-in-europe.
The Global Economy.com. 2022. "Human Rights and Rule of Law Index – Country Ranking." https://www.theglobaleconomy.com/rankings/human_rights_rule_law_index/Europe/.
The World Bank. "Worldwide Governance Indicators." http://info.worldbank.org/governance/wgi/Home/Reports.
The World Bank. 2022. "World Development Report 2022, Chapter 1. The Economic Impacts of the COVID-19 Crisis." The World Bank website. https://www.worldbank.org/en/publication/wdr2022/brief/chapter-1-introduction-the-economic-impacts-of-the-COVID-19-crisis.

Török, Gábor. 2012. "ha Habony Árpád lennék... A kettös beszédröl." *HVG*, March 19, 2012. Accessed June 5, 2022. https://hvg.hu/napi_merites/20120319_torok_gabor_kettos_beszed_habony.

Turtiainen, Suvi. 2019. "Unkari pitää Suomen tavoitetta sitoa EU-rahat oikeusvaltioperiaatteeseen turhana." *YLE Uutiset*, October 1, 2019. Accessed June 5, 2022. https://yle.fi/uutiset/3-10998236.

TVN24 Wybory prezydenckie. 2020. "Marszałek Sejmu Elżbieta Witek podała termin wyborów prezydenckich." June 3, 2020. Accessed May 29, 2022. https://tvn24.pl/wybory-prezydenckie-2020/wybory-prezydenckie-2020-nowy-termin-podany-przez-marszalek-sejmu-elzbiete-witek-4601061.

Walker, Brian, Lance Gunderson, Ann Kinzig, Carl Folke, Steve Carpenter, and Lisen Schultz. 2006. "A handful of heuristics and some propositions for understanding resilience in social-ecological systems." *Ecology and Society* 11, no. 1. https://www.jstor.org/stable/26267801?seq=2#metadata_info_tab_contents.

World Justice Project. 2021. "Rule of Law Index." World Justice Project website. https://worldjusticeproject.org/rule-of-law-index/global.

Zsiros Sándor. 2021. "Jourová: a bizottság tehetetlen a KESMA ügyében." *Euronews*, May 3, 2021. https://hu.euronews.com/my-europe/2021/05/03/jourova-a-bizottsag-tehetetlen-a-kesma-ugyeben.

Zubor, Zalán. 2020. "A tranzitzónák bezárása után is bizonytalan a menedékkérők helyzete Magyarországon." *Átlátszó,* May 26, 2020. https://atlatszo.hu/kozpenz/2020/05/26/a-tranzitzonak-bezarasa-utan-is-bizonytalan-a-menedek-kerok-helyzete-magyarorszagon/.

"2020. évi XII. törvény a koronavírus elleni védekezésrôl, Hatályos Jogszabályok." Wolters Kluwer. Accessed June 5, 2022. https://net.jogtar.hu/jogszabaly?docid=A2000012.TV.

"2021. évi I. törvény a koronavírus-vilagjárvány elleni védekezésrôl. Hatályos Jogszabályok." Wolters Kluwer. https://net.jogtar.hu/jogszabaly?docid=a2100001.tv.

"2022. évi VI. törvény szomszédos országban fennálló fegyveres konfliktus, illetve humanitárius katasztrófa magyarországi következményeinek elhárításáról." Wolters Kluwer. Accessed June 17, 2022. https://net.jogtar.hu/jogszabaly?docid=A2200006.TV&dbnum=1.

"2021. évi XCIX. törvény a veszélyhelyzettel összefüggő átmeneti szabályokról." Hatályos Jogszabályok, Wolters Kluwer. https://net.jogtar.hu/jogszabaly?docid=a2100099.tv.

"229/2018. (XII.5.) Korm. Rendelet a Közép-Európai Sajtó és Média Alapítvány nemzetstratégiai jelentôségûvé minôsítésérôl." Magyar Közlöny 2018/192, December 5, 2018. http://www.kozlonyok.hu/nkonline/MKPDF/hiteles/MK18192.pdf.

"1012/2020. (I.31.) Korm. Határozat a Koronavírus-járvány Elleni Védekezésért Felelôs Operatív Törzs felállításáról." Wolters Kluwer. https://net.jogtar.hu/jogszabaly?docid=A20H1012.KOR.

"128/2020. (IV. 17.) Korm. rendelet a veszélyhelyzet során teendő intézkedések keretében gazdálkodó szervezet működésének a magyar állam felügyelete alá vonásáról."

"289/2020. (VI. 17.) Korm. Rendelet a magyarországi székhelyű gazdasági társaságok gazdasági célú védelméhez szükséges tevékenységi körök meghatározásáról." Nemzeti Jogszabálytár. https://njt.hu/jogszabaly/2020-289-20-22.

"40/2020. (III.11) Kormányrendelet veszélyhelyzet kihírdetésérôl." Magyar Közlöny 2020/40. https://magyarkozlony.hu/dokumentumok/af0a665e93020a1bb69193ed9a8379f516854bf7/megtekintes.

3 State-Building, the EU, and the COVID-19 Pandemic

The Making of Healthcare Reform in Ukraine

Ryhor Nizhnikau

Introduction

Scholars often cite both crisis and external engagement to explain reforms in third countries. Crisis can trigger significant changes and permit the expansion of the role of external actors in institution-building. Academic literature on the EU's resilience-building specifically explores mechanisms and capacities for transformation in response to a crisis.

In recent years, Ukraine has consistently faced systemic challenges, which threatened both the state and society. This has been accompanied by a growing Western involvement in state-building, particularly aimed at preventing and dealing with crises. While Ukraine has proven to be more robust and resilient despite a myriad of vulnerabilities, including the weakness of state institutions and unresolved institutional malaises, its progress in institutional reforms has not been straightforward and often stumbled after initial successes.

This chapter investigates the role of the EU in the dynamic process of Ukraine's institutional transformation with a particular focus on the ongoing overhaul of the healthcare system. The EU has been an integral part of debates on the trajectory of Ukraine's reforms after the Euromaidan Revolution and during the pandemic crisis. It has been portrayed as a key transformative actor in the neighbourhood and one of the drivers of change. A long-term supporter and promoter of reforms in the neighbourhood, the EU's emphasis on resilience-building specifically aims to help partners address internal and external challenges. Such re-prioritisation of EU policies towards resilience-building – stronger governance, connectivity, and society – with its focus on reacting to emerging and ongoing crises, has increasingly reshaped EU engagement with its neighbours, including Ukraine.

In this respect, the focus on healthcare reform and the effect of both the pandemic and the EU's own response to the pandemic serves three purposes. First, it helps to analyse the dynamics of institution-building in Ukraine as well as other sources of transformative change. Healthcare provision is an integral part of the Ukrainian state's functions. Access to free healthcare is a right, which is guaranteed by the Constitution, and thus can be seen as a

DOI: 10.4324/9781003364870-4

core function of the Ukrainian state. Healthcare is something the state has had difficulties adequately providing in the past. The healthcare system has been corrupt, institutionally insolvable, and broken at all levels from medical education to procurement of medical provisions and service provision.

Second, this analysis contributes to the discussions of the EU's role in state-building and how the resilience strategy affects institution-building. Healthcare reform advanced beyond expectations prior to the pandemic's outbreak, even if it was dubbed 'the hardest' of the Ukrainian reforms (White Book 2019). Following a 20-year legacy of stalled reforms, when Ukraine's healthcare system functioned on the basis of the Semashko model (the Soviet-based healthcare system) that included centralised budgetary financing, hierarchical organisational structure, collusion, and corruption, Ukraine finally initiated a comprehensive reform in 2014. New structures, rules, or practices within the sector completely overhauled the healthcare system. New principles of medical care provision and financing, specifically the 'money follows the patient' concept, decentralised and linked medical care provision with the financing of medical services and transparent control over public expenditure.

Importantly, these healthcare reforms created synergies with decentralisation, anti-corruption, and public procurement reforms. Medical facilities have been transformed from budgetary institutions into communal or state-owned non-profit enterprises with more autonomy and control over their budgets. Local communities have been given the power to decide on the principles and resource allocation to their local healthcare units. Furthermore, new instruments and institutional innovations, such as the e-Health system, the National Health Service of Ukraine (NHSU), and a new state procurement agency 'Medical Prozorro' were established in 2018 and 2019, respectively. These advancements took place despite strong domestic opposition and limited original interest and involvement of external donors.

Finally, this chapter discusses how the pandemic crisis reshaped the EU's approach to Ukraine and Ukrainian reform dynamics. Until 2020, the healthcare sector was not at the top of the EU agenda. At this time, the EU was a core partner in the fight against the pandemic. Since the beginning of the pandemic, the EU invested significant resources in assistance to Ukraine and its healthcare sector, which coincided with the rise of resilience governance, which is at the forefront of EU external policies. In this respect, the juxtaposition of the Euromaidan Revolution and the political crisis in 2013–2014 and the Russian invasion of Eastern Ukraine and the annexation of Crimea with the pandemic crisis of 2020–2021 helps shed additional light on the reform dynamics and the EU's resilience-building strategy.

EU's Neighbourhood Policies: A Turn Towards Resilience Governance

Resilience-building strategies have been presented as a response to key challenges of EU neighbourhood policy. However, the EU continues to struggle to resolve its inherent contradictions. Since the introduction of the European Neighbourhood Policy (2004), the transformation of neighbouring countries has been at the core of EU foreign policy. The EU underlined the ambition to 'develop a special relationship with neighbouring countries, aiming to establish an area of prosperity and good neighbourliness, founded on the values of the Union and characterised by close and peaceful relations based on cooperation' (ENP Review 2015). To promote political and economic change, the EU relied on the external governance approach, which offered various incentives such as visa-free regimes, access to the EU market, and closer political integration in exchange for the import of EU rules. A reliance on positive and negative conditionality dominated the sectoral reforms as well and was combined with financial and technical assistance to create state capacities to implement EU rules.

Despite the EU's efforts, neither stability nor democratisation advanced. External threats and domestic vulnerabilities made the situation on the ground less stable and more challenging. The Russian war with Georgia, the Arab Spring, the war in Syria, the migration crisis, and the annexation of Crimea were all accompanied by domestic upheavals across the EU neighbourhood. The European Commission admitted its record of state-building, and democratisation was not very convincing (ENP Review 2015; Tocci 2020). The inability to instil change and a rise of instability across the neighbourhood led to a paradigm shift in EU foreign policy towards resilience-building.

The introduction of resilience-building at the core of EU foreign and development policies has been dubbed a new response to both security risks and stalling state-building in the region. Resilience as a form of governance focuses on promoting strategies of learning and adaptation to encourage societal actors to take responsibility and foster self-governance (Joseph and Juncos 2019). Three major innovations have been highlighted. First, the EU's resilience-building strategy aims to strike a balance between the promotion of stability and change to strike 'a middle ground between over-ambitious liberal peace-building and under-ambitious stability' (Wagner and Anholt 2016, 4). Resilience produces the capacity to absorb, react to, and respond to shocks and crises peacefully, as well as to promote incremental change and foster a 'stronger economy, stronger governance, stronger society, and stronger connectivity between the EU and partners' (EEAS 2019). In this respect, the ability to peacefully transform and adapt specifically emphasises that resilience is not about stability and the status quo.

Second, in contrast to external governance, resilience-building moves away both from state-centricity and EU-centricity, aiming to promote 'self-governance' in the neighbourhood (EEAS 2019), which requires the engagement of local actors and reliance on local knowledge and resources. Specifically, it recognises the importance of society in state-building, thus highlighting a transition from a top-down to a bottom-up approach in an ambition to 'blend top-down and bottom-up efforts' to enhance stability, which is 'rooted in local agency' and a shift towards 'greater flexibility and more tailored responses in dealing with rapidly evolving partners and reform needs' (the EU's Global Strategy 2016, 31). The shift towards inclusion of local actors in a flexible manner specifically empowers local non-state actors to take part in rulemaking and governance to contest and compete for the best governance solutions to local problems. The latter is specifically crucial given the chronic inabilities of the state to perform its functions and its capture by vested interests. In this respect, it considers state-building as an engagement between citizens and the state when seeking to identify 'mutual demands, obligations and expectations' (cf Maass 2020). The direct consequence of that is higher legitimacy and social trust, which positively affects the effectiveness of institutions (Stollenwerk, Börzel, and Risse 2021).

The literature, however, debates the construction and implementation of a resilience-building strategy and how much it has departed from its predecessor. It has been framed as a de-politicised capacity-building mechanism of enabling local solutions, relying on local communities and resources (Tocci 2017; Korosteleva and Petrova 2021). It is also considered an instrument of governance that allows to 'govern from a distance', which questions the extent of its departure from external governance, which 'unfolds as a hierarchal and top-down process' (Badarin 2021). The shift of the EU's focus from democratisation towards resilience-building has not necessarily changed the means and instruments of the EU's bilateral engagements. This raised more a question of continuity of EU policies than change and institutional perseverance in the partner states. Academic studies point to the path dependency of EU policies (Badarin and Schumacher 2020) and significant differences in the understanding of resilience, which create a mismatch between a strategy and its application to EU foreign policy (Joseph and Juncos 2019; Bargués and Morillas 2021). New initiatives, such as 20 Deliverables for 2020 and the Association Agendas, show that the EU still heavily relies on the logic of external governance and prioritises top-down transfer of EU rules to third countries. The resilience-building strategy incorporates the same principal means and mechanisms (conditionality, learning, and passive enforcement), which were previously used to promote the (in)direct uptake of EU rules (Tocci 2017).

The EU's responses to a crisis may add more confusion. While resilience strategy calls for the capacity-building of societies and communities rather than the state, a crisis may increase sharply the reliance on the state to respond to immediate threats. In this respect, a crisis may only stimulate cooperation with the state and hierarchisation of EU engagement, in which conditionality becomes a mechanism for exporting EU demands and solutions. Such an enhancement of the EU's reliance on elites and boosted capacities of institutions captured by vested interest may further reinforce the existing problem of access to power at the institutional level.

Following these debates, the efficiency of EU policies depends on its ability to grasp the roots of domestic governance malfunctions and connect with the endogenous sources of change. On the one hand, it requires moving away from top-down solutions and acknowledging that building resilience as well as institutional transformation is largely rooted in domestic processes, which are dependent on the dynamics of interactions and competition between local state and non-state actors (Nizhnikau 2021). On the other hand, EU policies should adjust to the domestic political context and its key challenges. The characteristics of domestic political institutions matter, underlying the types of risks and obstacles as well as the types of dominant change agents to emerge and strategies to pursue (Mahoney and Thelen 2015). In this respect, the inefficiency of EU policies can be explained by the inability of EU policies to address key impeding reform factors, namely paternalism and personalisation of domestic institutions, which distort power allocations among domestic stakeholders.

To achieve this, the EU can use resilience-building in three main functions: (1) a mechanism of empowerment of pro-reform collective action, (2) supporting the creation of new institutions by offering resources and expertise and political insulation, and finally (3) legitimising the new solution. First, the provision of resources to societal and community actors increases their capacity and possibility to participate in rulemaking. Empowerment is a vital mechanism to address the existing distortion of power and provide access to institution-building. It assists the process of searching for a new solution and facilitates both the contestation between various ideas and visions of institution-building and their subsequent realisation (Ostrom 2005). The provision of necessary resources can test the new solutions and help to show the efficiency of the new institutional solutions. The creation of necessary opportunities may help to lower the misbalance between society and the state, as well as increase the accountability of the latter (Myerson and Mylovanov 2014). EU expertise and knowledge can complement and extend existing models of institutional design.

Second, the EU's engagement affects the ability to form and sustain collective action. The collective action processes of institutional innovation are characterised by the collision of diverse and opposing actors, with each seeking to effect institutional change in order to achieve their own goals. Until the local solution proves its efficiency, the EU's endorsement and its conditionality can become an important motivator for local elites to participate. Similarly, the EU has the potential for fostering necessary conditions for key actors to design new institutions, which curtail the elite's structural power. Elites, who often exploit their privileged access to political and economic resources to control the state and the economy for the sake of private gains, often prevent the creation of new institutions or subvert their functioning. Insulating the local reform efforts and minimising veto possibilities, specifically through conditionality, has been proven to be a key instrument in the EU's hands, lowering the extent of discretion in institutional enforcement (Poteete 2014). EU officials on the ground have highlighted obstacles to reform to include 'unwillingness and resistance to change, gaps in legislation, insufficient funding, unsatisfactory professional standards, a lack of coordination between agencies' (EUAM Ukraine 2018, cf. Maass 2020).

Finally, the EU's participation can increase the legitimacy of both actors and institutions. Rules and institutions are to be legitimate among elites, stakeholders, and society, which makes legitimisation a core component of state-building activities. Legitimisation is crucial for overcoming existing mistrust between and within the elite, non-state actors, and society, which are forced to cooperate initially and allow the 'embedding' a new agency into the dominant system with a degree of autonomy (Evans 1995). As a part of legitimisation, the EU can particularly assist in ensuring compliance and enforcement of the new rule. Besides the provision of resources to guarantee enforcement, the EU's oversight can mitigate potential conflicts over the enforcement of new rules or contestation of their meaning. This helps to lower the uncertainty over a new solution and facilitate voluntary cooperation between various stakeholders and thus improving enforcement and monitoring of the new system through co-productive or co-governing mechanisms (Ostrom 2005).

In this respect, the reliance on local contexts, actors, and structures, which requires a significant investment of EU resources, does not necessarily help to address these problems. State and societal interests can often contradict each other. Henceforth, resilience-building should specifically target the discrepancies of power among domestic actors and support the endogenous sources of change and primarily the local attempts at constructing and improving the functionality of new institutions.

Healthcare Sector Reform after the Euromaidan Revolution

Ukraine's healthcare reform was primarily driven by a coalition of domestic stakeholders that utilised a system opening created by the Euromaidan Revolution. By 2014, Ukraine's healthcare system, inherited from the Soviet Union, was in deep crisis. At a cost of 7% of gross domestic product (GDP), it suffered from constant budget deficits, malfunctions, corruption, and low efficiency. As a service provider, it was deeply dissatisfactory and costly, even if free healthcare was guaranteed by the Constitution. The average Ukrainian covered some 45% of total health expenditure (Patients 2014). According to the World Bank (2020), informal payments reached 3.5% of GDP per year.

Numerous attempts by different governments with the assistance of international donors to reform the system with international assistance were short-lived and did not pass the pilot stage. Even though the system suited neither patients nor staff, it remained unchanged. Veto players that controlled formal and informal financial flows were seen as key roadblocks. Centralised specialised institutions controlled financial flows allocated for special financial services.

The Euromaidan was a trigger for systemic reform. The collapse of Yanukovych's regime created an opening for collective action to press for reforms. The new post-Yanukovych government endorsed new reforms, even if reluctantly due to financial problems and its focus on other more pressing issues.

Other factors that promoted healthcare reform included strong public pressure, as seen in the 72% of Ukrainians that supported health reform, along with the involvement of external actors as key financial contributors to Ukrainian financial and economic stability.

The role of external support has drastically risen since 2014. EU assistance initiated large-scale programmes, which advanced reforms in key good governance areas, such as public administration, the justice sector, rule of law, the fight against corruption, as well as civilian security sector reform. The Association Agreement (AA), which includes a wide programme of reforms in line with EU standards and norms, was endorsed as a symbol and a key practical instrument of transformation. This programme was further incapacitated by the establishment of the Support Group for Ukraine (SGUA) and sectoral initiatives such as the U-Lead as well as the EU Advisory Mission (EUAM) to assist with the implementation of reforms on the ground.

The primary driver of turning the opening into a reform opportunity was the mobilisation of previously excluded stakeholders, specifically patients' organisations, which later formed a reform coalition in the healthcare sector. Some of the networks were formed during the protests as a part of the Euromaidan's infrastructure. Some of the core actors emerged to address the sectoral problems, which were widely recognised by patients and doctors alike (Lekhan et al. 2015). For instance, the 'Patients of Ukraine' and 'Tabletochki' actively pushed forward the sectoral reform agenda. Having formed an open coalition, they launched a collective work to develop laws, support, control, and pressure the government. Some activists joined the government and the parliament. They also became part of the coalition of non-state organisations in the Reanimation Package of Reforms initiative and the EU-funded Reform Support Center of the Cabinet of Ministers as experts. This non-state organisation actively participated in the legislative work under the principle 'Nothing about us without us!'. Their work included advocacy, information pressure, and monitoring of progress, with a particular focus on media and external donors. The organisations, which supported patients dependent on state supported medication, were particularly engaged with the changes in the procurement system (Patients 2016).

A coalition of governmental and non-governmental actors became a key vehicle of legislative work, which allowed the coalition to address major peculiarities and problems in Ukraine's legal, financial, and administrative systems. In August 2014, the Ministry of Health launched work on National Strategy on Healthcare Reform (MOZ 2019), which aimed to outline the contours of the strategic overhaul of the system. Upon public request, the Strategic Advisory Group (SAG) was formed of leading Ukrainian experts who worked in international organisations, the public sector, and business, along with international experts to develop and present the National Health Reform Strategy for Ukraine for 2015–2020. The priority areas were outlined jointly by the government of Ukraine and independent experts to include major non-state initiatives (IRF 2014).

At the end of 2014, SAG presented the National Health Reform Strategy for Ukraine for 2015–2020, which envisioned a transformation of the healthcare system into state-owned or municipal enterprises, the establishment of the National Healthcare Financing Agency responsible for procurement of healthcare services along with the public health system, and a new procurement mechanism. In mid-2015, the SAG prepared key draft laws including the draft on the autonomy of healthcare facilities. Bill No. 6327 'On State Financial Guarantees for Providing Medical Services and Medications' introduced a new model for financing health services. Bill No. 6604 'On Amending the Budget Code of Ukraine to Support the State Financial Guarantees for Providing Medical Services and Medications' outlined the rules of distribution of expenses between the budget in line with the new model for financing primary care and the public health system. Both draft bills were adopted only in 2017. In 2016, the Cabinet of Ministries of Ukraine approved the 'Concept of Reforming of the Healthcare Financing' (Patients 2017).

Before the laws were submitted and passed in the Verkhovna Rada, during 2015–2016, key stakeholders (patients, doctors, heads of medical institutions, local governments, and local administrations) in all regions of the country were consulted in two stages. This process involved over 7,5 thousand people to make amendments to the draft laws and action plans and subsequent changes were developed for implementing the laws (MOZ 2019).

The EU played a supporting role, primarily because unlike the anti-corruption or civilian security sector reforms, the healthcare sector was a marginal priority. The EU had no interest in direct rule transfer, which also allowed local solutions to flourish. The Chapter of the AA on public health included general provisions such as developing cooperation in the public health field and raising the level of public health safety as well as protection of human health.

The EU's role had two key elements, which particularly aimed at supporting bottom-up initiatives financially and politically as well as helping to overcome the counteraction of the opponents of the reform. First, EU assistance became an instrument of empowerment for the pro-reform actors in the healthcare sectors, which were allowed to set up new initiatives. The EU's funding allowed the creation of a SAG on healthcare, which allowed domestic pro-reform groups to access both government decision-making and EU expertise. This permitted the consideration of various healthcare system models of the EU and neighbouring countries, which have been in 'the same situation as Ukraine now but have already changed the system quickly and efficiently' (Ushinina and Sytnik 2016). It also lured the government's interest. Crucially, Ukrainian government officials particularly eyed the 214 million dollars pledged by the World Bank, with the EU's support, to conduct the reform. For the reformers and the veto players alike, the perspective of receiving the grant overweighed any other risks, including the inclusion of opponents in the institution-building process. However, only a minor fraction of this funding was dispersed at an early stage, which would remain a source of frustration in the government, but also an incentive to continue institution-building. Second, the EU served as a benchmark for the reform initiatives, emphasising its support for the reform's guiding principles of autonomy, transparency, access, and efficiency. The main principle of the reform was not new and included provisions from the previously tested external reform initiatives, such as the project of the World Bank healthcare reform before the Euromaidan (Yakovenko 2018).

Initial reform progress quickly stalled as the new regime stabilised itself. Even if the outline of the reform was presented in January 2016 and approved in November by the Cabinet of Ministers of Ukraine in Resolution No. 1013-r, institution-building was delayed for over a year due to resistance from key veto groups. The unreformed Ministry of Health and the parliamentary committee on healthcare were two key obstacles. The new Minister, Oleh Musiy, was not able to fire his deputies in the ministry who were appointed by Oleksandr Yanukovych. This blocked major ministerial functions, such as the procurement of medicines. Musiy's successor, Oleksandr Kvitashvili, faced similar problems, which led to his demands that the parliament fire him after just several months on the job (Gorchinskaya 2015). In the first two and a half years of its work (2014–2017), the health committee passed only four laws (Twigg 2017). The combination of Western and public pressure allowed to break the deadlock. The coalition of non-state actors actively monitored and challenged the government, contesting the veto players in the healthcare sector, government, and parliament (EASO 2021). The EU's endorsement of the reform and the pressure on the government helped to secure the involvement of President Petro Poroshenko and Prime Minister Volodymyr Groysman to unblock the reform. Western engagement particularly helped to cut domestic debates about the best healthcare solutions and principles and to legitimise the decentralised and autonomy-driven solution under public control (Yakovenko 2018, 7). The result of constant public pressure was an increased inclusion of pro-reform actors in the government, a clean-up at the Ministry of Health, and more pro-reform actors in the government more generally. This included the head of the Patients of Ukraine Olga Stefanyshyna as a deputy minister and later activist Ulyana Suprun as a minister in 2016 after a dozen of candidates declined to take the job (Kovtonyuk 2017).

It took 22 attempts to pass key healthcare reform legislation in the Verkhovna Rada (NV.ua 2019). In 2017, parliament finally adopted the key laws 'On Government Financial Guarantees of Medical Care' and 'On Improving Affordability and Quality of Medical Services in Rural Areas', which alongside the governmental decrees created a new framework and principles for healthcare financing (White Book 2019). In 2018, the NHSU was established to act as a public agency responsible for contracting health service providers. The implementation of the reform was divided into two parts. During the first stage, which began in April 2018, the focus fell on the primary healthcare system, the introduction of new standards, and the launch of the Medical Guarantees Programme.

EU assistance in other sectoral reforms allowed the healthcare sector to build upon other reforms and created necessary institutional synergies with other key reforms, such as decentralisation, public administration (PAR), and public procurement reforms. Decentralisation emboldened reform planners to transfer responsibilities and resources to the local level. The medical subvention was introduced in 2015, which allowed local authorities to manage subordinated facilities more effectively (White Book 2019). The U-Lead programme specifically financed regional projects on how to learn and efficiently use new powers. Under the programme, 309 local councils were supported since 2016 in local and regional development. The PAR created mechanisms of transparent and merit-based hiring that were used in the selection of new staff for new institutions.

Similarly, the public procurement reform facilitated the emergence of medical procurement systems. Before that, however, the EU created capacities to limit the power of key monopolists by transferring pharmaceutical procurement over to UNICEF, the United Nations Development Program, and Crown Agents (UK). Buying medicines through international organisations brought transparency and eliminated corrupt intermediaries, reducing prices dramatically for vaccines and other drugs before the Medical Prozorro was set in place. The State Enterprise 'Medical Procurement of Ukraine' was made the only national agency in charge of centralised procurement of quality medicines and medical devices for state funds in October 2018. Under the management of the Ministry of Health of Ukraine, Medical Procurement of Ukraine is organisationally autonomous and uses the experience and institutional innovation of the Prozorro reform.

After the legislation was passed, the re-making of the relations between the state and medical establishments and patients and healthcare facilities began. The legal status of medical establishments was changed to public enterprises subordinated to local authorities, which was a precondition to receive budget allocations from the NHSU. Similarly, patients were allowed to start signing contracts with family doctors of their choice, which guaranteed a certain income to the latter. The Ministry of Health and new institutions went through transparent competitive hiring processes, which brought new cadres from the private and civil society sectors to run the five new policy directorates established by the new legislation. Each of the civil servants went through six difficult stages during the hiring competition, with some only passing the second or third time (Kovtonyuk 2019).

Only at this stage did institutions receive significant external capacity-building support. USAID funded improvements for the new hiring process at the Ministry. WHO's grant of 215 million dollars was unlocked to help improve service delivery, as well as enhance the efficiency of the healthcare system. WHO's Biennial Collaborative Agreement (BCA 2022) funded the realisation of Ukraine's national health policies and plans. BCA was also supportive of the health sector's ongoing reforms and policies on decentralisation – the concept of local self-governance reform and territorial organisation of power. The EU offered policy recommendations to improve new institutions and recommendations on strengthening the national health emergency preparedness and response system.

Zelensky's Government, Reforms, and the Pandemic

Prior to the pandemic's outbreak, Volodymyr Zelensky's governance showed more continuity than change from his predecessors. Upon his election, dubbed 'an electoral revolution', he pledged sweeping reforms to 'break the system', clean up the corrupt elite, defeat the oligarchy, and modernise the state. A victory of his party 'Servant of the People' in the parliamentary elections in August 2019 offered the means necessary to further reforms. It allowed for the establishment of control over the Verkhovna Rada and the government and started the promotion of legislative changes in the so-called 'turbo-regime' in autumn 2019. This included the introduction of several long-delayed economic, political, and security laws, such as the law on the land market and the new labour code.

Zelensky's agenda to rebuild the state fit the EU's resilience-building agenda. The EU was presented as the benchmark for reforms, seen as part and parcel of the European integration agenda. The EU's 20 Deliverables for 2020 included a set of goals aimed to strengthen both the state and society. This constituted intentions to increase civil society participation and governance reforms, including strengthening the rule of law and anti-corruption mechanisms and the implementation of key judicial reforms (EEAS 2017). The new government quickly affirmed its commitment to further implementation of both the AA and IMF stand-by programmes. Ukraine's dependence on external funding also created additional leverage for the EU. Following Western demands, the work of the High Anti-Corruption Court and the National Agency on Corruption Prevention was unblocked. In June 2020, after the parliament approved the so-called 'anti-Kolomoisky law', forbidding the return of nationalised banks to former owners, the IMF granted Ukraine a new loan of five billion dollars. The change of government did not affect the pace of the reform progress though. The same governance challenges remained, and it was not long before the Zelensky team returned to the path of reform imitation and turned its full attention to presidential power-building, which included the re-subordination of state agencies and appointing loyalists to key positions.

Attempts to embed state executive agencies and regulatory bodies in the presidential vertical of power intensified (BTI 2022). Zelensky actively expanded his influence over security and law enforcement agencies. The Office of the President, explicitly or implicitly, by means of new legislative initiatives, started to interfere in the functioning of key state agencies, including newly established ones. A number of appointments were made with dubious selection processes when the authority of the selection commission was ignored or legal criteria were not met (for instance, in the selection process of the new head of the Special Anti-Corruption Prosecutor's Office). The judicial reform was paralysed. The law on the State Bureau of Investigations was changed in the president's favour. Since the SBI was rebooted in December 2019 and its head illegally fired, it has been chaired by presidential interim appointees in violation of the law (Nizhnikau 2021).

Healthcare reform was equally affected by these developments. It was endorsed by donors and the public. By autumn 2020, over 30 million people signed (healthcare) declarations. Eighty-seven percentage of the population showed satisfaction with primary healthcare (National Health Index 2020). Ninety-seven percentage of regional medical institutions were reorganised into communal institutions, and 90% of hospitals applied for contracts with the National Health Service in preparation for the second stage of the reform. Zelensky's presidency did not prioritise healthcare reform, but taking into account the wide acclaim and approval of the first stage of the healthcare reform, he showed initial support. His criticism of the healthcare reform in the presidential debates created an uproar in civil society and sparked harsh criticism from 50 leading organisations (Nv.ua 2019). However, the active remaking of state institutions opened an opportunity to roll back the reform. In early 2020, Zelensky established an interim working group of 'exceptional doctors' on health system reform to analyse medical reform progress (NV.ua 2021), which included a number of notorious reform opponents (Kovtonyuk 2020). As Decree No. 55/2020 stated, 'based on the results of this analysis, the working group should make proposals for the further reform of domestic medicine: on financing, improving the training system and professional development of doctors and other medical workers, raising salaries, and providing scientific support to the healthcare system'. A number of opponents of the healthcare reform, represented inter alia by the head of the Ministry of Health Stepanov and the head of the parliamentary health commission Radutsky, became a part of Zelensky's team, while some key proponents of the reform were fired.

The COVID-19 pandemic only furthered the challenge to sustain and continue the reform. Healthcare became a primary issue in political infighting in the middle of a major crisis, all while the second stage of the reform was to be launched on April 1, 2020, to reorganise the secondary level of healthcare. The government was ill-prepared to identify the spread of COVID-19 and responded inefficiently in the initial stages of the pandemic. The pandemic recorded over 1 million registered cases and over 18,000 deaths during 2020 (Shevtsova 2020). Among the myriad of shortcomings, there was a lack of equipment, qualified specialists, and necessary facilities and resources such as testing labs or personal protective equipment. There was also inadequate compensation to medical staff for the risk of working in these conditions. As a result, the media reported that medical staff either quit or faced life-threatening conditions.

The government shifted the blame to the ongoing reform. Zelensky's orders and anti-reform statements put pressure on its continuation. The claim that

'Ukraine's healthcare needs a real reform' and a requirement to overhaul the major principles of the ongoing reform allowed the new leadership of the Ministry of Health to begin a major revision. Minister Stepanov rejected the second stage of the reform, as not 'a real reform', which 'doesn't foresee anything good either for doctors or patients [...] [and bring] the disastrous consequences for Ukrainians' (UNIAN 2020). Following Zelensky's call to resolve the funding issues and amend the existing mechanism, an attempt to overturn the financial aspect of the reform and take under control the financial flows, undermining the autonomy of both the NHSU and Medical Prozorro system (UNIAN 2020).

The second stage of the reform was postponed. Minister Stepanov and the head of the health committee Radutsky called to change the funding principle and return the old distribution of funds. A disinformation campaign to undermine the legitimacy and public support was launched, in which false information was distributed (Vox Ukraine 2022). Both Zelensky and Stepanov repeated fake information that the reform would lead to the firing of '50,000 medical workers and the closure of 332 hospitals'. In early May 2020, Zelensky said the pandemic showed that the reform 'failed' and left the country 'medically naked' (Zelensky 2020). Stepanov and the Rada's health committee called to reorganise the reform. The Minister of Health blocked key appointments including public competition for a new head of NHSU. The confirmation of the public committee to oversee the new health sector institutions was delayed (Twigg 2020). The Minister of Health was accused of corruption on non-transparent medical tenders (Odintsova 2020) and suspended medical procurement via the official mechanism.

President Zelensky triggered special attention to the public health system, which created additional system bottlenecks to the decision-making system. Zelensky twice changed the ministers of health in the space of just three weeks in March and formed eight different executive commissions to fight the virus. He added to an institutional confusion. In March, he tasked eight oligarchs with coordinating efforts to tackle the pandemic in different regions, which further complicated a delineation of roles and responsibilities between central and regional governance as well as the Ministry of Health and the sanitary service. This also complicated a delineation of policymaking and executive functions among those institutions (Piven and Habicht 2022).

The pandemic was also used as a reason to suspend the main elements of the PAR, such as hiring practices for civil servant positions and the provisions of the Medical Prozorro. The latter led to paralysis of the system for two months due to scandals, after which the Ministry of Health suspended the work of the specialised enterprise and took over its procurement functions. During this period of blocking purchases through Medical Prozorro the Ministry significantly overpaid the suppliers (Antac 2020). In May, the Verkhovna Rada simplified the procurement procedure for the purposes of COVID-19, which led to a spike in dubious tenders. Funds to fight the pandemic were allocated for road construction and law enforcement. Eventually, the Constitutional Court was approached to cancel the healthcare reform because it prevented fighting the pandemic (NV.ua 2021).

State resilience-building turned into an EU priority. Thirty million euros were proportionally allocated for the Eastern Partnership countries to purchase necessary supplies and strengthen the health system's capacity to respond to the outbreak. The EU Initiative for Health Security offered capacity-building activities on preparedness for epidemiologists and frontline health staff and reinforced crisis management mechanisms. In June 2020, the EU offered a support package of 190 million euros and in July 2020 announced the allocation of 1.2 billion euros of macro-financial assistance. Germany disbursed a 150-million-euro loan for the healthcare sector. The World Bank allocated additional 135 million dollars to scale up Ukraine's health sector response to the COVID-19 pandemic. Ukraine was assisted with important hospital upgrades and reforms. Thirty-five million dollars were allocated for COVID-19 emergency response activities. External partners invested heavily in technical and operational support of the Ministry of Health to prepare and implement the national COVID-19 Strategic Preparedness and Response Plan 'to rapidly detect, diagnose and prevent the further spread of the virus, and ensure the continuity of essential services and systems during the outbreak' (BCA 2022). The external help was vital in implementing vaccination, tracing infections, and re-establishing institutional facilities (Piven and Habicht 2022).

The government's failure was mitigated by the mobilisation of civil society, which redirected its efforts on the fight against the pandemic. Civil society substituted for the state, when needed, collecting necessary resources, raising awareness, spreading reliable information, and fostering community development to respond to emerging needs (Shapovalova 2020). It collected data and monitored the government's actions including deficiencies in preparedness and ineffective public spending on the fight against the pandemic. The pressure on the government increased as the involvement of the broader civil society including main anti-corruption non-governmental organisations (NGOs) and advocacy coalitions in the healthcare sector grew. External assistance to civil society was specifically redirected to pandemic-related activities, which profoundly enhanced their involvement in the healthcare sector.

Overall, the crisis allowed civil society to expand its networks, build social capital, and build partnerships. Their increased role in combination with the dependence of Ukraine on external support helped to prevent a major reform rollback in the healthcare sector. Conditionality was embedded in major support packages. The continuation of the health reform was a part of the negotiation of the IMF programme, and a part of the EU, World Bank, and WHO conditionality. In June 2020, the IMF approved an 18-month Stand-by Arrangement (SBA) of five billion dollars, in which an audit of medical procurement under the COVID-19 programme was included as a condition. The EU's offer of a direct contribution to healthcare reform, including through a financial contribution to the WHO, targeted the capacity-building of the ongoing reform. In November 2020, the Ministry of Health and the WHO signed a Cooperation Agreement to continue rolling out reforms and the development and implementation of strategies and reforms of health financing. The growth of external involvement led to the establishment of the Health Financing Sectoral Working Sub-Group as a coordination platform in January 2021 between international partners and local state and non-state stakeholders, which discussed legislative and operational steps (USAID 2021). Healthcare reform continued even if slower than originally planned. By 2022, the medical guarantees programme became fully operational, which was specifically set to reduce 'catastrophic' out-of-pocket spending on healthcare (Bredenkamp et al. 2022). Most of the specialised medical care facilities have signed a contract with the NHSU for the provision of healthcare services, which has been paying for the delivery of medical services, including four new packages of services for patients with COVID-19 (Panasytska and Ivantsova 2021).

Conclusion

Healthcare reform as a state-building process in Ukraine is a work in progress. Since 2014, steady progress has been recorded despite political resistance and critical conditions. Ukraine has considerably overhauled the main institutional premises of its healthcare sector, developed new infrastructure, and slowly rearranged the relations between the state, service providers, and patients. There is much work still ahead. The success of this reform depends on the continued improvement of the legal framework to address new challenges and fix reoccurring issues, as well as the development of new institutions and their capacities, such as NHSU.

This chapter discussed healthcare reform and its drivers, particularly emphasising the role of the EU in the institution-building stage and during the pandemic crisis. It finds that the key drivers of healthcare reform are endogenous, motivated by a dynamic contestation between various groups for rights and resources. The healthcare reform was born primarily out of domestic demand and developed in clashes between various stakeholders and their competing visions of state-building and healthcare reform. In this context, external involvement has been vital to advance change by means of facilitating, empowering, and enforcing reform.

The EU's role in Ukraine's healthcare reform can serve as an example of how resilience-building strategies can work. Societal resilience and its focus on adaptive change for the resilience of institutions for self-governance possess the necessary capabilities to turn the EU into an instrument of change. The EU can facilitate political competition and empower existing networks and organisations to engage in institution-building. Overall, the EU and other donors provided resources, built capacities of actors and institutions, served as a benchmark, and broke political deadlocks in crucial moments. At the same time, this case also hints at how the contradictions of external involvement in institution-building can be potentially resolved. First, resilience-building and reliance on local context, actors, and resources require the creation of necessary conditions for disadvantaged domestic actors to achieve relative autonomy to enable them to design their own rules for self-governing. In Ukraine's healthcare reform, the EU used its involvement to negate the existing gap in power and resources between domestic stakeholders and provided political insulation to the new institutions and pro-reform actors to prove the efficiency and sustainability of new solutions. The latter has been simplified by a lack of initial interest in the overhaul of the healthcare system, which created an opportunity for the bottom-up forces to take the lead in the reform process.

Second, the conflict and challenge of balancing state and societal resilience can increase during times of crisis and potentially stall and even reverse reforms. External attention to mitigating the immediate effects of the pandemic and prioritisation of capacity-building of the state can backfire on proposed institutional change. In this respect, the pandemic crisis brought rather a counter-reform momentum in Ukraine's healthcare sector. Yet, it was short-lived primarily due to a presence of a strong local coalition in support of continuing the reform, which was also decisive in affecting the stance of external donors and mobilising them to continue the push for change.

References

Alcaro, Riccardo, and Nathalie Tocci. 2021. "Navigating a COVID World: The European Union's internal rebirth and external quest." *The International Spectator* 56, no. 2: 1–18.

ANTAC. 2020. "100 days of procurement: How the ministry of health, the ministry of internal affairs and others used the pandemic for millions' corruption schemes." June 23, 2020. https://antac.org.ua/en/news/100-days-of-quarantine-procurement/.

Badarin, Emile. 2021. "Politics and economy of resilience: EU resilience-building in Palestine and Jordan and its disciplinary governance." *European Security* 30, no. 1: 65–84.

Badarin, Emile, and Thomas Schumacher. 2020. "Projecting resilience across the Mediterranean.". In *Building Resilience across the Mediterranean*, edited by Eugenio Cusumano and Stefan Hofmaier, 63–86. Basingstoke: Palgrave Macmillan.

Bargués, Pol, and Pol Morillas. 2021. "From democratization to fostering resilience: EU intervention and the challenges of building institutions, social trust, and legitimacy in Bosnia and Herzegovina." *Democratization* 28, no. 7: 1319–1337.

Bredenkamp, Caryn, Elina Dale, Olena Doroshenko, Yuriy Dzhygyr, Jarno Habicht, Loraine Hawkins, Alexandr Katsaga, Kateryna Maynzyuk, Khrystyna Pak, and Olga Zues. 2022. *Health financing reform in Ukraine: progress and future directions.* World Bank Publications. https://apps.who.int/iris/handle/10665/357171.

BTI. 2022. "Ukraine Country Report 2022." https://bti-project.org/en/reports/country-report/UKR.

EASO. 2021. "Ukraine FFM report – healthcare reform and economic accessibility 2021." European Asylum Support Office. https://www.ecoi.net/en/file/

local/2045259/2021_02_EASO_MedCOI_Ukraine_FFM_report_healthcare_system_and_economic_accessibility.pdf.

EEAS. 2017. "A strategic approach to resilience in the EU's external action." JOIN(2017) 21 final, 7 June. Brussels: European Commission.

EEAS. 2019. "Eastern partnership -20 deliverables for 2020 focusing on key priorities and tangible results." https://ec.europa.eu/neighbourhood-enlargement/sites/default/files/eap_20_deliverables_for_2020.pdf.

ENP Review. 2015. "Review of the European Neighbourhood Policy." JOIN (2015)50 final, 18 November. Brussels: European Commission.

European Commission. 2022. "EU factsheet – EU solidarity with Ukraine." https://ec.europa.eu/commission/presscorner/detail/en/fs_22_650.

European Neighbourhood Policy. 2004. Communication from the Commission. Strategy Paper. Brussels, 12.5.2004 COM(2004) 373. https://neighbourhood-enlargement.ec.europa.eu/system/files/2019-01/2004_communication_from_the_commission_-_european_neighbourhood_policy_-_strategy_paper.pdf

Evans, Peter. 1995. *Embedded Autonomy: States and Industrial Transformation.* Princeton: Princeton University Press.

Gorchinskaya, Aleksandra. 2015. "Ukrainskiy patsiyent. Chto uspel za 10 mesyatsev ministr Sandro, kotoromu ne dayut ni uyti, ni ostat'sya" *Novoe Vremya*, October 1, 2015. https://nv.ua/publications/idi-domoj-lechis-tam-kto-i-zachem-tormozit-provedenie-medreformy-71775.html.

IRF. 2014. "Strategic Advisory Groups: Promoting reforms in Ukraine." June 19, 2014. https://www.irf.ua/en/spriyannya_reformam_v_ukraini_rozpochinayut_robotu_strategichni_doradchi_grupi/.

Joseph, Jonathan, and Ana E. Juncos. 2019. "Resilience as an emergent European project? The EU's place in the resilience turn." *JCMS: Journal of Common Market Studies* 57, no. 5: 995–1011.

Korosteleva, Elena, and Irina Petrova. 2021. "Community Resilience in Belarus and the EU response." *Journal of Common Market Studies* 59, no. 1, 124–136.

Kovtonyuk, Pavel. 2017. "Pavel Kovtonyuk o sryve medreformy: Na metallolom vremya nashli."

Kovtonyuk, Pavel. 2019. "Konflikt v Minzdrave". *Novoe Vremya*, 1 October 2019. https://biz.nv.ua/experts/konflikt-u-moz-uryad-ne-povinen-zdavati-svojih-50045619.html

Kovtonyuk, Pavel. 2020. "Medreformu gotovyatsya svorachivat'. Za mesyats do nachala." *Novoe Vremya*, February 25, 2020. https://biz.nv.ua/experts/medreforma-otmenyaetsya-kto-i-pochemu-ee-peresmatrivaet-pavel-kovtonyuk-novosti-ukrainy-50072115.html.

Kyiv School of Economics. 2019. "White Book 2019." https://kse.ua/community/stories/to-buy-white-book-on-reforms/.

Lekhan, Valery, Volodymyr Rudiy, Maryna Shevchenko, Dorit Nitzan, and Erica Richardson. 2015. "Ukraine: Health system review." *Health Systems in Transition* 17, no. 2: 1–153.

Maass, Anna-Sophie. 2020. "The Actorness of the EU's state-building in Ukraine-before and after Crimea." *Geopolitics* 25, no. 2: 387–406.

Mahoney, James, and Kathleen Thelen, eds. 2015. *Advances in Comparative-Historical Analysis*. Cambridge: Cambridge University Press.

MOZ. 2019. "MOZ Ukrayiny zasterihaye kandydativ u prezydenty vid poshyrennya feykiv." April 18, 2019. https://moz.gov.ua/article/news/moz-ukraini-zasterigae-kandidativ-u-prezidenti-vid-poshirennja-fejkiv.

Myerson, Roger, and Timofiy Mylovanov. 2014. "Fixing Ukraine's fundamental flaw." *Kyiv Post,* March 7, 2014. https://www.kyivpost.com/article/opinion/op-ed/fixing-ukraines-fundamental-flaw-338690.html.

National Health Index. 2020. "Health Index. Ukraine – 2019: Results of the National Survey." *International Renaissance Foundation.* http://health-index.com.ua/HI%20Report%202019%20eng.pdf.

Nizhnikau, Ryhor. 2021. "Ukraine's half-hearted reforms: What needs to change in the West's approach?". FIIA Briefing Paper 307. https://www.fiia.fi/sv/publikation/ukraines-half-hearted-reforms.

NV.ua. 2019. "My shokirovany': Obshchestvennyye organizatsii prizvali Zelenskogo ob'yasnit' pozitsiyu otnositel'no medreformy." https://nv.ua/ukraine/politics/my-shokirovany-obshchestvennye-organizacii-prizvali-zelenskogo-obyasnit-poziciyu-otnositelno-medreformy-50017734.html.

NV.ua. 2021. "Ombudsmen Denisova poprosila KSU otmenit' medreformu Suprun." https://nv.ua/ukraine/politics/ksu-prosyat-otmenit-medicinskuyu-reformu-suprun-novosti-ukrainy-50134287.html.

Odintsova, Anastasiia. 2020. "Korruptsionnyy skandal vo vremya pandemii". *Novoe Vremya.* 21 April 2020. https://nv.ua/ukraine/politics/moz-popal-v-korrupcionnyy-skandal-v-svyazi-s-neprozrachnoy-zakupkoy-zashchity-dlya-medikov-novosti-ukrainy-50083466.html

Ostrom, Elinor. 2005. *Understanding Institutional Diversity.* Princeton: Princeton University Press.

Panasytska, Oleksandra, and Anastasiia Ivantsova. 2021. "New packages and more money: What has been changed in the medical reform in 2021." *Vox Ukraine*, April 22, 2022. https://voxukraine.org/en/new-packages-and-more-money-what-has-been-changed-in-the-medical-reform-in-2021/.

Patients. 2014. "Ukraine is in TOP-5 countries with the lowest level of satisfaction with health care services." September 16, 2014. https://patients.org.ua/en/2014/09/16/ukrayina-u-p-yatirtsi-krayin-svitu-z-najnizhchim-rivnem-vdovolenosti-medichnimi-poslugami/.

Patients. 2016. "The draft concept of system of state procurement of medicine." March 14, 2016. https://patients.org.ua/en/2016/03/14/the-draft-concept-of-system-of-state-procurement-of-medicine/.

Patients. 2017. "Pediatrician Drags Medical Reform through the Verkhovna Rada." October 12, 2017. https://patients.org.ua/en/2017/10/12/pediatrician-drags-medical-reform-through-the-verkhovna-rada/.

Piven, Nataliia, and Jarno Habicht. 2022. "Ukraine country snapshot: Public health agencies and services in the response to COVID-19." *WHO Website*, March 28, 2022. https://eurohealthobservatory.who.int/news-room/articles/item/ukraine-country-snapshot-public-health-agencies-and-services-in-the-response-to-covid-19.

Poteete, Amy R. 2014. "How far does evolution take us? Comment on Elinor Ostrom's: Do institutions for collective action evolve?" *Journal of Bioeconomics* 16: 91–98.

Shapovalova, Natalia. 2020. "The Coronavirus Crisis as an Opportunity in Ukraine." *Carnegie Europe website*, December 7, 2020. https://carnegieeurope.eu/2020/12/07/coronavirus-crisis-as-opportunity-in-ukraine-pub-83144.

Shevtsova, Maryna. 2020. "Covid-19 Pandemic Case Study: Ukraine, Boell Foundation." December 2020. https://us.boell.org/sites/default/files/2020-12/20201209-HB-papers-ukraine-A4-01.pdf.

Stollenwerk, Eric, Tanja A. Börzel, and Thomas Risse. 2021. "Theorizing resilience-building in the EU's neighbourhood: Introduction to the special issue." *Democratization* 28, no. 7: 1219–1238.

Tocci, Nathalie. 2017. "From the European security strategy to the EU global strategy: Explaining the journey." *International Politics* 54: 487–502.

Tocci, Nathalie. 2020. "Resilience and the role of the European Union in the world." In *Resilience in EU and International Institutions*, 25–43. Routledge.

Twigg, Judyth. 2017. "Ukraine's Health Sector Sustaining Momentum for Reform." *CSIS Website*, August 18, 2017. https://www.csis.org/analysis/ukraines-health-sector.

Twigg, Judyth. 2020. "Ukraine's Healthcare System is in Critical Condition Again." *Atlantic Council Website*, July 21, 2020. https://www.atlanticcouncil.org/blogs/ukrainealert/ukraines-healthcare-system-is-in-critical-condition-again/.

UNIAN. 2020. "Zelensky Creates Interim Working Group on Health System Reform to Analyze Medical Reform Progress by March 1." https://en.interfax.com.ua/news/general/642795.html.

USAID. 2021. "USAID Health Reform Support." https://pdf.usaid.gov/pdf_docs/PA00XDTV.pdf

Wagner, Wolfgang, and Rosanne Anholt. 2016. "Resilience as the EU Global Strategy's New Leitmotif: Pragmatic, Problematic or Promising?" *Contemporary Security Policy* 37, no. 3: 414–430.

WHO. 2022. "Biennial Collaborative Agreement (BCA) 2022–2023." https://www.who.int/ukraine/our-work/biennial-collaborative-agreement-(bca)-2022-2023.

WHO. 2022. "Health Financing Reform in Ukraine: Progress and Future Directions: Overview." June 24, 2022. https://www.who.int/europe/publications/i/item/WHO-EURO-2022-5657-45422-65003.World Bank. 2020. "Reforms in the Health Sector in Ukraine." https://thedocs.worldbank.org/en/doc/796791611679539176-0090022021/original/ReformsintheHealthSectorinUkraine.pdf.

Yakovenko, Igor. 2018. "Healthcare Reform in Ukraine: Initial Results Pending." November 2018. https://library.fes.de/pdf-files/bueros/ukraine/15504-20190614.pdf.

Zelensky, Volodymyr. 2020. "Statystyka zakhvoryuvan' na COVID-19 v Ukrayini daye nam nadiyu na maybutnye". Facebook watch, 4 May 2020. https://www.facebook.com/watch/?v=2525245104392517

4 Bad Governance in Times of Exogenous Shocks

The Case of the COVID-19 Pandemic in Russia

Vladimir Gel'man

Exogenous Shocks, Resilience, and Russia during the Pandemic

The analysis of exogenous shocks – that is, unexpected and very strong one-time negative impacts on political, economic, and societal systems due to the effects of exogenous factors – provides unique opportunities for social research. It enables scholars to relatively quickly identify and explain trends and processes which might be barely noticed and/or poorly explained under 'normal' conditions, over long periods of time (Rosenfeld 2018). Exogenous shocks, on the one hand, may serve as trigger events for degradation and further decay of some previously existing institutions and practices and, on the other hand, may provide incentives for certain innovative solutions in various policy areas in spite of Schumpeterian 'creative destruction'. In this regard, scholars discuss various patterns of resilience of states and economies (Benedikter and Fathi 2017; Thoren and Olsson 2018; Ungar 2018), with an emphasis on its mechanisms. They focus on three major modes of resilience: adaptive (capacity to absorb exogenous shocks), proactive (capacity to reduce vulnerability to potential exogenous shocks in the future), and transformative (capacity to increase efficiency after certain changes driven by exogenous shocks) (Obrist, Pfeiffer, and Henley 2010). In many ways, the COVID-19 pandemic came as an exogenous shock for various states and nations in terms of their economies, welfare, and public health systems. This is why research into their resilience is worth detailed exploration (Boin, McConnell, and Hart 2021; Linkov, Keenan, and Trump 2021) and further systematic cross-national analysis.

When discussing exogenous shocks, one should avoid the tendency (popular among journalists and pundits) to equate them with 'black swans' (Taleb 2007) – sudden and heavily destructive phenomena which cannot be countered by any institutions and mechanisms of governance. They irreversibly damage the socio-economic order as a whole, similar to the pandemic of bubonic plague in Europe in the mid-fourteenth century. Rather, the response of various states to exogenous shocks in most instances is a logical effect of previously existing institutions and mechanisms of governance. Under new stresses and contradictions from exogenous shocks, these institutions

DOI: 10.4324/9781003364870-5

demonstrate their strengths and weaknesses in coping with increasing challenges. The response of the Soviet state to the exogenous shock of a major decline in global oil prices in 1985–1986 may serve as a prime example of this phenomenon. Former Russian prime minister Yegor Gaidar rightly pointed out that the Soviet mechanisms of governance were poorly adjusted for conducting key policy changes under worsening conditions. At the same time, the formal and informal political constraints, which emerged during the 1950s–1980s in the Soviet Union, did not allow the political leadership to revise its social and economic promises and obligations without transformation of policy priorities. As a result, the response of Soviet leaders to exogenous shock was very inefficient and provoked a shift to an ill-considered and inconsistent macroeconomic policy, which, alongside numerous other factors, greatly contributed to the decline and subsequent collapse of the Soviet state (Gaidar 2010, especially Chapter V). In a more general sense, the effects of exogenous shocks on systems of governance are to a great degree dependent upon the main features of previously existing institutions and mechanisms of governance. The response of states to exogenous shocks also heavily depends upon the priorities of major political and economic actors, their use of available resources, and their strategies for coping with crises. From this perspective, the COVID-19 pandemic, which affects practically all countries in the world, became a kind of 'perfect storm' which established a basis for cross-national comparison of responses by different states (including post-Communist ones) to exogenous shocks, and of variations in their resilience (Laruelle et al. 2021; Arkturk and Lika 2022).

Overall, the success and failure of various countries in combatting the COVID-19 pandemic have been explained through the mutual impact of state capacity (with regard to the infrastructural power of the state) (Mann 1984), legitimacy, political leadership, and public health policies (Fukuyama 2020).[1] The quality of democracy also became an important constraint for excess mortality during the COVID-19 pandemic (Jain, Clarke, and Beaney 2022). For many, including developed countries, the existing conditions of their national healthcare systems turned out to be the weakest link, if not a bottleneck. Hospitals across the globe struggled to cope with excess pressures during a surge of infections (especially in some European countries, like Italy, that had high shares of aged residents, the most vulnerable to the pandemic). Some political leaders, such as Jair Bolsonaro in Brazil or Donald Trump in the United States, underestimated the severity of the COVID-19 threat, responded to the pandemic challenge sluggishly, and behaved inconsistently, ineffectively, and often irresponsibly vis-à-vis pandemic threats. In certain countries, such as Sweden, alternative strategies of pandemic response chosen by politicians and state officials have also contributed to their dubious performance. In Russia, however, all these components of state response to the pandemic were heavily affected by the consequences of bad governance, which had emerged and consolidated well before the COVID-19 pandemic (Gel'man 2022).

From the viewpoint of initial conditions, Russia had strong potential for a relatively efficient response to the COVID-19 crisis. A relatively low population density, large distances between major cities, and not particularly high domestic or international transport connectivity (except for major urban hubs and trans-border areas) created the potential for a slow spread of the virus across the country. A relatively developed public health infrastructure and large number of medical personnel also made successfully combatting the pandemic possible. Moreover, COVID-19 reached Russia fairly late relative to other major European states, so Russia had enough time to prepare for the crisis. In addition, Russian citizens were much more tolerant of the coercive actions imposed by the state than their European counterparts and did not openly object to the government's actions. Although the infrastructural state capacity and quality of public health services in Russia were rather imperfect, these problems were not crucial in terms of response to the pandemic. Nevertheless, Russia found itself on the list of developed countries with the highest excess mortality rates, which was mostly driven by COVID-19. According to some expert statements, by the end of 2021, excess mortality in Russia exceeded one million, although this data (based upon population registers) may be rather incomplete (Giattino et al. 2022).

However, apart from these preconditions, Russia's response to the pandemic was mostly driven by the political and policy priorities of its leadership. Unlike in most countries in the world (both developed and developing), the lives and health of Russian citizens were not prioritised by the authorities and were considered relatively unimportant vis-à-vis preservation of the political and economic status quo. As the doctor Alexander Myasnikov, the spokesperson in charge of state information management during the pandemic, openly stated in his speech on Russian TV: 'Those who are supposed to die will die'.[2] This reasoning was not based only on cynicism but also reflected the strategic considerations of the Russian authorities. Unlike in many democracies, under authoritarian conditions human losses themselves did not challenge the preservation of the political regime and the mechanisms of governance (Jain, Clarke, and Beaney 2022). This is why they were considered to be of secondary importance at best. The Kremlin perceived risks not from the pandemic as such but rather from the political disequilibrium it could cause, at least in the short term. Political and policy priorities of Russia's leadership coincided with incentives, which were driven by the institutions and mechanisms of bad governance. These incentives, in turn, affected the response of state actors during the pandemic.

Priorities, Institutions, and Incentives

Political and policy priorities aimed at the preservation of the previous status quo irrespective of exogenous shocks may be considered as a manifestation of adaptive resilience instead of proactive and transformative forms of resilience. In case of the COVID-19 pandemic in Russia, these priorities became clearly visible during the first wave of the pandemic. At the exact time when COVID-19 reached Russia, its leadership prioritised other issues than dealing with the pandemic, as it was driven by the nature of Russia's political regime. At that moment, a large-scale revision of the Russian constitution was in full swing, with a handful of amendments approved by the parliament in March 2020 designed to allow Putin to retain power in Russia until 2036. As the Russian regime built its legitimacy in the eyes of its citizens on the basis of voters' support for an undemocratic leader, a quasi-plebiscitary 'popular vote' was set for April 2020 to formalise these changes with a demonstration of citizens' approval of the constitutional amendments and of the continuity of Putin's rule (Yudin 2020). It comes as no surprise that the constitutional amendments turned out to be priority number one for the Kremlin. Had the pandemic not happened, this plan would most likely have been successfully implemented. Predictably, the pandemic was initially perceived by the Russian authorities as just a minor bump on the road to the main goal of preserving political power through extending the presidential term. However, the scale of the infection surge forced the Kremlin to postpone the upcoming approval of constitutional amendments until a later date. This unexpected and unwanted change in the Kremlin's political strategy and its search for new legitimation of Putin led to Russia's late and largely inefficient response to the pandemic challenge. In the end, the 'popular vote' conducted in July 2020 amid the pandemic was probably the most massive and shameless instance of fraudulent voting in Russia's post-Communist history. Using various means, ranging from large-scale workplace mobilisation of voters (mostly public sector employees) (Frye, Reuter, and Szakonyi 2014) to routine ballot box stuffing and delivering entirely fake results, the Kremlin reached its target. Before the 'popular vote', the Kremlin's mouthpieces openly declared that their goal was to cement the status quo for as long as possible and to demonstrate to all Russians that everything in the country would remain the same.[3]

This kind of adaptive resilience implies that prospects for Russia's development (including the lives and health of its citizens) were sacrificed for the sake of the political interests of the ruling groups (Rogov 2021), and to a large degree, it determined the approach of Russia's leadership to the pandemic. As long as the constitutional 'popular vote' required a large-scale mobilisation of the coercive resources of the state apparatus, combatting the pandemic was a task of secondary importance in the eyes of state officials. This is why in the wake of the pandemic outbreak, many necessary steps came with delays and were guided by the political motivations of Russia's authorities. The first stimulus package for the economy was approved only in May 2020 and used about 1.5% of the GDP (which was highly insufficient by the standards of developed countries) (Guriev 2020). As for state compensations for Russian citizens, they were fairly limited and mostly driven by considerations of buying the loyalty of voters: before the constitutional plebiscite, families with children received one-off payments of 10,000 rubles (about 127 euro) per child. Also, rather than making any bold moves in the wake of the outbreak, Putin refused to announce a state of emergency or a major lockdown. Instead, he officially declared a 'week off' at the end of March 2020 and then extended it several times up until May 2020 (the same trick was repeated once again in May 2021, during a new outbreak of the pandemic).

Nevertheless, even after the constitutional plebiscite in July 2020, the Kremlin pursued the same strategy of state response to the pandemic. On the one hand, Russia's authorities aimed to minimise budgetary expenditures and, on the other hand, to avoid unpopular measures, such as lockdowns or forced vaccination of Russian citizens. Overall, during the second and later waves of the pandemic, the Kremlin attempted to somehow wait out the troubles that had befallen Russia due to an exogenous shock and transfer responsibility for resolving multiple problems to the cabinet of ministers, to regional authorities, and to the public health system. This minimalist approach to state spending was mostly focused on support for large state-owned companies rather than for small and medium businesses, let alone individual Russian citizens, the decline of whose real incomes did not much bother the government over the course of the pandemic (Rogov 2021). In other words, the Russian government's response to exogenous shock followed the logic of 'privatisation of gains and nationalisation of costs', which is a typical way of dealing with many issues under conditions of bad governance (Gel'man 2022). In turn, Russian citizens, while facing this approach by the Kremlin, barely followed government-imposed pandemic-related restrictions or even tended to defy them in one way or another. At the same time, sanctions for violations of these restrictions implemented by Russian law enforcement agencies were applied very selectively, if not arbitrarily. As a result, the spiral of state regulations unwound further: the density of these regulations increased, but their quality remained poor. State restrictions became less and less effective, and their implementation was of little help in combatting the pandemic.

Russian authorities acted in a similar way during the pandemic with regard to development and promotion of the Russian vaccine against COVID-19, which had certain potential for becoming a 'success story' of Russia but in the end did not greatly contribute to the preservation of lives and health of Russian citizens. Nevertheless, the Russian authorities put major efforts into developing Russia's own COVID-19 vaccine. Thanks to over-concentrating the resources necessary to develop and produce a vaccine and a rush to launch it, Russian authorities proudly registered a vaccine, labelled Sputnik V (official title Gam-COVID-Vac), in August 2020, earlier than other similar products by global pharmacological companies such as Pfizer or Johnson and Johnson. Such an extraordinary hasty approval of Sputnik V was met with criticism in the mass media and discussions in the expert community about whether approval was justified in the absence of robust scientific research confirming safety and efficacy (Cole 2020; Ilyushina and Pleitgen 2020). Despite these concerns, in February 2021, an interim analysis from the trial was published in *The Lancet*, the major global medical journal, indicating

91.6% efficacy without major side effects (Logunov et al. 2021). In many ways, Sputnik V's launch was perceived by Russian authorities as a great advancement. However, its trajectory became not dissimilar to some other short-lived 'success stories' in Russia, including the Soviet space programme of the 1950s–1960s (Gel'man 2022, Chapter 6).

Similar to the promotion of the Soviet space programme in the international arena as a foreign policy tool, Russia attempted to use the supplying of new anti-COVID medicine as a tool of aggressive 'vaccine diplomacy', demanding major concessions from several member states of the European Union for priority supply of the vaccine. Russia's vaccine-related pressure on governments in countries like Slovakia and the Czech Republic, aimed at changes in their policies towards Russia, caused major political scandals (Charouz 2021; Higgins 2021). Some other countries faced delays in procuring Russian vaccines. Second, and most important, the domestic campaign of vaccination largely failed. Russia had officially started vaccination with Sputnik V as early as December 2020 (the use of foreign vaccines was not permitted in Russia). However, by the end of 2021, only 45% of Russians had received at least one dose of the vaccine – a much lower share than in most developed countries. The Russian authorities paid little attention to persuading citizens to be vaccinated, while state propaganda aimed at discrediting the European and American experience of combatting the pandemic (including vaccination efforts abroad) intentionally or unintentionally spread many nonsensical ideas about the pandemic and therefore disoriented many ordinary Russians. Only in June 2021, when a new outbreak of COVID-19 caused a new spike in the number of victims, did the government seek to increase the vaccination rate at least among public sector employees and service sector workers. These belated measures barely helped to combat the pandemic in Russia. The potential 'success story' failed because the Kremlin perceived the Russian vaccine not as a medicine aimed at combatting the pandemic but rather as an instrument of soft power aimed at promotion of Russia's position in the international arena. At the same time, Russian authorities refused to allow the use of foreign vaccines within the country, driven by the rationale of a protectionist economic policy, and insisted on mutual recognition of Russian vaccines in the EU and vice versa. Although Sputnik V was mostly considered a bargaining chip in the global spread of Russia's influence, the results of this aggressive international promotion did not meet the Kremlin's desires. In the end, Russian attempts to conquer international vaccination markets had limited success, as Sputnik V failed to receive quick approval by American and European regulators and soon was nearly forgotten internationally. This is how Russia's comparative advantage, which has its own vaccine-producing industry, turned into a major deficiency. One can imagine that without such an industry, Russian authorities could have been forced to buy Pfizer or other foreign vaccines and pay more attention to the vaccination of their citizens. However, the chances to convert the potential 'success story' of Sputnik V into a more efficient Russian response to the pandemic have been lost.

The macro-level incentives, driven by the political and policy priorities of the Russian leadership, were complemented by micro-level incentives for state officials and personnel of public health organisations within the framework of top-down hierarchical governance, known in Russia as the 'power vertical'. These incentives resulted from the 'overregulated state' in Russia (Paneyakh 2013), which contributed to inefficient combatting of the pandemic. The awkward combination of high density and poor quality of state regulations in the field of public health eventually put directors of hospitals as well as front-line doctors and nurses between a rock and a hard place. They have had to minimise risks of being fired by their superiors, if not prosecuted by law enforcement agencies, for any real or imagined wrongdoings. Meanwhile, the ongoing ill-designed 'optimisation' of public health facilities in Russia, aimed at making huge conglomerates of big hospitals at the expense of local medical centres (especially in small towns and rural areas), has only aggravated the situation, making medical personnel even more vulnerable vis-à-vis their superiors (Novkunskaya 2020, Chapter 2). This is why loyally following any directives from their superiors, who in turn are interested in whitewashing statistics and portraying a rosy picture of successfully combatting the pandemic, remains the only available strategy for almost every worker in the Russian public health system. The hierarchy of the 'power vertical' transmitted these incentives from the top to the bottom, thus aggravating the situation, as minimising responsibility for inefficiency in combatting the pandemic became a key priority for governing public health amid the COVID-19 outbreak. To put it bluntly, the priority interests of all public health actors were related to reporting, which could help to avoid potential conflicts with state watchdogs, rather than to preserving the lives and health of fellow Russian citizens.

At the same time, the rise of the 'information autocracy' (Guriev and Treisman 2019) in Russia – a regime based upon extensive use of lies as a tool of its dominance – has proved to be a double-edged sword under the conditions of the pandemic. It provides strong incentives for intentional distortion of information and production of Kremlin-desired good numbers at all layers of the state hierarchy, ranging from regional governors and city mayors to directors of local hospitals, etc. (Kalashnikov 2020). It is no wonder that the major package of anti-crisis measures adopted in Russia in late March 2020 included, *inter alia*, criminalisation of fake news regarding the pandemic and imposition of strict control over the spread of unwanted information on the ground. Doctors and nurses across Russia were at risk of being fired, if not prosecuted, and shared information with journalists and independent observers only under conditions of anonymity (Safonova 2020). When the meaninglessness of official Russian statistics on the number of infected people and of pandemic-related casualties was demonstrated by experts, who used advanced quantitative techniques of analysis, these disclosures caused a furious reaction from Russian state officials and vicious counterattacks against international media (Burn-Murdoch and Foy 2020; Meyer 2020).

The response of the Russian state was an additional change in regulations aimed at further decreasing official numbers and obscuring the real picture (Litavrin, Frenkel, and Skovoroda 2020). From this perspective, Russia's rulers followed the practices of the Soviet Union, as Soviet officials tended not to disclose bad news regarding major negative trends. This practice had a devastating effect during the Chernobyl nuclear disaster in 1986 when Soviet leaders attempted to conceal information. They publicly acknowledged the nuclear accident after a major delay – Soviet officials acted only after the spread of alarming news in the West (Plokhy 2019). Although reliance upon distorted information was not helpful in combatting the pandemic, the power vertical, which prioritised loyalty over efficiency, most probably pursued other goals than the health of Russian citizens, and the media provides evidence of Russian state officials passing the blame in the midst of the pandemic (Rustamova and Pertsev 2020).

Russian State Actors during the Pandemic

Which state actors were involved in combatting the COVID-19 pandemic in Russia, and why was their performance during the crisis so inefficient? Ultimately, the authority to combat the coronavirus was de facto entrusted to the chief executives of Russia's regions (Smyth et al. 2020). They gained rights and responsibilities to handle problems caused by the pandemic, including regulating work, travel, and services and preparing medical facilities for the influx of patients. Administrative decentralisation in itself could have been a justified measure during the pandemic. Russia is a very diverse country, and the scale of the problems caused by the coronavirus varied greatly between the provinces.

Yet the entire mechanism of governance in Russia was insufficient for the country to provide an effective response to the pandemic crisis at the regional level. First and foremost, many provinces had limited amounts of resources to resist the pandemic, while transfers from the federal budget reached regional coffers with a major delay. Second, the conditions of the overregulated state caused a failure by both federal and regional governments to provide the resources needed to deal with the consequences of the pandemic (due to the risk of being accused of misusing state funds) (Gilev and Dimke 2021). Third, the power vertical was not designed to deal with such crises, as apart from delivering required voting results at any cost and avoiding mass protests, the regional and local officials' objective was to achieve targets imposed in a top-down manner, measured as percentage points of performance indicators against previous years (Paneyakh 2014). Therefore, it is hardly surprising that during the pandemic the governors of some Russian regions provided official reports to the Kremlin of nearly the same and apparently fabricated numbers of cases and (mostly unsuccessfully) attempted to hide excess mortality data. The only major exception was the city of Moscow, which has an immense amount of resources and which was a priority area for combatting the pandemic (given both the political importance of the nation's capital and the salience of the pandemic in a megapolis with 12 million residents). This is why the Moscow city government responded to the pandemic more proactively. It imposed a partial lockdown during the initial outbreak of the disease, increased the number of special medical facilities, and offered extra payments from the city budget to elderly Muscovites. However, the case of Moscow was truly unique. Most of Russia's regional authorities more or less replicated the federal approach to combatting the pandemic, having limited resources and facing numerous institutional barriers due to the conditions of the 'overregulated state'.

At the same time, the approach of the Russian state leadership was flawed in institutional terms on the medical front nationwide. Unlike in many developed countries, responsibility for combatting the pandemic was transferred not to the Ministry of Health or any other specialised state agency in charge of medical affairs but to the state watchdog agency Rospotrebnadzor, primarily responsible for numerous regulations in the consumer market. This agency (which set sanitary norms and had broad discretion over punishment for their violation) had previously gained a notorious reputation for being involved in the politically motivated ban on food imports from 'unfriendly' countries such as Georgia. A comparative analysis of performance of state regulators in Russia convincingly demonstrated that Rospotrebnadzor was relatively inefficient vis-à-vis other state watchdog agencies (Kuchakov 2020). Meanwhile, the Kremlin prioritised manual control through the top-down chain of command and adherence to formal rules and regulations over combatting the outbreak of COVID-19. This is why transferring responsibility to Rospotrebnadzor was a preferable solution in the eyes of state leadership. While public health agencies are based on a two-tier system of subordination (most hospitals are subordinated to and funded by subnational authorities, and the federal ministry performs functions of coordination), Rospotrebnadzor is based on the strict top-down hierarchy of its own power vertical. It was perceived by the government as an organisation that could implement top-down orders without consulting other agencies. This is why the government nominated the head of Rospotrebnadzor, Anna Popova, to be in charge of all regulatory actions taken by the state during the pandemic. The territorial branches of this agency became veto actors in the regions regarding the pandemic, as governors were instructed to get its approval on all related actions, and it gained discretion and funding without bearing any responsibility for public health performance. According to journalists' reports, Popova received carte blanche from the top leadership, and her political patron, the deputy prime minister Tatyana Golikova, counselled Popova at the beginning of the pandemic to act such that, in their words: 'Everything will be all right and afterwards you will not be ashamed (before superiors)' (Barabanov, Soshnikov, and Reuter 2020). Unsurprisingly, the impact of Rospotrebnadzor on combatting the pandemic was hardly productive: it contributed to distortion of information within the hierarchy of the power vertical and stimulated a passive adaptive reaction to the crisis by state officials and medical personnel and often aggravated the situation in the regions because of multiple cases of overregulation (especially during the initial outbreak of the pandemic). Indeed, it became nearly useless in resolving numerous problems in the public health system. This approach was as if the Russian authorities had entrusted the extinguishing of a fire not to professional firefighters but to fire inspectors who were in charge of monitoring the presence of fire extinguishers.

All in all, the nationwide coordination of various state agencies during the outbreak of the pandemic remained the weakest link in governance in Russia. There were several bodies in charge of this task, including the operational headquarters of the government, led by Golikova, a special task force of the State Council, led by Mayor of Moscow Sergey Sobyanin, and the top political leaders – President Vladimir Putin and Prime Minister Mikhail Mishustin. In fact, the responsibility for combatting the pandemic was unevenly and ineffectively distributed between several state officials, and there was no one who would take actual leadership during the crisis. In Russia, in the 2020s, there was a lack of top officials who could perform similar to the Soviet deputy prime minister Boris Shcherbina, who relatively successfully took on such a role during the Chernobyl nuclear disaster in 1986 and was able to diminish the most pernicious consequences of the tragedy (Plokhy 2019). When Putin self-isolated during the outbreak of the pandemic, the shortage of effective managerial leadership in Russia became highly visible. Such a shortage was a side effect of bad governance in Russia even under routine conditions, but in a situation of pandemic-related exogenous shock, its negative effects became extraordinary.

To what extent were political risks caused by the outbreak of the pandemic – such as a major decline in public support for Putin and for the Russian political regime itself, or the rise of mass protests – a real threat for the Kremlin? I would argue that these risks were greatly overestimated from the very beginning of the COVID-19 pandemic in Russia, to a major degree being fuelled by the constitutional plebiscite. The mass political support of governments in many developed countries, which put major efforts into genuinely combatting the pandemic and provided financial support to business and to citizens, resulted in quite the opposite picture. Political support of some leaders and governments sometimes even temporarily increased in spite of the 'rally around the flag' phenomenon, although some democratically elected governments later on were punished by voters during the next round of polls. Even a certain decline in Putin's approval rate, which was observed during the first outbreak of the pandemic, was a short-term phenomenon and not a critical one for maintenance of the political status quo in Russia (Zavadskaya and Sokolov 2020). Moreover, one can imagine that more serious financial support for Russians by the government as a more proactive approach by the authorities to combatting the pandemic (especially before in the wake of mass vaccination) could have contributed to stronger political support for the status quo. Meanwhile, in the wake of the outbreak, no serious socio-economic protests were observed in Russia during the pandemic, and mass rallies and protests in this period were driven by other causes. The weakness of mass mobilisation in Russia did not only result from the threat of increasing state repressions. As previous research has demonstrated, in the context of Russian authoritarianism, socio-economic crises and decline in real incomes contribute to falling protest intentions and orientations of Russian citizens. Rather, they are more inclined to protest not during periods of severe crises, but when hard times are over, and mass expectations for the future are more positive (Semenov 2020).

Regardless, the combination of the priorities of Russia's political leadership, inefficient institutions, and contradictory incentives provided by state actors very negatively affected Russia's response to exogenous shock during the COVID-19 outbreak. Russian authorities at all levels of the power vertical acted sluggishly and lost many opportunities to combat the pandemic more successfully. At the same time, similar to Russia's crises in the 1990s (Javeline 2009), shifting the blame to various state agencies and regional actors and dividing responsibility between them has served as an efficient instrument for maintenance of the political status quo at a time of crisis.

Lessons from the Pandemic: Exogenous Shocks, Resilience, and Involution in Russia

The Russian response to the outbreak of the COVID-19 pandemic may be regarded as a clear case of adaptive resilience to exogenous shock. Such a response was driven not only by structural socio-economic conditions but mostly by the strategic choices of Russia's political leadership. The Russian authorities were able to preserve and strengthen their rule without losing control over the political order or much by way of financial and political resources. Yet this goal was achieved at the cost of heavy losses for Russia's human capital (and, to a much lesser degree, for Russia's economy) (Rogov 2021). This approach to responding to exogenous shocks excludes both measures for reduction of vulnerabilities to new exogenous shocks (proactive resilience) and changes in governing the state aimed at increasing its efficiency (transformative resilience). The Kremlin intentionally moved these possible solutions off the menu of options for Russia. Rather, the conservative adaptation to consequences of exogenous shock demonstrated by Russia during the pandemic was an instance of involution. This was defined by American sociologist Michael Burawoy as 'an alternative to both "revolution" and "evolution". It implies profound degeneration the opposite of accumulation' (Burawoy 1996, 1109). It is a kind of defensive inward turn of previously existing institutions and practices, aimed at preventing major changes to the previous political and socio-economic order or, at least, at minimising the effects of these changes. Burawoy, who observed and analysed a public response to market reforms in the Russian provinces during the 1990s, considered involution to be a major mechanism for adaptation of Russian society to the hardships of economic transition (Burawoy 1996, 2001). He believed that instead of the transformation of the Russian economy and society towards a new economic order, involution contributed to conservation of many old pathologies of Russian society and aggravation of new problems. Although many assessments made by Burawoy at that time were somewhat contradictory and/or lost their relevance during the economic boom of the 2000s, his observations and comments make sense for analysis of Russia's response to exogenous shocks in a broader perspective.

Why has involution, as the experience of the pandemic tells us, become the main, if not the only, mechanism of resilience in Russia, while any other varieties of response to exogenous shocks visibly remain off the agenda for the country? Of course, the self-interests of ruling groups and other actors, who tend towards avoiding major losses in the short term, played an important role in strategic choices under conditions of bad governance, with its institutions and incentives. But the choice of risk-aversive strategies under high uncertainty (Kahneman, Slovic, and Tversky 1982) in Russia is also based upon the previous experience of dissatisfaction and disillusionment after transformative responses to exogenous shocks in the late 1980s (Gaidar 2010) and especially in the 1990s. Judging by this experience, it is no wonder that Russia's response to exogenous shocks related to exhaustion of sources of economic growth (Rogov 2021) and its possible major recession after the 2022 invasion of Ukraine is most likely to be involutionary. The problem is that involution is not only unproductive as a response to numerous socio-economic challenges, especially due to the pernicious consequences of exogenous shocks, but it may also only aggravate problems and postpone inevitable solutions, which may become more painful over time. This postponement means that Russia's limited potential for proactive and transformative resilience may diminish over time, and its vulnerability to new exogenous shocks (perhaps of a different nature than those of the pandemic) will only increase.

One might expect that the problems of the poor quality of governance in Russia will not disappear after the pandemic – rather, they are set to become much more salient, especially in the wake of the Russian invasion of Ukraine in 2022. Although the immediate losses of many Russians during the outbreak of COVID-19 due to the Russian state's inefficient response to pandemic-related exogenous shock are significant, long-term losses and their consequences are even more important. Sooner or later, Russian rulers as well as many Russian citizens will have to pay the bills which were issued as a result of the exogenous shocks.

Notes

1 Here and in the following sections, I rely upon analysis presented in a previous publication (Gel'man 2022, Chapter 7).

2 See "Doktor Myasnikov: komu polozheno umeret' – pomrut". May 20, 2020. Accessed April 18, 2022. https://www.youtube.com/watch?v=wztfLJLUSWc.

3 See Popravki v konstitutsiyu zatsementiruyut polozhenie Rossii, zayavil Peskov, *RIA Novosti*, June 20, 2020. Accessed April 18, 2022. https://ria.ru/20200620/1573236667.html.

References

Aktürk, Şener, and Idlir Lika. 2022. "Varieties of resilience and side effects of disobedience: Cross-national patterns of survival during the coronavirus pandemic." *Problems of Post-Communism* 69, no. 1: 1–13.

Barabanov, Ilya, Andrey Soshnikov, and Svetlana Reuter. 2020. "Ona byla tikhaya-tikhaya: Kto takaya Anna Popova, vozglavivshaya bor'bu s koronavirusom v Rossii." *BBC Russian Service*, May 29, 2020. Accessed April 18, 2022. http://www.bbc.com/russian/features-52775158.

Benedikter, Roland, and Fathi Karim. 2017. "What is a resilient society?" *International Policy Digest*, September 17, 2017. Accessed April 18, 2022. https://intpolicydigest.org/2017/09/17/what-is-a-resilient-society/.

Boin, Arjen, Allan McConnell, and Paul Hart. 2021. *Governing the Pandemic: The Politics of Navigating a Mega-Crisis*. London: Springer Nature.

Burawoy, Michael. 1996. "The state and economic involution: Russia through a China lens." *World Development* 24, no. 6: 1105–1117.

Burawoy, Michael. 2001. "Transition without transformation: Russia's involutionary road to capitalism." *East European Politics and Societies* 15, no. 2: 269–290.

Burn-Murdoch, John, and Henry Foy. 2020. "Russia's Covid death toll could be 70 per cent higher than official figure." *The Financial Times* May 11, 2021.

Charouz, Ladislav. 2021. "Can the Czech Health Minister Have His Cake and Eat It Too?" *The New Federalist*, April 14, 2021. Accessed April 18, 2022. http://www.thenewfederalist.eu/can-the-czech-health-minister-have-his-cake-and-eat-it-too-a-game-of?lang=fr.

Cole Brendan. 2020. "Putin's World-Beating COVID Vaccine Faces Doubts from Doctors and Russians." *Newsweek*, December 8, 2020. Accessed April 18, 2022. http://www.newsweek.com/russia-putin-sputnik-v-coronavirus-vaccine-kremlin-1553136.

Frye, Timothy, Ora John Reuter, and David Szakonyi. 2014. "Political machines at work voter mobilization and electoral subversion in the workplace." *World Politics* 66, no. 2: 195–228.

Fukuyama, Francis. 2020. "The pandemic and political order." *Foreign Affairs* 99, no. 4: 26–32.

Gaidar, Yegor. 2010. *Collapse of an Empire: Lessons for Modern Russia*. Washington, DC: Brookings Institution Press.

Gel'man, Vladimir. 2022. *The Politics of Bad Governance in Contemporary Russia*. Ann Arbor: University of Michigan Press.

Giattino, Charlie, Ritchie Hannah, Roser Max, Ortiz-Ospina Esteban, and Hassel Joel. 2022. "Excess Mortality during the Coronavirus Pandemic (COVID-19)." *Our World in Data*, February 14, 2022. Accessed April 18, 2022. https://ourworldindata.org/excess-mortality-covid.

Gilev, Aleksei, and Dimke Daria. 2021. "'No time for quality': Mechanisms of local governance in Russia." *Europe-Asia Studies* 73, no. 6: 1060–1079.

Guriev, Sergei. 2020. "Kak Vladimir Putin proigral koronavirusu." *Internetproekt.com*, June 29, 2020. Accessed April 18, 2022. http://internetproekt.com/novosti/item/688326-sergey-guriev-o-tom-kak-putin-proigral-koronavirusu.

Guriev, Sergei, and Daniel Treisman. 2019. "Informational autocrats." *Journal of Economic Perspectives* 33, no. 4: 100–127.

Higgins, Andrew. 2021. "Slovakia Claims a Bait-and-Switch with the Russian Vaccines it Ordered." *The New York Times,* April 8, 2021. Accessed April 18, 2022. http://www.nytimes.com/2021/04/08/world/europe/slovakia-coronavirus-russia-vaccine-sputnik.html.

Ilyushina, Mary, and Frederik Pleitgen. 2020. "Reality Bites for Putin's Much-Hyped COVID-19 Vaccine, as Concerns over Efficacy and Safety Linger." *CNN*, October 27, 2020. Accessed April 18, 2022. http://edition.cnn.com/2020/10/27/health/russia-coronavirus-vaccine-sputnik-v-reality-check/index.html.

Jain, Vageesh, Jonathan Clarke, and Beaney Thomas. 2022. "Association between democratic governance and excess mortality during the COVID-19 pandemic: An observational study." *Journal of Epidemiology Community Health* 76, no. 10: 853–860.

Javeline, Debra Lynn. 2009. *Protest and the Politics of Blame: The Russian Response to Unpaid Wages*. Ann Arbor: University of Michigan Press.

Kahneman, Daniel, Stewart Paul Slovic, and Amos Tversky eds. 1982. *Judgment under Uncertainty: Heuristics and Biases*. Cambridge: Cambridge University Press.

Kalashnikov, Sergei. 2020. "Lipetskii gubernator poprosil podchinennykh popravit' statistiku po koronavirusu". *Kommersant*, May 25, 2020. Accessed April 18, 2022. http://www.kommersant.ru/doc/4356084.

Kuchakov, Ruslan. 2020. "Reforma kontrol'no-nadzornoi deyatel'nosti v Rossii v 2016–2019: promezhutochnye itogi (St. Petersburg: Institute for the Rule of Law, European University at St. Petersburg)." Accessed April 18, 2022. https://enforce.spb.ru/images/analytical_review/irl_reform_results.pdf.

Laruelle, Marlene, Mikhail Alexseev, Cynthia Buckley, Ralph S. Clem, J. Paul Goode, Ivan Gomza, Henry E. Hale et al. 2021. "Pandemic politics in Eurasia: Roadmap for a new research subfield." *Problems of Post-Communism* 68, no. 1: 1–16.

Linkov, Igor, Jesse M. Keenan, and Bemjamin D. Trump, eds., 2021. *COVID-19: Systemic Risk and Resilience*. Cham: Springer.

Litavrin, Maksim, David Frenkel, and Egor Skovoroda. 2020. "Vesnoi kak minimum v 7 regionakh sil'no vyrosla smertnost', i ofitsial'nye dannye po koronavirusu eto ne ob'yasnyayut." *Mediazona*, June 30, 2020. Accessed April 18, 2022. http://zona.media/article/2020/06/30/mortality.

Logunov, Denis Y., Inna V. Dolzhikova, Dmitry V. Shcheblyakov, Amir I. Tukhvatulin, Olga V. Zubkova, Alina S. Dzharullaeva, Anna V. Kovyrshina et al. 2021. "Safety and efficacy of an rAd26 and rAd5 vector-based heterologous prime-boost COVID-19 vaccine: An interim analysis of a randomised controlled phase 3 trial in Russia." *The Lancet* 397, no. 10275: 671–681.

Mann, Michael. 1984. "The autonomous power of the state: Its origins, mechanisms and results." *European Journal of Sociology/Archives Européennes de Sociologie* 25, no. 2: 185–213.

Meyer, Henry. 2020. "Experts Question Russian Data on COVID-19 Death Toll." *Bloomberg.com*, May 13, 2020. Accessed April 18, 2022. http://www.bloomberg.com/news/articles/2020-05-13/experts-question-russian-data-on-covid-19-death-toll.

Novkunskaya, Anastasia. 2020. "Professional Agency and Institutional Change: Case of Maternity Services in Small-Town Russia. PhD dissertation, University of Helsinki."

Obrist, Brigit, Constanze Pfeiffer, and Robert Henley. 2010. "Multi-layered social resilience: A new approach in mitigation research." *Progress in Development Studies* 10, no. 4: 283–293.

Paneyakh, Ella. 2013. "The overregulated state." *Social Sciences* 45, no. 1: 20–33.
Paneyakh, Ella. 2014. "Faking performance together: Systems of performance evaluation in Russian enforcement agencies and production of bias and privilege." *Post-Soviet Affairs* 30, no. 2–3: 115–136.
Plokhy, Serhii. 2019. *Chernobyl: History of a Tragedy*. London: Penguin.
Rogov, Kirill, ed. 2021. "Zastoi-2: Posledstviya, riski i al'ternativy dlya rossiiskoi ekonomiki (Moscow: Liberal'naya missiya)." Accessed April 18, 2022. https://liberal.ru/wp-content/uploads/2021/04/zastoj-2.pdf.
Rosenfeld, Richard. 2018. "Studying crime trends: Normal science and exogenous shocks." *Criminology* 56, no. 1: 5–26.
Rustamova, Farida, and Pertsev Andrey. 2020. "Dazhe slovo 'karantin' starayutsya ne upotreblyat'. Kak president i pravitel'stvo perekladyvayut drug na druga otvetstvennost' v bor'be s koronavirusom." *Meduza.io*, April 1, 2020. Accessed April 18, 2022. http://meduza.io/feature/2020/04/01/dazhe-slovo-karantin-starayutsya-ne-upotreblyat.
Safonova, Kristina. 2020. "My vse boimsya – i rukovodstvo, i vrachi." *Meduza.io*, April 21, 2020. Accessed April 18, 2022. http://meduza.io/feature/2020/04/21/my-vse-boimsya-i-rukovodstvo-i-vrachi.
Semenov, A. 2020. "Nerovnyi ritm: Dinamika gotovnosti k ekonomicheskim protestam v Rossii (1996–2019)." *Economicheskaya sotsiologiya* 21, no. 4: 107–124.
Smyth, Regina, Sharafutdinova Gulnaz, Timothy Model, and Aiden Klein. 2020. "The Russian Power Vertical and the COVID-19 Challenge: The Trajectories of Regional Responses." *PONARS Policy Memos*, N 646. Accessed April 18, 2022 https://www.ponarseurasia.org/the-russian-power-vertical-and-the-covid-19-challenge-the-trajectories-of-regional-responses.
Taleb, Nassim Nicholas. 2007. *Black Swan: The Impact of the Highly Improbable*. New York: Random House.
Thorén, Henrik, and Olsson Lennart. 2018. "Is resilience a normative concept?" *Resilience* 6, no. 2: 112–128.
Ungar, Michail. 2018. "Systemic resilience: Principles and processes for a science of change in context of adversity." *Ecology and Society* 23, no. 4. Accessed April 18, 2022. https://doi.org/10.5751/ES-10385-230434.
Yudin, Grigory. 2020. "Edinstvennyi ili nikakoi: Chego khochet ot plebiscite Putin i chto mogut sdelat' opponenty." *Republic.ru*, June 11, 2020. Accessed April 18, 2022. http://republic.ru/posts/96942.
Zavadskaya, Margarita, and Boris Sokolov. 2020. "The Linkages between Experiencing COVID-19 and Levels of Political Support in Russia." *PONARS Policy Memos*, N 677. Accessed April 18, 2022. http://www.ponarseurasia.org/linkages-between-experiencing-covid-19-and-levels-of-political-support-in-russia/.

5 Authoritarian Responses to Protest Participation During COVID-19

The Russian Case

Eemil Mitikka

Introduction

Restrictions introduced during the COVID-19 pandemic were widely received as a serious assault on individual freedoms. Concerns about using pandemic restrictions as an excuse to repress oppositional voices are especially relevant in authoritarian countries like Russia where anti-establishment voices were curbed long before the pandemic (Lamberova and Sonin 2022; Laruelle et al. 2021). However, did the Kremlin exploit pandemic restrictions to repress anti-governmental political protests during COVID-19? If yes, were these measures targeted against certain political protests more clearly than others?

From social and individual freedom perspectives, the dilemma of imposing COVID-crisis-related social distancing policies is that although these restrictions were seen as an essential measure in tackling the pandemic, they also restrict many fundamental rights, such as freedom of assembly. These concerns are real in any society because pandemic restrictions could also be used as a tool to restrict the activities of undesired opposition and anti-governmental social movements. This is especially relevant in authoritarian countries where security officials are often used extensively to keep civil society under control. Indeed, there were concerns about repressive uses of epidemic regulations already in early stages of the pandemic (Diamond 2020). Later research indicates that pandemic restrictions have also been used in practice to suppress the political opposition in Russia (Lamberova and Sonin 2022).

This chapter offers an overview of how the Russian establishment responded to political protests in Russia during COVID-19. More specifically, I showcase how the Russian authorities instrumentalised pandemic restrictions to curb oppositional movements during the pandemic. Russia is a relevant case study for this kind of examination because while the level of authoritarian repression has steadily increased during the last decades, two major anti-governmental protest waves took place precisely at the height of the COVID-19 pandemic in 2020–2021: the Khabarovsk Krai protests and protests supporting Alexei Navalny. I use both local and national level research data to display that the Russian authorities have used COVID-19 social distancing measures inconsistently, selectively, and arbitrarily to

DOI: 10.4324/9781003364870-6

respond to these anti-governmental protest movements. The main argument of this chapter is that while the Russian authorities have used repressive measures in holding back both these protests, their response has been generally much harsher with Alexei Navalny's support protests compared to the Khabarovsk Krai protests. Moreover, Russian authorities also more frequently instrumentalised pandemic legislation to penalise and curb Navalny protests compared to the latter protests.

The chapter proceeds as follows: first, there is a brief overview of the two aforementioned major protests in 2020–2021. Next, the Russian authorities' responses to public gatherings related to political protest during COVID-19 are introduced. After that, the research data and methods used in this research are presented. The next section answers the research question about the differences in the legal responses of the Russian authorities to the Khabarovsk Krai and Alexei Navalny's support protests. The chapter concludes by discussing the relevance of these findings in studying political protest in contemporary Russia.

Background: Political Protest during the Pandemic in Russia

Russia has become increasingly authoritarian since President Putin's first term in the 2000s (Coppedge et al. 2022). Therefore, one could assume that the recent COVID-19 pandemic should limit people's eagerness for oppositional mass gatherings, as participation in anti-government protests has become increasingly risky. Moreover, the chances of contracting COVID-19 are lower when people practise social distancing. Thus, practising social distancing and avoiding public gatherings would make sense not only from a social but also from an individual perspective. Against this background, it is interesting that some of the largest mass protests in the history of post-Soviet Russia occurred during the last few years and the COVID-19 pandemic. Figure 5.1 depicts the number of protests with over 10,000 participants in Russia during 2011–2021. In the plot on the left, the vertical axis captures the number of participants in distinct protest events (marked with scatter points) and horizontal axis captures the date of the protest. The plot on right in Figure 5.1, in turn, zooms in for the protests with over 10,000 participants in 2020–2021, that is, during the COVID crisis.

It is possible to draw a few insights from Figure 5.1. Firstly, in spite of growing repression (see, e.g. Coppedge et al. 2022), participation in political protests has not decreased in Russia. Secondly, some of the biggest political protests have taken place during COVID-19, or during 2020–2021. Thirdly, the largest political protests in this time period dealt with support for popular political figures: Boris Nemtsov, Sergei Furgal, and Alexei Navalny. It is important to note that since calculating the exact number of protest participants is hard or even impossible, these numbers are naturally only rough estimates of protest participation in Russia during the last decade. Nevertheless, they indicate that the size of protests during COVID-19 is significant

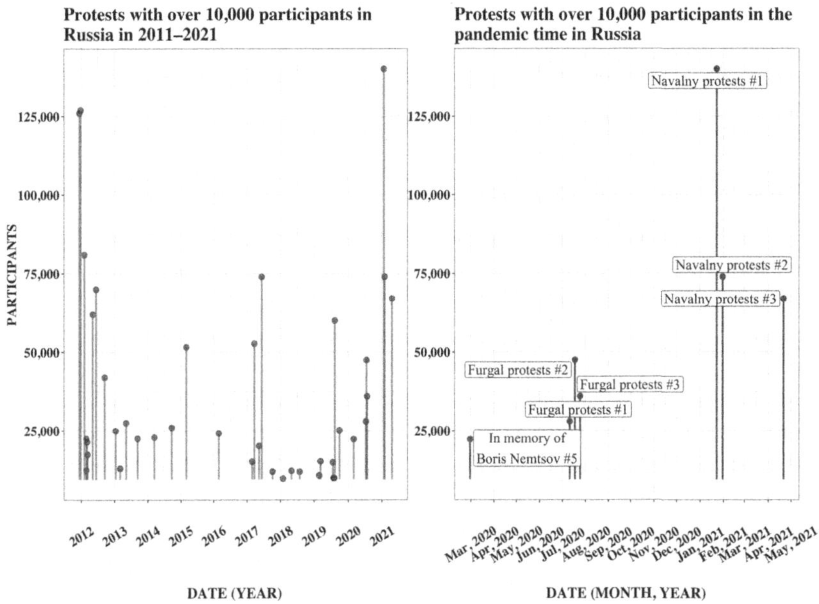

Figure 5.1 Development of mass protests in Russia in 2011–2021. Data source: Rogov and Shukyurov (2021).

Source: Author's creation

even if observed in a longer time frame. Moreover, it has been argued that the contradiction between social policy promises, 10 years of stagnation in living standards before the COVID-19 crisis, and limited investment in health care raised protest potential in Russia before the pandemic (Laruelle et al. 2021). In addition, polling data on Putin's support are in line with raising protest moods in Russia since his approval ratings stagnated after the 2018 pension reform protests until the 2022 Russian war of aggression in Ukraine. Moreover, according to some estimates, Putin's approval ratings even reached a historic low during the pandemic in 2020 (Levada-tsentr 2022; Snegovaya, Volkov, and Goncharov 2020).

This observation raises the question of how the Russian authorities then reacted to these protests. Were COVID-19 measures intended to curb anti-governmental political unrest in Russia? If yes, did these measures differ between protests? Answering these questions is important because it might help us understand the social context for political protest in authoritarian countries such as Russia in times of exogenous shocks akin to the COVID-19 pandemic.

The next section of this chapter gives a brief overview of the overall response of the Russian authorities to public gatherings during 2020–2021. As the commemoration protest march in honour of Boris Nemtsov was arranged in February 2020 when there were no social distancing restrictions yet and COVID-19 was not yet widespread in the country, I focus on protests dealing with Sergei Furgal and Alexei Navalny. However, before proceeding to the response of Russian authorities, the two protests that will be utilised are briefly introduced.

Protest in Support of Sergei Furgal

Besides Navalny-related protests, another noteworthy protest movement in 2020–2021 in Russia was the support protests for the dismissed and imprisoned Governor of Khabarovsk Krai, Sergei Furgal. In 2018, the Liberal Democratic Party of Russia's (henceforth: LDPR) candidate Furgal was elected against all odds as Governor of Khabarovsk Krai in the Russian Far East. Furgal outbid the incumbent and United Russia's candidate Vyacheslav Shport in a landslide victory during the second round of Russian gubernatorial elections. What makes the Furgal case intriguing is that although a member of LDPR, Furgal represented the so-called Russian 'systemic opposition'. He later became a popular politician among the local public, for example, due to his progressive social policies and cutting costs in local public administration (DVHAB.RU 2018; AiF 2019; Gardner 2019; Varlamov 2020). Furgal doubled the provision for the assignment of new teachers, extended benefits for families with many children, ordered to raise the living wage of pensioners, and issued an order according to which the inhabitants of the northern region of the Krai would get substitutes for buying airline tickets to Khabarovsk (Varlamov 2020). On 9 July 2020, Furgal was arrested over the killings of business rivals in 2004–2005. However, the public of the Khabarovsk Krai viewed these accusations as fabricated and already on 11–12 July 2020 there were 10,000–12,000 protesters (according to the police estimates) on the streets of Khabarovsk demanding the release of and a fair trial for Furgal (Lokhov 2020; TASS 2020). The large protests kept going for months and some experts estimated that as many as 5% of the residents of the city of Khabarovsk went to the streets to support the dismissed governor (Rogov 2021b, 13).

What made the Furgal protests exceptional is that even as these protests took place outside of Moscow or St. Petersburg, they managed to mobilise a large number of people. Despite their anti-Kremlin claims, these protests were in support of a politician who was 'an insider' in Russia's political system. Prior to his duty as governor, Furgal served as a member of the Legislative Duma of the Khabarovsk Krai in 2005–2007 and as a member of the State Duma (representing the LDPR) in 2007–2018 (Rosbalt 2020). Thus, unlike many other popular opposition political figures in Russia, Furgal was not a representative of an anti-governmental opposition organisation and did not come from the fringes of the Russian political system.

The Furgal protests started on 11 July 2020, and there were still protest events related to the case in September 2021. However, the protest peak was most prominent in the Summer of 2020 and lasted about 1 month; already in August 2020, there were signs of declining interest in protests (Komarov 2020).

Protest in Support of Alexei Navalny

Alexei Navalny is arguably the most well-known Russian opposition politician in Russia and internationally. He had been challenging the Kremlin by running for office at different administrative levels in Russia and by heavily criticising the Russian political system on various social media platforms. Navalny is widely known for his investigatory videos on political corruption in Russia, posted on his YouTube channel (Naval'nyy 2022; Dollbaum, Lallouet, and Noble 2021; Rogov 2021a, 84).

In August 2020, Navalny was poisoned with a Novichok nerve agent during a flight from Tomsk to Moscow and was evacuated to a hospital in Berlin later in September 2020 (BBC News 2020; The Moscow Times 2020). On 17 January 2021, he returned to Russia and was immediately arrested at passport control. The day after, Navalny called his supporters to go to the streets and support him. On 19 January 2021, in turn, the Navalny team's investigative film 'A Palace for Putin' was released. Many famous people spoke out in defence of the oppositionist and calls for protest actions began to spread on social networks (Meduza 2021). Soon after, thousands of people went to the streets to show support for the detained opposition politician and to protest against Putin's rule (Goryashko and Zotova 2021; Roth 2021). It is also noteworthy that these protests took place amidst COVID-19 and the so-called 'political coma' that the quarantine year of 2020 caused in Russia (Arkhipova, Zakharov, and Kozlova 2021, 31).

The Navalny protests started on 23 January 2021 and lasted a little over 2 months. On 21 April 2021, there were still protests related to the Navalny case in 109 cities across Russia. According to conservative estimates, in 15 of these cities more than 1,000 people participated in these protests (MBKH 2021). After this, mass protests related to the case declined.

The Kremlin's Response to COVID-19 and Political Protests in Russia

As mentioned at the beginning of the chapter, there were realistic worries that social control of political leaders over the citizens would increase with COVID-19 social distancing measures (Lamberova and Sonin 2022). Another concern with restrictions akin to social distancing measures is that such restrictions would stay in use even after they would not be needed or when they would still have little effect from an epidemiological point of view (Gebrekidan 2020). In Russia, the Kremlin's response to the pandemic was that President Putin delegated responsibility for handling the crisis to regional authorities (Lamberova and Sonin 2022, 6). This decision seems like a rational response at first sight as regional authorities may be considered likely to have a better picture of the local COVID-19 situation than the Kremlin. In relation, it is likely that rather than showing confidence in regional governors, Putin wanted to shift the blame from himself to regional leaders in case of the pandemic was unsuccessfully managed (Åslund 2020; King 2020).

In theory, regional administrations were supposed to be accountable for monitoring social distancing policies and public gatherings in Russia during the COVID-19 crisis. Yet, there is evidence suggesting that social distancing policies and other COVID-19 policies related to mass gatherings were politically motivated rather than based on preventing the spread of COVID-19. For example, regarding restrictions on freedom of assembly during COVID-19, several laws restricting civil rights and freedoms were passed at once by the State Duma in December 2020. A State Duma deputy Dmitry Vyatkin proposed six pieces of legislation, the so-called Vyatkin package, that provided stricter legislation for Federal Law on how rallies could be organised and proposed changes to the Code of Administrative Offences as well as to the Criminal Code. Changes to the Federal Law on rallies from the Vyatkin package included banning foreign and anonymous funding of public events, obliging organisers of rallies to change the location of rallies when proposed by the authorities, obliging journalists to wear press badges, prohibiting journalists from wearing masks during public events, extending the time period for authorities to offer a response to proposed public events, banning rallies close to buildings of the 'emergency response services' (including the police and the FSB), limiting agitation for participation in a public event, and offering courts discretion to recognise solo demonstrations or picket lines as unauthorised public events after the fact (OVD-Info 2022b).

Changes to the Code of Administrative Offences from the Vyatkin package, in turn, included an introduction of the right to prosecute journalists for the illegitimate wearing of press badges under Article 212.1 of the Criminal Code ('Law on Mass Riots'). In case of repeated violations, liability can be assigned to the rallies' organisers and donors for violating regulations regarding the prohibition of foreign and anonymous funding of rallies. Harder punishments can also be applied under articles 19.3 ('Law on Failure to Follow Lawful Order of The Authorities') and 20.2 ('Law on Violations in Organising Public Gatherings') of the Code of Administrative Offences on the defiance of a police officer's legitimate order and on the violation of rules for holding a public event (Code of Administrative Offences 2022; Criminal Code 2022; OVD-Info 2022b).

Finally, changes to the Criminal Code introduced by Vyatkin included amendments to Article 267 ('Law on Putting Out of Commission Transport Vehicles or Communications'), which provide liability for deliberate transport blocking, if these acts create a threat to the life, health, and safety of citizens, or threaten destruction or damage to property of natural and/or legal persons (Criminal Code 2022; OVD-Info 2022a,b). The watchdog organisation OVD-Info raised concerns that with the new amendments, the arbitrary use of criminal liability is possible even for formal violations that may not result in severe negative consequences. Moreover, Article 213 of the Criminal Code ('Law on Hooliganism') was amended in a way that allows application of this article in the case of a gross violation of public order 'with the use or threat of violence against citizens'. As 'threat of violence' is a very broad and ambiguous term, there were concerns that this article could be applied arbitrarily in various situations, whether the 'threat of violence' is actual or not. In addition, the second part of 'Law on Hooliganism' was extended also to the actions of a 'group of persons' including unorganised groups and groups with no previous concert (ibid.).

Arguably the most well-known example of the application of epidemiological legislation is the so-called 'sanitary case' (*sanitarnoe delo*), a legal action against ten opposition politicians and dissidents in the aftermath of January 2021 protests in support of imprisoned opposition politician Alexei Navalny. In this legal case, Russian authorities accused the Navalny support protesters of violating legislation on assemblies and pandemic distancing rules. Soon after these protests, the Moscow police opened criminal proceedings in connection with an alleged crime for 'violating sanitary and epidemiological rules' (Article 236.1 of the Criminal Code, violation of this Criminal Code carries a penalty of up to 2 years of imprisonment). According to Amnesty International (2021), the Moscow police, the Investigative Committee of Russia, and the Office of the Prosecutor General claimed that protesters 'did not keep social distance or wear masks' and that the outbreak of COVID-19 was averted due to 'coordinated actions of law enforcement personnel that prevented close contact between present citizens'. The criminal investigation of the 'Sanitary Case' also concluded that by publishing social media posts calling for public protests, the individuals in question 'committed incitement' to crime under Article 236.1 of the Criminal Code (ibid.). Officials also claimed that these social media posts resulted in the protest participation of 19 people who were legally required to self-isolate because of positive COVID-19 tests in Moscow, thus putting at risk others who attended (Kramer 2021).

Besides the 'sanitary case', there were later examples of targeted COVID-19 restrictions against opposition politicians. In June–July 2021, UEFA European Football Championship games were played in 11 countries, with one of the host countries being Russia. Before the games began, there were concerns that the Delta-variant of COVID-19, which was detected in Russia, would spread to other countries when football tourists returned home – a scenario that eventually occurred (Teivainen 2021). Despite these worries, the football games were organised as planned in St. Petersburg, while all oppositional protests were banned (Durnovo et al. 2021, 112). Moreover, quarantine measures are suspected to have been imposed at least partly as a strategy to limit civic activities in Russia (Luhn 2020; Laruelle et al. 2021, 6). Indeed, in July 2021, the head of Navalny's campaign team in Murmansk, Violetta Grudina, was hospitalised in a COVID-19 ward at the decision of the Murmansk district court at health authorities' request due to an alleged COVID-19 infection, although she recently received a negative COVID-19 test from a clinic certified by the same authorities (The Barents Observer 2021). Grudina herself cited that the reasons behind this forced hospitalisation were completely political since the ruling party United Russia was afraid to lose its supermajority in the State Duma in the 2021 elections in September. She also called herself the first 'medical prisoner' in history (Collinson 2021). Indeed, quarantine measures are suspected to have been imposed at least partly as a strategy to limit civic activities in Russia (Luhn 2020; Laruelle et al. 2021, 6).

Russia also promoted the implementation of facial recognition in Moscow at the beginning of the crisis. Although this system was later strained under the growing crisis and the Moscow authorities abandoned it in favour of a low-tech 'social monitoring' application (Laruelle et al. 2021, 6), this is yet another example of how the Russian authorities used the pandemic to tighten their grip on the population.

Natalia Lamberova and Konstantin Sonin (2022), in turn, establish that the Russian authorities often underreport deaths from COVID-19 and arrest political activists due to political motives. They also show that repression complements propaganda, as the number of arrests increased the extent of information manipulation. Lamberova and Sonin demonstrate that the political composition of regional parliaments has been connected to repressive measures of the Russian authorities during the COVID-19 crisis, as a larger share of seats held by United Russia in regional parliaments is linked with a higher probability to ban public meetings (ibid.). They argue that especially Article 6.3 of the Administrative Code of Russian Federation ('Violation of the Law in the Area of Securing the Sanitary-and-Epidemiological Well-Being of the Population', see Code of Administrative Offences 2022) was extensively used to repress political protests.

But how did the repressive measures described above reflect on the Russian authorities' response to political protest during COVID-19 in light of legislative measures? Did Russian authorities instrumentalise legislation to curb political protests during COVID-19? My research here indicates that the answer is yes. However, before moving to actual analysis, the data and methods of this research are presented in the next section.

Data and Methods

The primary data for my examination come from the Russian non-governmental organisation (NGO) OVD-Info. This NGO monitors the abuse of legal power in Russia and has been operating since 2011. OVD-Info runs a round-the-clock hotline where people can report when they consider they have been mistreated by officials. The organisation also offers legal assistance and juridical services, publishes reports, and conducts investigative legal projects focusing on the abuse of power. This chapter focuses on stories published on OVD-Info's webpage section ('Express News' henceforth: News Section). To compare how Russian COVID-19 policies relate to mass protests and gatherings, I used the time-series data from the COVID-19 stringency index of the Oxford COVID-19 Government Response Tracker (Hale et al. 2021).

In OVD-Info's News Section, the NGO gathers stories and news about the misuse of power in Russia (OVD-Info 2022a). Technically, articles in the News Section consist of a header, time and place of the event, and text (the actual story/news). Additionally, OVD-Info reports which paragraphs of Russian laws are related to these stories. They also give tags and specific themes to each News Section item. Table 5.1 exemplifies the contents included in OVD-Info's news coverage. Although these data do not offer a complete and all-encompassing picture of how the Russian establishment reacted to mass protests during the pandemic, they serve as a robust indicator of pandemic politics related to oppositional mass gatherings in Russia during COVID-19. For example, these data indicate which legislative measures have been used and/or were relevant at different points in time to related mass protests. Accordingly, we can use these data to examine the quantitative and

Table 5.1 Example case from the dataset (OVD-Info 2021)

Header	*In St. Petersburg, the police detained an activist due to a picket*
Time	01.06.2021, 13:39
Place	St. Petersburg
Text	In St. Petersburg, the police detained Ekaterina Mistryukova due to a picket held near the metro station 'Yelizarovskaya' on 25 May supporting Roman Protasevich and Sofia Sapega, who was arrested in Belarus. She informed OVD-Info about this herself. Now the activist is being taken to police station No. 10. Evgeny Kheifits, a lawyer from OVD-Info, came to assist her. 17:57 A protocol was drawn up against the detainee under the article on organising an uncoordinated rally (part 2 of article 20.2 of the Code of Administrative Offences), the picketer and the lawyer from OVD-Info are waiting for a court decision on the protocol. • On May 31, Moscow police detained an activist who walked out with a poster in support of Sofia Sapega to the building of the Ministry of Foreign Affairs. She was released with a promise to appear. • On May 23, the plane on which Belarusian journalist and former editor-in-chief of the NEXTA Telegram channel Roman Protasevich flew to Vilnius made an emergency landing in Minsk at the request of the Belarusian authorities; together with Protasevich, they detained his girlfriend, Russian Sofia Sapega. Criminal cases were opened against both, allegedly for organising mass riots. The international community imposes various sanctions against Belarus.
Paragraphs	Part 2 of the Article 20.2 of Code of the Russian Federation on Administrative Offences
Tags	Detention, picket, police department
Themes	Freedom of assembly

qualitative differences in legal response to the Furgal and Navalny protests. In other words, how often and what kind of legislation was applied to stunt these protests.

The primary research data used here consist of 14 variables and 9,188 observations (the full list of variables is available in Appendix 1). The raw version of my secondary research data, that is, the data for the COVID-19 stringency index of the Oxford COVID-19 Government Response Tracker, consists of 906 variables and 187 observations. However, after filtering for the Russian Federation COVID-19 stringency data, the data consist of three variables: country name, date, and stringency index.

The COVID-19 stringency index subset data for Russia used here cover the period from 1 January 2020 to 21 June 2022 and reports the overall stringency index for the COVID-19 restrictions in Russia ranging from 0 to 100, where 0 = 'Least stringent' and 100 = 'Most stringent'. This index is calculated based on information about school, public transport, and workplace closings, as well as cancellations of public events, restrictions on public gatherings, requirements to stay home, restrictions on internal movement, international travel controls, and public information campaigns (for details, see Hale et al. 2021; OxCGRT 2022). Like the OVD-Info News Section data, the COVID-19 response tracker is a rough estimator of COVID-19 restrictions in Russia during 2020–2021. However, since this index consists almost entirely of social distancing measures, it serves as a robust indicator of fluctuations in social distancing policies during the period of interest.

Analysis

To answer my research question on how the Russian authorities deployed COVID-19 policies to curb political protest movements related to the Sergei Furgal and Alexei Navalny protests, I use the means of descriptive statistics. At the beginning of my study, I separated the legal clauses from each other so that only the 'parent law' is present in the final examination. For example, if the OVD-Info News' story contained the following legal paragraphs: 'Paragraphs: part 1 of the Criminal Code 282.2, part 2 of the Criminal Code 282.2' ('Law on Organising Extremist Organization'), I removed the parts 'Paragraphs: part 1' and 'part 2', and separated this row into two identical rows containing only the text '282.2 of the Criminal Code'. This way I could find out what type of legal measures were mentioned most often during COVID-19 according to OVD-Info.

Figure 5.2 offers an overview of the most frequently mentioned legal paragraphs in OVD-Info's News Section during 2020–2021. Interestingly, the most often mentioned paragraphs are related to mass gatherings and protests. For example, 20.2 Administrative Code, which is the most often mentioned clause, refers to the 'Law on Violation of the Established Procedure for Organising or Holding a Meeting, Rally, Demonstration, Procession or Picketing'. 282.2 Criminal Code, in turn, is a 'Law on Organising the

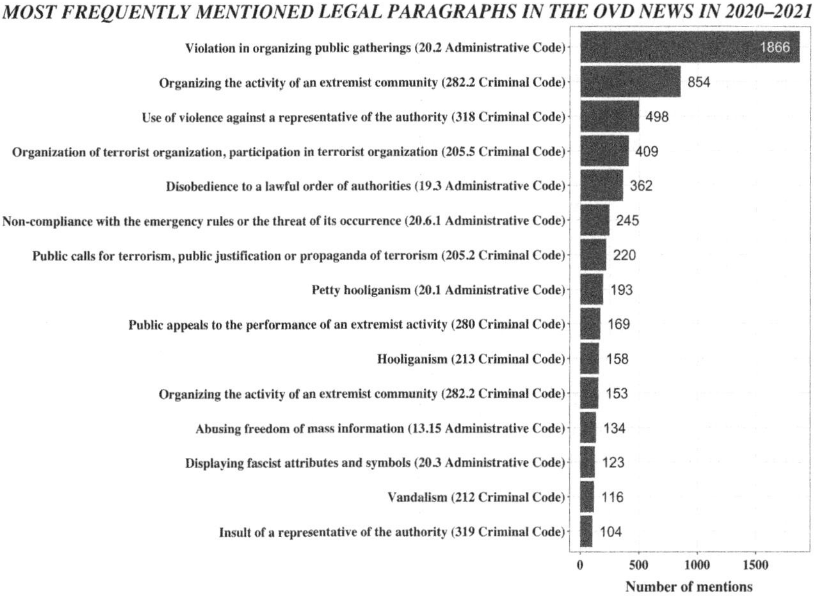

Figure 5.2 Most frequently mentioned legal paragraphs in the OVD-Info News Section during 2020–2021.

Source: Author's creation

Activities of an Extremist Organization', and 318 Criminal Code refers to 'Use of Violence Against a Representative of Authority'. Overall, legal paragraphs on mass protests, resisting the authorities, and terrorism/extremism seem to dominate OVD-Info's News Section data during 2020–2021.

Nine out of the 15 most frequently mentioned legal paragraphs in the OVD-Info data represent criminal legislation, which generally consists of harsher punishments compared to administrative offences. For example, violations of 20.2 Administrative Code may result in a fine or minor administrative arrest, whereas violating the 'Law on Organising Extremist Community' or section 282.2 of the Criminal Code could result in 3 years in prison (Criminal Code 2022). Moreover, laws that were amended by the so-called Vyatkin package introduced earlier in this chapter also often occurred in the most frequently mentioned legal paragraphs in OVD-Info's News Section. For example, 20.2 and 19.3 of the Administrative Code hold the first and fifth place in overall mentions of legal paragraphs in 2020–2021. These observations are in line with the concerns of legal experts about the increasingly arbitrary use of legal charges amended within the framework of the Vyatkin package (Amnesty International 2020; OVD-Info 2022b). The 'Law on Hooliganism', or 213 of the Criminal Code, which was part of the Vyatkin package, is also mentioned frequently in the OVD-Info News Section. To recap, this law was amended so that instead of including only 'gross violations of public order', it also includes 'a threat' of such violations and the definition of 'group of persons' engaging in hooliganism was broadened to include any group of citizens violating public order. The maximum punishment for 'hooliganism' is up to 7 years in prison, which indicates the severity of this law.

To find out which kind of themes occurred most often in the OVD-Info News Section during 2020–2021, a similar data manipulation process was conducted with the 'tags' variable, as with the legal paragraphs mentioned above. Figure 5.3 depicts 15 of the most used tags. Again, many frequently used tags relate to mass gatherings, political protests, and extremism. Interestingly, both Alexei Navalny and Sergei Furgal are also frequently used as tags. This is significant because the actual number of tags related to their support protests might be even larger, as such frequently mentioned tags as 'extremist organisation' (Navalny) and 'governor' (Furgal) are likely to be linked to them as well. The 'coronavirus' tag also appears often. Taken together, these observations give further grounds to narrow the examination of political protests related to Furgal and Navalny.

There were still over 262 unique legal paragraphs after the above-mentioned data manipulation process, where the legal paragraphs were separated to include the 'parent laws' only. Hence, further reduction of the dimensions of data selection was undertaken to make more mutually exclusive categorisations for the separate laws to see what kind of legislative measures were used

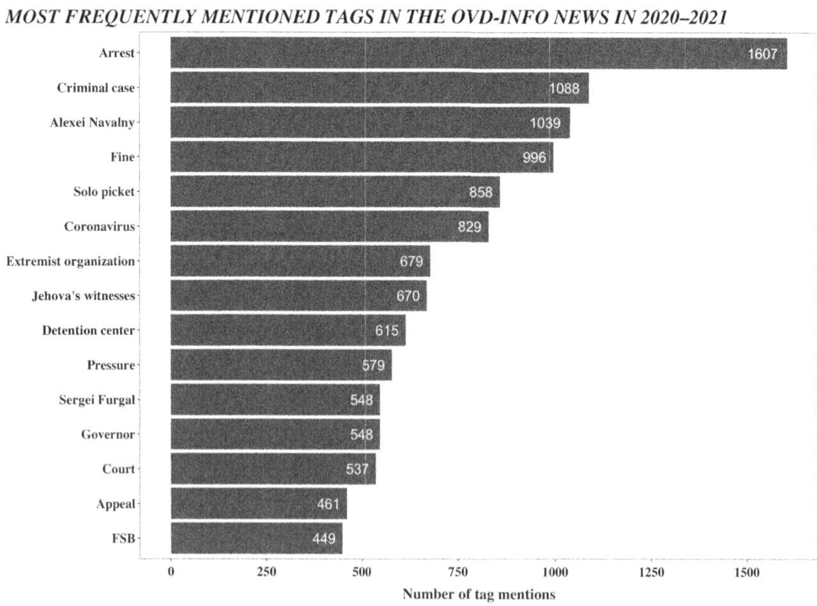

Figure 5.3 Most frequently mentioned tags in the OVD-Info News Section during 2020–2021.

Source: Author's creation

most often at different times during 2020–2021 in Russia. This was done by categorising the laws cited based on the legal paragraphs they represent. As a result, 13 different types of legal charges were detected:

1. Terrorism/extremism
2. Public gatherings
3. Resisting authorities
4. Freedom of speech-related laws (or abusing freedom of speech)
5. Violence
6. Pandemic distancing
7. Foreign agent/undesired organisation
8. Charges of treason
9. Other
10. Drug crimes
11. Migration violations
12. Abuse of power
13. Electoral malpractice (or election laws)

In the following section, the different responses from the Russian authorities to protests for Furgal and Navalny are examined more closely.

How Did Russian Authorities Instrumentalised COVID-19 Restrictions to Respond to Political Protest?

To answer the question of whether the Russian authorities responded similarly to the Furgal protests and Navalny protests, I examined the Furgal and Navalny-related OVD-Info News Section data from 2020 to 2021 and observe which legal categories were mentioned most frequently. This was done by only analysing news containing tags that refer to Sergei Furgal or Alexei Navalny. The lemmatised keywords 'furgal' and 'khaba' were used for Sergei Furgal and 'naval' for Alexei Navalny to include only news related to these events. After filtering, there were altogether 13 unique news tags to be included in my examination (see Appendix 2 for details).

Figure 5.4 depicts the quantity of most frequently mentioned legal charges for Furgal and Navalny-related news. As we can see from the figure, Navalny-related legal charge mentions exceed the number of Furgal-related mentions. Besides quantitative differences, there was also a clear qualitative difference between the legal paragraphs mentioned. Seven out of the 15 most frequently mentioned legal paragraphs with Furgal are administrative offences, whereas the same number with Navalny is only four. That is, legal paragraphs mentioned with Navalny tags are more often from criminal legislation, where punishments are as a rule harsher compared to administrative offence violations.

Moreover, all the laws amended by the Vyatkin package – 20.2 and 19.3 of the Administrative Code, 267 and 213 of the Criminal Code – are present in

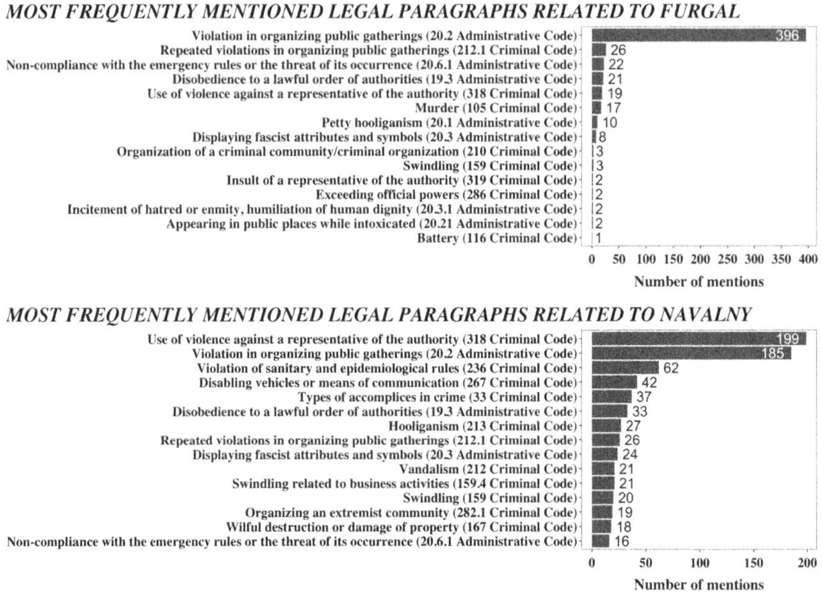

Figure 5.4 Most frequently mentioned legal paragraphs related to Sergei Furgal and Alexei Navalny.

Source: Author's creation

the most frequently mentioned legal paragraphs associated with the Navalny tags. However, the administrative offences amended by the Vyatkin package (20.2 and 19.3 of the Administrative Code) are most often mentioned with the Furgal-related OVD-Info News Section items. Based on this evidence, it seems that the major legislative restrictions related to freedom of assembly introduced during the COVID-19 pandemic have been largely instrumentalised and targeted against certain political actors in Russia. In addition, some criminal legislation-related legal paragraphs related to Furgal are likely to be rather connected to Furgal himself, than to those protesting against his imprisonment. For example, all the mentions of sections 105 (Murder) and 159 of the Criminal Code (Swindling), dealing with murder and business fraud prosecutions, are in reference to Furgal personally, and not against protesters. Lastly, the law on violating sanitary and epidemiological rules (section 230 of the Criminal Code) is mentioned only in relation to Navalny-related news, but it is virtually absent from news dealing with Furgal.

Similar differences are present when legal charge mentions are examined through a more qualitative lens. Figure 5.5 shows the share of legal paragraph mentions with Furgal and Navalny by types of legal charges.

The share of the differences in the volume of legal charges between Furgal and Navalny is likely explained by the size of these protests. For instance, according to some estimates, the biggest Navalny protests gathered

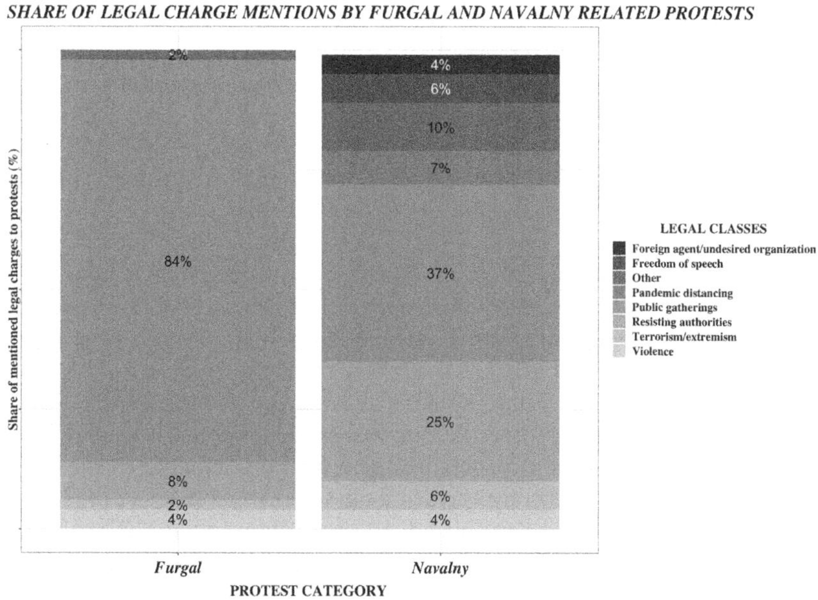

Figure 5.5 Share of legal charge mentions related to Sergei Furgal and Alexei Navalny.
Source: Author's creation

approximately 140,000 participants, while the largest Furgal protests gathered approximately 47,500 participants (Rogov and Shukyurov 2021). These figures exemplify how Navalny protests were a nationwide movement, whereas Furgal protests were more centralised in Khabarovsk Krai and the Russian Far East. Still, based on the data used here, it seems that the Russian authorities responded more strictly to the Navalny protests compared to the Furgal protests. For example, looking at the relative share of different legal categories applied to these protests reveals that Furgal supporters were accused mainly of violating laws on public gatherings, while Navalny supporters were accused also of engaging in terrorism/extremism, resisting public authorities, violating pandemic distancing rules and laws on freedom of speech, and functioning as foreign agents. Therefore, participation in pro-opposition protests supporting Navalny was riskier compared to the Furgal case since most of the terrorism/extremism legal charges present in the data belong to the Criminal Code of Russia, while the majority of public gathering legal charges belong to the Code of the Russian Federation on Administrative offences. The maximum punishment for the former, in turn, is on average much more severe than the latter. For instance, criminal legislation linked to Navalny and terrorism/extremism in the OVD-Info News Section included paragraphs:

- 282.1 (Organising an Extremist Community),
- 280 (Public Appeals to the Performance of an Extremist Activity),

- 205.2 (Public Calls for Terrorist Activities, Public Justification of Terrorism or Propaganda of Terrorism),
- 207 (Knowingly Making a False Communication About an Act of Terrorism),
- 283.3 (Financing Extremist Action), and
- 355 (The Development, Manufacture, Stockpiling, Acquisition or Sale of Mass-Destruction Weapons) of the Criminal Code.

The maximum punishment for the above-mentioned legal breaches is multiple years in prison. Thus, their deterrence effect is also likely to be stronger compared to minor administrative offences more often linked to the protests that were in support of Furgal.

Another factor that could explain the harsher response to the Navalny support protests compared to the Furgal support protests is that the latter may have come more as a surprise to the Kremlin compared to the former. For instance, prior to Navalny's return from Germany to Russia, the Kremlin announced that it would be 'obliged' to detain him in case he returned to Russia (The Moscow Times 2021). Navalny and his team, in turn, agitated for protest in their 'Putin's Palace' video, where Navalny's investigative team revealed the secret luxury life of Putin (BBC News 2021). As mentioned previously, Furgal was an insider of the official political system and therefore the public outcry related to his imprisonment might have been a surprise to the Kremlin. Moreover, since the Furgal support protests took place before Navalny's, the Russian authorities might have co-opted new ways for dealing with oppositional protests during COVID-19. For example, the legal reforms of the Vyatkin package were introduced in late 2020, only a bit before the Navalny support protests took place. Therefore, it is possible that they also reflect the Russian authorities' overall reaction to the Furgal protests, although answering this question is outside of the scope of this chapter.

Polls on Furgal and Navalny protests indicate that Russians sympathised significantly more with participants of the Furgal protests compared to participants of the Navalny protests. According to the Levada-tsentr (2021), almost 50% of Russians had a positive attitude towards the participants of the Furgal protests, while only approximately one-fifth of the respondents related positively to participants of the Navalny protests. Also, the share of respondents having a negative attitude towards the Navalny protesters is more than twice as large compared to the Furgal protesters. These results may indicate that expressing supportive views towards the Navalny protests was socially riskier than supporting the Furgal protests. On the other hand, greater negative public perceptions towards the Navalny protests might have given the Kremlin more political leeway in punishing the participants of these protests compared to the Furgal protests. In other words, punishing participants of the Navalny protests might have been politically less costly for the Kremlin's popular support in Russia than punishing Furgal protesters.

Yet, what if Navalny supporters were breaking the law more frequently and severely compared to Furgal protesters? Could non-political aspects related to these protest events, such as the pandemic situation, play a more decisive role in the Russian government's response to these protests than politics of repression? The existing evidence suggests that this is hardly the case. Figure 5.6 shows how these protest events relate to pandemic restrictions in Russia. As the figure illustrates, the overall COVID-19 restriction stringency index was a lot higher in July 2020, when the largest Furgal protests took place compared to January–April 2021, when the Navalny protests took place. In fact, the value of the stringency index was below the pandemic mean for most of the time during the Navalny protests, while it was at a high level during the Furgal protests. Yet, there are virtually no legal charges for violating pandemic distancing rules with Furgal protests, whereas Navalny protesters faced legal charges for violating the pandemic distancing legislation regardless of the pandemic situation. Lastly, the Pearson correlation between the COVID-19 stringency index and the legal paragraph mentions dealing with pandemic distancing and public gatherings is low, 0,19.

Besides the data represented in Figure 5.6, there is additional evidence suggesting that the actual pandemic situation and public health were hardly

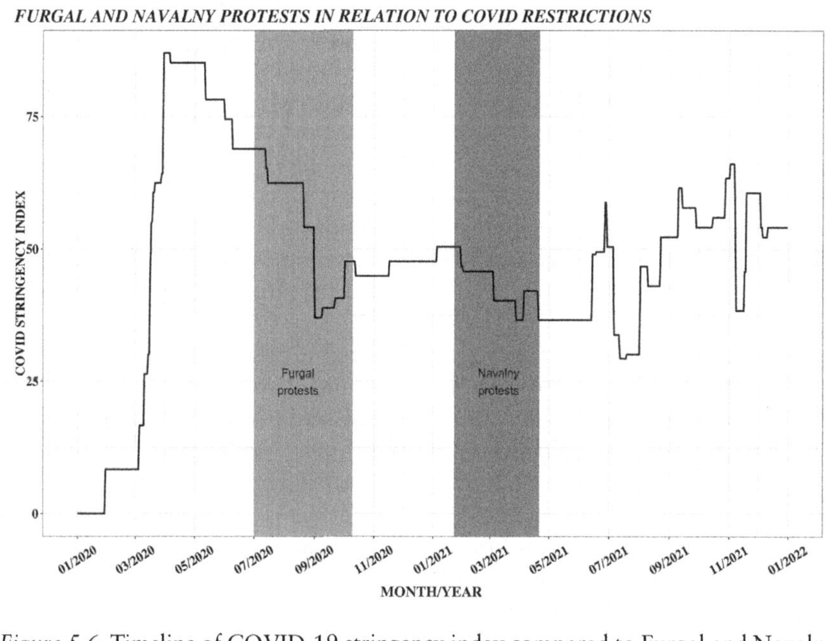

Figure 5.6 Timeline of COVID-19 stringency index compared to Furgal and Navalny protests.

Source: Author's creation

decisive factors regarding the response of Russian authorities to protests. For instance, official COVID-19 statistics indicate that the pandemic situation in Khabarovsk Krai was worse at the beginning of July 2020 compared to many other areas in Russia. According to the Rospotrebnadzor (The Federal Service for the Oversight of Consumer Protection and Welfare), the average daily growth rate of COVID-19 infections in Khabarovsk Krai was 1,9%, while in the rest of Russia it is only 1,1%. Moreover, Furgal himself demanded stricter social distancing measures and punishments for violating these measures at the beginning of July 2020 before his arrest (Kokurin 2020a). Accordingly, after Furgal's arrest on 9 July 2020, the vice chairman on social issues of Khabarovsk Krai, Yuri Minaev, pleaded a day before the Furgal support protests that the residents of the Krai should refrain from public gatherings to prevent the spread of the pandemic (Kokurin 2020b). Yet, the Furgal protesters did not face charges for breaking pandemic distancing rules according to the data presented here.

Discussion

The evidence presented in this article suggests that the pandemic restrictions have been widely targeted and used as a political weapon during the COVID-19 pandemic in Russia. This is showcased by what kind of legal consequences and/or threats the participants of two major COVID-19 era oppositional protest movements, the Furgal protests and the Navalny protests, faced after they participated in these movements. But why were the Kremlin's responses to these protests so asymmetric?

One obvious answer is the scale of these protests. Although the Furgal protests brought, relatively speaking, a large number of the Khabarovsk Krai citizens to the streets, they were still more regional compared to the Navalny protests. As noted at the beginning of this chapter, the 2021 Navalny protests are cited as one the biggest anti-Kremlin protest movement in the history of post-Soviet Russia. Moreover, it is estimated that they gathered participants in over 100 Russian cities (Rogov 2021b).

A second important factor contributing to the Russian authorities' response to these two political protests is linked to what kind of political characters Furgal and Navalny are. As mentioned earlier in the chapter, Furgal was a 'systemic' politician with a long career in the official political system of Russia, whereas Navalny was operating largely outside the official political framework and on social media platforms. Thus, Furgal became a 'black sheep' for the Kremlin only after he beat United Russia's candidate in the 2018 regional elections (Rosbalt 2020). Navalny, in turn, had been a *persona non grata* to the Kremlin for years already due to his anti-corruption disclosure videos and the oppositional network he and his team built over the years. The Navalny team's disclosure video 'Putin's palace' likely affected Putin's political reputation at least with some Russians.

Another relevant factor in the differing responses from the Russian authorities is the temporal difference between the protests. The Furgal protests started in July 2020, while the Navalny protests began in January 2021. Because of the 6-month time difference between the protest beginnings, the Kremlin had time to update its strategies for responding to oppositional protest movements and learn from the 'mistakes' made in their response to the Furgal protests. Moreover, although the pandemic had already been ongoing for months in July 2020, in January 2021 Russian authorities were half a year more experienced with pandemic politics and the tools that could be used to target undesirable social movements.

The Furgal and Navalny protests exemplify that large oppositional protest movements can exist also in authoritarian countries. Accordingly, these protests also indicate that people living in authoritarian societies can rise against those in power and speak against politics they dislike, even in times of global pandemic. Yet, from the individual protest participant's perspective, the arbitrariness and asymmetry in the reactions of authorities result in a situation where it is very hard to anticipate the risks of engaging in oppositional political participation.

Although we can obtain a robust overview of the Kremlin's response to COVID-19 era oppositional mass protests by examining the descriptive frequencies of the OVD-Info News Section related to the Furgal and Navalny protests, examination here does not reveal to what extent these legal charges were or were not realised. This is a limitation of this research. To answer this question, future research could examine how well the information available from Russian officials matches OVD-Info's News Section data on the topic. Moreover, a closer examination of the OVD-Info News Section's contents might reveal interesting qualitative differences in the Kremlin's response to these protest movements. Another possible future line of research on the topic would be to interview participants of these protest movements: how did they perceive the response of the Russian authorities to these protests? Are these perceptions in line with the findings of this article?

Evidence presented in this chapter suggests that while anti-governmental political protest is possible in authoritarian countries like Russia, the risks of participating in contentious politics are higher compared to democratic countries. This and the fact that a leading Russian oppositional politician was jailed (Meduza 2022) may partly explain why there have been so few anti-war political protests in Russia after Russia's full-scale attack on Ukraine in February 2022.

Acknowledgements

I would like to extend my sincere thanks to Finnish Foundation for the Support of Strategic Research (STRATU) for funding this research and Aleksandra Rumiantseva for sharing the OVD-Info research data with me.

References

AiF. 2019. “Sergey Furgal: ‘Gosdolg Khabarovskogo kraya budet sokrashchat'sya.’” December 24, 2019. https://hab.aif.ru/money/sergey_furgal_gosdolg_habarovskogo_kraya_budet_sokrashchatsya.

Amnesty International. 2020. “Vladimir Putin podpisal zakony iz ‘paketa Vyatkina’. Kakiye ugrozy sozdayut dlya prava na svobodu sobraniy novyye initsiativy rossiyskikh vlastey, ob"yasnyayet Amnesty International.” December 30, 2020. https://eurasia.amnesty.org/2020/12/30/vladimir-putin-podpisal-zakony-iz-paketa-vyatkina-kakie-ugrozy-sozdayut-dlya-prava-na-svobodu-sobranij-novye-inicziativy-rossijskih-vlastej-obyasnyaet-amnesty-international/.

Amnesty International. 2021. “Russia: Activists Detained under Absurd ‘Sanitary’ Charges for Social Media Posts in Support of Public Protest.” April 23, 2021. https://www.amnesty.org/en/documents/eur46/4027/2021/en/.

Arkhipova, Aleksandra, Aleksey Zakharov, and Irina Kozlova. 2021. “Protestnaya Mobilizatsiya – 2021: Kto Vyshel Na Mitingi i Pochemu.” In *God Naval'nogo – Politika Protesta v Rossii 2020–2021: Strategii, Mekhanizmy i Posledstviya*, edited by Kirill Rogov, 31–55. Liberal'naya missiya — Ekspertiza. Vypusk 14. Moskva: FOND “LIBERAL'NAYA MISSIYA.”

Åslund, Anders. 2020. “Responses to the COVID-19 Crisis in Russia, Ukraine, and Belarus.” *Eurasian Geography and Economics* 61, no. 4–5: 532–545. https://doi.org/10.1080/15387216.2020.1778499.

BBC News. 2020. “Alexei Navalny: ‘Poisoned’ Russian Opposition Leader in a Coma.” August 20, 2020. https://www.bbc.com/news/world-europe-53844958.

BBC News. 2021. “Alexei Navalny: Millions Watch Jailed Critic’s ‘Putin Palace’ Film.” January 20, 2021. https://www.bbc.com/news/world-europe-55732296.

Code of Administrative Offences. 2022. “Code of Administrative Offences of the Russian Federation No. 195-FZ of December 30, 2001.” https://www.wto.org/english/thewto_e/acc_e/rus_e/wtaccrus58_leg_63.pdf.

Collinson, Sarah, dir. 2021. *Fearless: The Women Fighting Putin*. Documentary. Hardcash Productions.

Coppedge, Michael, John Gerring, Carl Henrik Knutsen, Staffan I. Lindberg, Jan Teorell, Nazifa Alizada, David Altman, et al. 2022. “V-Dem [Country–Year/Country–Date] Dataset V12.” Varieties of Democracy (V-Dem) Project. March 12, 2021 https://doi.org/10.2139/ssrn.3802627.

Criminal Code. 2022. “The Criminal Code of the Russian Federation No. 63-FZ of June 13, 1996.” https://www.wto.org/english/thewto_e/acc_e/rus_e/wtaccrus58_leg_63.pdf.

Diamond, Larry. 2020. “Democracy Versus the Pandemic,” August 24, 2020. https://www.foreignaffairs.com/articles/world/2020-06-13/democracy-versus-pandemic.

Dollbaum, Jan Matti, Morvan Lallouet, and Ben Noble. 2021. *Navalny: Putin’s Nemesis, Russia’s Future*. London: Hurst Publishers.

Durnovo, Grigoriy, Ivan Kas’yanenko, Grigoriy Okhotin, Nataliya Smirnova, Denis Shedov, and Tat’yana Uskova. 2021. “Repressii i Repressivnyye Tekhnologii -2021: Ot Sderzhivaniya k Unichtozheniyu.” In *God Naval'nogo – Politika Protesta v Rossii 2020–2021: Strategii, Mekhanizmy i Posledstviya*, edited by Kirill Rogov, 96–120. Liberal'naya missiya — Ekspertiza. Vypusk 14. Moskva: FOND “LIBERAL'NAYA MISSIYA.”

DVHAB.RU. 2018. "Furgal Sokratil Pensii Chinovnikam Khabarovskogo Kraya — Novosti Khabarovska." December 19, 2018. https://www.dvnovosti.ru/khab/2018/12/19/92654/.

Gardner, Yuliya. 2019. "Ekonomnoye nebo (AviaPort)." AviaPort.Ru. March 14, 2019. https://www.aviaport.ru/digest/2019/03/14/579763.html.

Gebrekidan, Selam. 2020. "For Autocrats, and Others, Coronavirus Is a Chance to Grab Even More Power." *The New York Times*, March 30, 2020. https://www.nytimes.com/2020/03/30/world/europe/coronavirus-governments-power.html.

Goryashko, Sergey, and Nataliya Zotova. 2021. "Den′ vserossiyskogo protesta: kak proshli aktsii v podderzhku Naval′nogo – Novosti na russkom yazyke." *BBC News Russkaya sluzhba*. January 23, 2021. https://www.bbc.com/russian/live/news-55779010.

Hale, Thomas, Noam Angrist, Rafael Goldszmidt, Beatriz Kira, Anna Petherick, Toby Phillips, Samuel Webster, et al. 2021. "A Global Panel Database of Pandemic Policies (Oxford COVID-19 Government Response Tracker)." *Nature Human Behaviour* 5, no. 4: 529–538. https://doi.org/10.1038/s41562-021-01079-8.

King, Kelsey. 2020. "Pandemic and Protests: Key Drivers of Russia's Increased Threat Perception." September 24, 2020. https://www.csis.org/blogs/post-soviet-post/pandemic-and-protests-key-drivers-russias-increased-threat-perception.

Kokurin, Boris. 2020a. "V Khabarovskom kraye gubernator potreboval ser′yezno uzhestochit′ nakazaniya dlya narushiteley protivoepidemicheskikh mer." hab.kp.ru. July 3, 2020. https://www.hab.kp.ru/daily/27151.5/4246882/.

Kokurin, Boris. 2020b. "Situatsiya s koronavirusom v Khabarovskom kraye: yesli rost zabolevayemosti prodolzhitsya, nam snova pridetsya sest′ na karantin." hab.kp.ru. July 10, 2020. https://www.hab.kp.ru/daily/27154.5/4250775/.

Komarov, Dmitriy. 2020. "Za Mesyats Interes k Khabarovskim Protestam i Delu Furgala Upal Pochti v Pyat′ Raz." September 22, 2020. https://web.archive.org/web/20200922113619/https://www.znak.com/2020-08-27/za_mesyac_interes_k_habarovskim_protestam_i_delu_furgala_upal_pochti_v_pyat_raz.

Kramer, Andrew E. 2021. "In Russia, a Virus Lockdown Targets the Opposition." *The New York Times*, March 19, 2021. https://www.nytimes.com/2021/03/19/world/europe/russia-covid-opposition.html.

Lamberova, Natalia, and Konstantin Sonin. 2022. "Information Manipulation and Repression: A Theory and Evidence from the COVID Response in Russia." *SSRN Scholarly Paper*. July 29, 2022. Rochester, NY. https://doi.org/10.2139/ssrn.4174501.

Laruelle, Marlene, Mikhail Alexseev, Cynthia Buckley, Ralph S. Clem, J. Paul Goode, Ivan Gomza, Henry E. Hale, et al. 2021. "Pandemic Politics in Eurasia: Roadmap for a New Research Subfield." *Problems of Post-Communism* 68, no. 1: 1–16. https://doi.org/10.1080/10758216.2020.1812404.

Levada-tsentr. 2021. "Sluga naroda: Kak Sergei Furgal popal v chislo podhodyaschikh dlya rossiyan kandidativ v prezidenty." https://www.levada.ru/2020/08/07/sluga-naroda-kak-sergej-furgal-popal-v-chislo-podhodyashhih-dlya-rossiyan-kandidatov-v-prezidenty/.

Levada-tsentr. 2022. "Odobreniye organov vlasti." 2022. https://www.levada.ru/indikatory/odobrenie-organov-vlasti/.

Lokhov, Petr. 2020. "V Khabarovske proshel samyy massovyy miting v istorii goroda — v zashchitu arestovannogo gubernatora Sergeya Furgala. Glavnoye." Meduza. July 11, 2020. https://meduza.io/feature/2020/07/11/v-habarovskeproshel-samyy-massovyy-miting-v-istorii-goroda-v-zaschitu-arestovannogo-gubernatora-sergeya-furgala-glavnoe.

Luhn, Alec. 2020. "How Coronavirus Helps Putin." POLITICO (blog). March 18, 2020. https://www.politico.eu/article/how-coronavirus-covid19-outbreak-helps-russian-president-vladimir-putin/.

MBKH. 2021. "Na aktsii 21 aprelya vyshli ot 51,3 tysyachi do 120 tysyach chelovek." MBKH media — novosti, teksty, video, podkasty (blog) (blog). April 22, 2021. https://mbk-news.appspot.com/news/naakcii/.

Meduza. 2021. "Aktsii za Naval'nogo. Kak eto bylo Mitingovala vsya Rossiya. Zaderzhany boleye trekh tysyach chelovek (eto rekord). V Moskve proshli stolknoveniya grazhdan i politsii." Meduza. 2021. https://meduza.io/live/2021/01/23/mitingi-v-podderzhku-alekseya-navalnogo-hronika.

Meduza. 2022. "Why Don't Russians March on Moscow? Resisting the Unpopular Draft Requires Coordination, Says the Political Scientist Vladimir Gelman." Meduza. September 27, 2022. https://meduza.io/en/feature/2022/09/27/why-don-t-russians-march-on-moscow.

Naval'nyy, Aleksey. 2022. "Aleksey Naval'nyy - YouTube." 2022. https://www.youtube.com/.

OVD-Info. 2021. "V Peterburge politseyskiye zaderzhali aktivistku iz-za piketa." June 1, 2021. https://ovd.news/express-news/2021/06/01/v-peterburge-policeyskie-zaderzhali-aktivistku-iz-za-piketa.

OVD-Info. 2022a. "Ekspress-novosti." 2022. https://ovd.news/express-news.

OVD-Info. 2022b. "Legislative Restrictions of Freedom of Assembly at the End of 2020." 2022. https://reports.ovdinfo.org/legislative-restrictions-freedom-assembly-end-2020.

OxCGRT. 2022. "Oxford COVID-19 Government Response Tracker." 2022. https://covidtracker.bsg.ox.ac.uk/.

Rogov, Kirill. 2021a. "Delo Naval'nogo: Predposylki, Strategii i Itogi Protivostoyaniya." In *God Naval'nogo – Politika Protesta v Rossii 2020–2021: Strategii, Mekhanizmy i Posledstviya*, edited by Kirill Rogov, 70–95. Liberal'naya missiya — Ekspertiza. Vypusk 14. Moskva: FOND "LIBERAL'NAYA MISSIYA."

Rogov, Kirill, ed. 2021b. *God Naval'nogo – Politika Protesta v Rossii 2020–2021: Strategii, Mekhanizmy i Posledstviya*. Liberal'naya missiya — Ekspertiza. Vypusk 14. Moskva: FOND "LIBERAL'NAYA MISSIYA".

Rogov, Kirill, and Aby Shukyurov. 2021. "Protesty 2021 Goda i Protestnoye Desyatiletiye 2011–2011 Gg. Dinamika i Otsenki Chislennosty." In *God Naval'nogo – Politika Protesta v Rossii 2020–2021: Strategii, Mekhanizmy i Posledstviya*, edited by Kirill Rogov, 56–95. Liberal'naya missiya — Ekspertiza. Vypusk 14. Moskva: FOND "LIBERAL'NAYA MISSIYA."

Rosbalt. 2020. "Politolog: Furgal stal «beloy voronoy» srazu, kak tol'ko vyigral vybory vopreki vole Kremlya." July 9, 2020. https://www.rosbalt.ru/piter/2020/07/09/1852861.html.

Roth, Andrew. 2021. "Tens of Thousands Protest in Russia Calling for Navalny's Release." *The Guardian*, January 23, 2021. https://www.theguardian.com/world/2021/jan/23/alexei-navalny-supporters-join-protests-across-russia.

Snegovaya, Maria, Volkov Denis, and Goncharov Stepan. 2020. "The Coronavirus Could Hit Putin Most of All." *Foreign Policy (blog)*. June 5, 2020. https://foreignpolicy.com/2020/06/05/coronavirus-vladimir-putin-russia/.

TASS. 2020. "V Khabarovske Prokhodit Vtoraya Nesanktsionirovannaya Aktsiya v Podderzhku Sergeya Furgala." July 12, 2020. https://tass.ru/obschestvo/8944761?utm_source=en.wikipedia.org&utm_medium=referral&utm_campaign=en.wikipedia.org&utm_referrer=en.wikipedia.org.

Teivainen, Aleksi. 2021. "Over 200 Infections Linked to Euro 2020 Detected in Finland." *Helsinki Times*. June 28, 2021. https://www.helsinkitimes.fi/finland/finland-news/domestic/19478-over-200-infections-linked-to-euro-2020-detected-in-finland.html.

The Barents Observer. 2021. "Violetta Grudina Faces Court-Approved Forced Hospitalization." *The Independent Barents Observer*. July 15, 2021. https://thebarentsobserver.com/en/democracy-and-media/2021/07/violetta-grudina-faces-court-approved-forced-hospitalization.

The Moscow Times. 2020. "Navalny Taken Off Ventilator as Novichok Recovery Continues – German Hospital." September 14, 2020. https://www.themoscowtimes.com/2020/09/14/navalny-taken-off-ventilator-as-novichok-recovery-continues-german-hospital-a71437.

The Moscow Times. 2021. "Russia Warns 'Obliged' to Detain Kremlin Critic Navalny on Return." January 14, 2021. https://www.themoscowtimes.com/2021/01/14/russia-says-obliged-to-detain-navalny-upon-return-a72611.

Varlamov, dir. 2020. Narodnyy Gubernator: Pochemu Lyudi Polyubili Furgala i Progonyayut Degtyarëva? https://www.youtube.com/watch?v=OKtgwWdZ44g.

Appendix 1

Description of the research data

Variable	*Explanation of the variable*
Index	URL address of news' index
Header	Title of news
Text	Text of news
Publication date	Publication date of news
Region	Region where the news' events took place
Themes	Themes of the OVD-Info News, four distinct categories: 1 System 2 Political pressure 3 Freedom of speech 4 Freedom of assembly
Legal	Legal paragraphs relevant to news
Tags	Tags related to news
Stories	Stories related to news, e.g. "foreign agents", "Alexei Navalny"
Stories URL	URL address of stories
Location	Location of the news' event

Appendix 2

Unique tags related to Furgal and Navalny protests

Furgal tags (English)	*Furgal tags (Russian)*	*Navalny tags (English)*	*Navalny tags (Russian)*
Furgalmobile	Фургаломобиль	Alexei Navalny	алексей навальный
Sergei furgal	сергей фургал	Staff of Navalny	штаб навального
Khabarovsk	Хабаровск	"Freedom to Navalny!"	«свободу навальному!»
		Navalny live	навальный live
		Supporter of Navalny	сторонник навального
		Navalny	навальный
		Action in support of Navalny	акция в поддержку навального
		Oleg Navalny	олег навальный
		Supporters of Navalny	сторонники навального
		Yuliya Navalnaya	юлия навальная
		Actions in support of Navalny	акции в поддержку навального

6 Survival and Adaptation of Small Business in Russia

A Double Blow of Bad Governance and the Pandemic

Diana Kurtametova and Anna Tarasenko

Small Business, Politics and Governance in Russia: Academic Debate and Research Questions

It has been argued that small entrepreneurs and businesses, including small- and medium-sized enterprises (SMEs) in times of prolonged crisis, especially economic crisis, may suffer from downturns because of their limited financial resources (Vargo and Seville 2011). Indeed, the 2020 crisis, triggered by the outbreak of COVID-19 led to a decrease in entrepreneurial and SME activities in the short and long terms. This decrease was explained by the crucial role SMEs play in the creation of innovative products and workplaces, as well as their role in stimulating gross domestic product (GDP) growth in market economies. Despite reasonable expectations about the downsizing of SME activity in Russia under similar circumstances, this research demonstrates the opposite. How does Russia's non-democratic context and bad governance affect the survival of SMEs? The empirical analysis of Russian regions provides us with the opportunity to scrutinise the effect.

Some studies describe the role of investment to support SMEs, as well as focus on creating favourable conditions for enterprises that were engaged in innovative activities (Hud and Hussinger 2015). Naudé (2020, 1) claimed that during the COVID-19 pandemic 'entrepreneurship, as reflected in the start-up of new firms and the growth of existing firms, particularly SMEs, have been severely curtailed'. Governments today have many financial and regulatory tools to support the survival and maintenance of SMEs, including fiscal, monetary, and tax policies aimed to assist individual entrepreneurs in doing business (Gourinchas et al. 2020).

As the Russian federal government claims, favourable conditions for doing business have been supported to increase the contribution of small enterprises to the country's GDP. The goal is to increase this contribution to 32.5% by 2024 (Passport of the national project 'Small and Medium Enterprises and Support for Individual Entrepreneurial Initiatives' 2018). There were various government financing schemes to provide credits to SMEs introduced before the pandemic. For example, grants from the state budget and private investment were allocated to SMEs in this sphere as government contracts.

DOI: 10.4324/9781003364870-7

However, evidence suggests that since 2016, there has been a decrease in the number of SMEs by 6–10% annually in Russia (Razumovskaia et al. 2020). As a result, the share of SME credit in total business was only 12.6% in 2019, which is lower than their contribution to Russia's GDP (22%) and is half the OECD average (25%) (Chunikhin 2020; Pedraza 2021, 38). This indicator sums up the overall share of small enterprises, making no difference between regions, in some of which this indicator may be even less. Overall, the challenges of SMEs have been divided into two large groups.

The first deals with bureaucratic procedures and excessive regulation for SMEs. These regulations include, for example, a complex list of required documentation, i.e., issuing permits and their multiplicity, non-transparency of land acquisition procedures, urban planning documentation, setting the land rent, etc. Russian small enterprises often face problems while opening and doing business which, in turn, inhibit entrepreneurial activity. A number of authors (Barinova, Stepan, and Yulia 2018) emphasised the necessity of effective legal and state regulatory policy in this sector of the Russian economy to survive business activity and stimulate SME growth. In contrast, some research has indicated (Kuzmin, Vinogradova, and Guseva 2019) that the Russian context has had various advanced institutional factors for business development, differing from region to region. However, most of the challenges for Russian SMEs are associated with regulatory policy and a national complex bureaucratic and legislative structure. The bad governance approach (Gel'man and Zavadskaya 2021) helps to describe these numerous aspects of failing state regulation.

The second group is associated with financial support for small companies, from insufficient levels of subsidies and grant aid to the ineffectiveness of tax legislation and unpredictability of tax policy (Chunikhin 2020). It has been proven that expenditures on technological innovations and investments in research and development in science, education, and the private sector, which is focused on innovative products and services, stimulate growth in all sectors of the economy (Kaneva and Untura 2019). Therefore, increasing investment in the innovative activities of entrepreneurs in the field of high-tech and intellectual services contributes to both a qualitative change in the population's life and the growth of national GDP. In the case of Russia, one can observe a decline in production and investments. These factors directly impact Moscow's overall small business policy, which includes cutting down subsidies aimed at business activity in Russia's regions. In turn, there is a lack of sufficient resources to assist small businesses, especially in the high-tech sector, which requires significant financing from regional budgets.

There is one specific aspect of the COVID-19 crisis which also matters for understanding SME survival and adaptation. Most scholars have claimed that in contrast to the global financial crisis of 2008, in which banks and large companies were supported by the European governments more than small businesses, the current political agenda is focused on support for SMEs (Juergensen, Guimón, and Narula 2020). A similar situation is unlikely to be true for the case of Russia where SMEs traditionally face modest governmental attention in terms of support, capacity building, and facilitation of a positive environment for development. First, SMEs are not the main taxpayers in Russia and their survival might not be among the priorities of the federal and regional authorities during such a big crisis as a pandemic. Second, big business as the most reliable employer in Russia is expected to keep the population satisfied and deliver votes for incumbents (Panov and Ross 2013). SMEs are less reliable in this sense and usually are not involved in political machine-building in Russian regions. The specificity of small- and medium-sized businesses is that they operate in spheres of an economy that are highly dependent on the mobility of the population. The pandemic crisis with its limitation on the mobility of the population hit SMEs significantly.

Explaining the survival and adaptation of SMEs during the pandemic is a challenging task complicated by the specifics of the Russian context. Considering the problematic environment for SME activity in Russia, we treat the large external shocks of the COVID-19 pandemic as a crash test of existing political and socio-economic models of cooperation, as well as of the effects of governmental regulations. We consider if the pre-pandemic relations and models of cooperation between government and SMEs remained robust during the pandemic.

We focus on two considerations. First, the activities of SMEs in Russia were associated with excessive regulation of monitoring agencies, neglect of SMEs' hardships, and modest state support. We aim to see whether the pandemic reshaped policies towards SMEs and principal-agent relations. Second, national governments reacted differently to the crisis, either supporting the population or providing major support to employers. What response did the Russian government demonstrate? Looking at these two characteristics of policy measures will not only help to see the inner dynamic but also situate the Russian case in a global context.

There are two research questions we pose in light of the academic debate. First, we ask how the pandemic influenced SMEs' survival and adaptation in Russian regions. Second, what explains the entrepreneurial activity, adaptation, and survival of small- and medium-sized businesses in Russian regions during the COVID-19 pandemic? The study combines qualitative and quantitative methods of data analysis. In order to respond to the first question, we scrutinise governmental measures and SME responses by analysing qualitative data and research as well as descriptive statistics. We utilise the concept of an incentive structure to study policy measures introduced by the principal to ensure certain behaviour from agents. Regression analysis is employed to respond to the second research question. We approach SME activity and their survival from several perspectives, measuring them via the workforce involved, turnout, the number of officially registered entities, and SMEs per capita. By employing the principal-agent framework, we demonstrate specific relations between the authorities and SMEs which impact the reaction of SMEs towards policy measures introduced by the federal government in response to the COVID-19 pandemic. The detailed methodological design is further explicated in the section below.

The data collected to compare Russian regions with the help of regression analysis enables testing hypothesis regarding the role of socio-economic context. Electoral statistics as well as specific data on hi-tech workplaces in SMEs and unemployment helped to elaborate counter-intuitive hypotheses and contribute to broader debates on the role of structural and political contexts.

The Structure of Incentives in Principal-Agent Relations between the Federal Government and SMEs: Assumptions and Hypotheses

We employ principal-agent theory as a broader theoretical framework to study how the principal (the national and regional governments) impacts agents (SMEs) to ensure their survival in all Russian regions. We draw from assumptions and arguments offered by this theoretical framework to explain and interpret the effect of the pandemic crisis occurring alongside political and socio-economic contexts as well as policy measures introduced by the government on SMEs' adaptation and survival (Miller 2005).

We draw on the main arguments of a principal-agent theory to frame the empirical analysis, significantly considering the effect of outcome-based incentives employed by the principal to ensure policy compliance and the phenomena of information asymmetry. The interpretation of the principal-agent problem in policy studies treats the chief executives as the principal and corresponding public, non-profit, or private actors as agents (Batley 2004). Scholars typically see the principal as having several functions: setting policy goals, creating incentives to ensure compliance with set goals, and monitoring their implementation. In political science literature, citizens are treated as the principals and ultimate beneficiaries of a policy on behalf of whom politicians (agents) act. In the context of Russia, citizens are deprived of the role of principals and lack the ability to control and punish agents (federal and regional politicians) because of the constrained elections. Thus, the central government is seen as the principal who initiates a policy, while responsibility for its implementation is forced on regional authorities who act to encourage certain behaviours from agents (SMEs). Despite the pandemic being a national crisis that did not affect principal-agent relations in Russia, regions indeed became more flexible in how they applied different policy instruments (Busygina and Filippov 2020).

To ensure compliance, the principal creates incentives for agents. We utilise the notion of an **incentive structure** to differentiate between various policy measures introduced by the principal during the rise of the pandemic in Russia. There are two types of incentives: supportive and restrictive. The supportive incentives involved those which encouraged business activities of SMEs under such challenging circumstances as the pandemic. These incentives include the reduction of excessive monitoring as well as moratoriums on bankruptcy and various penalties. Restrictive incentives aimed at preventing the spread of COVID-19 among the population. The restrictive measures were directed towards general regulations of everyday life and included regional lockdowns, social distancing, and other public health-related requirements (masks and gloves, obligatory temperature measurement of employees, etc.). As a rule of thumb, one could expect that these measures would harm SME activities since they target employees, their work routine, and entrepreneurial costs. There were, however, other restrictive measures which impact on SME activity might be different. In particular, various lockdown regimes encouraged an increase in demand for SME services from the population and compensated for additional costs that arose out of the pandemic. For example, demand increased for online purchases, delivery and catering, nursing (especially for the elderly), and private medical care.

In order to stimulate certain behaviour of SMEs, the federal government initiated a number of policy measures. Policy goals in the context of the pandemic included either direct support for the population and simultaneous restrictions of business activity or stimulation of business to escape a dramatic economic downturn. While the support was initiated from the principal itself, the implementation of restrictions was imposed on regional authorities. Therefore, the Russian federal government, acting as the principal, seemed to pursue both policy goals and delegation of responsibilities. We look at two main tools available to the principal to ensure compliance of agents, i.e., SMEs, which compose the incentive structure. These tools include various monitoring instruments and policy tools to allocate costs and rewards (Sharafutdinova 2010). *The first tool*, monitoring, is aimed at holding agents responsible for policy implementation. It is widely recognised in the literature that monitoring is costly for a principal and as a rational actor, it seeks cheaper options. As a result, the principal inclines to monitor the outcome of the agent's performance instead of its actual action (Miller 2005). The evolution of technocratic governance in Russia (Huskey 2010) demonstrates how monitoring tools and multiple regulatory agencies previously encouraged the development of outcomes utilising audit procedures (Power 2000).

The case of governmental regulation of SME activity represents one of the key dilemmas of autocracies. On the one hand, there is a need for an autocrat to demonstrate a capacity to arrange an effective performance of government. The key to SME development is a relatively comfortable business environment, safe investment schemes, and conducive socio-economic conditions. On the other hand, constrained elections and suppression of independent mass media and civil society in Russia deprive the principal of a natural tool for monitoring agents' performance. This limits tools of monitoring to solely outcome-based incentives enabled via bureaucratic instruments. One of the outcomes is the empowerment of monitoring agencies whose performance is believed to encourage effective policy implementation (Gilev and Dimke 2021). As a result, the activity of monitoring agencies brings about excessive regulation, counteracting the initial intention to encourage SME performance through a comfortable business environment.

The second tool attempts to reduce risks and losses caused by policy implementation. There are three ways a principal might deal with these issues. As Knight and Shi (1999, 14) demonstrate, a principal can either take all risks or transfer them to the agent. In both cases, the agent will have fewer incentives to implement policy. Alternatively, risks can be shared, having a positive effect on the agent's commitment. In the Russian case, the second and the third options with some modifications are applied. The selective encouragement and support for limited regional agencies developed as part of technocratic negotiations where outcome-based monitoring became the agent's 'currency' in lobbying for budget support and preferences.

Taking into consideration these theoretical arguments, three main hypotheses about the impact of policy measures on SMEs during the COVID-19 pandemic are formulated. The first three hypotheses derive from theoretical expectations related to the incentive structure created by the principal to ensure compliance of agents, i.e., certain behaviour of SMEs. First, policy measures, including monetary and other forms of support introduced by the federal government, will be considered risk-reduction tools employed by the principal. We expect financial support (loans) to positively correlate with SME entrepreneurial activity and survival.

Second, as many experts demonstrated, online sales became popular during lockdowns due to the growing demand for service delivery (Chernova and Neklyudova 2021). Therefore, the innovative potential in a given region could affect the adaptation of SMEs to this demand. We hypothesise that investments in a given region could play an important role in SME survival for two reasons. By default, we expect that the more investments attracted in a given region, the better it is for the development of the economy of a given region which is conducive to SME activity. Similarly, the cost of innovations, private investments, and high-tech workplaces could act as proxies for a conducive business environment in a given region. It might also signal a lack of (or at least not severe) excessive regulation of executive and monitoring agencies of business activity. These considerations lead us to hypothesise that the more private investments, money allocated for innovations, and high-productive workplaces in a given region, the more SMEs will survive the pandemic crisis.

Third, the efficiency of the government is directly felt by the population via the situation in the labour market. Employment policy in Russia proved to be one of the pillars of the social policy which ensures the legitimacy and political stability of incumbents (Gimpelson, Kapelyushnikov, and Lukyanova 2010). Therefore, the federal and regional governments strive to retain a certain level of employment by supporting half-time working contracts and through similar insecure methods to keep employees from ending up unemployed. There are political and social benefits gained thanks to this employment policy (Gimpelson and Kapelyushnikov 2014). Following this policy, the federal government offered compensation to private companies which kept their employees during the pandemic. The COVID-19 pandemic appeared to be a test for this policy. Adherence to this policy would require financial support to employers in addition to direct support for the population. The hypothesis can be formulated that the higher the level of employment, the more chances there are for SME survival. The role of the grey market should be taken into account, as will be discussed below.

Fourth, it has been proved that political support and demonstration of loyalty towards federal and regional incumbents is an essential part of the contract between the federal and regional levels of governance in Russia. In the long perspective, this contract downplays the government's performance and policy achievements. In the short perspective, it is utilised by regional authorities to negotiate and attract additional financial resources and support in a given region. Therefore, the political business cycle proved to be a good predictor for some policies in Russian regions. Incumbents aiming to be re-elected tend to mobilise the electorate via networks of regional and local elites, including small- and medium-sized businesses (Orttung 2004; Starodubtsev 2014). As a result of this electoral strategy, SMEs could benefit from the distribution of federal financial transfers fuelled during electoral campaigns in Russian regions (Sharafutdinova and Turovsky 2017). We hypothesise that elections, run in 2020 at the regional level, would trigger long-existing redistributive mechanisms of federal transfers, and this budget influx might stimulate entrepreneurial activities of SMEs. Thereby, in Russian regions where either gubernatorial or parliament elections took place, we expect a bigger number of SMEs and stronger performances than in regions where there were no elections. In addition, we consider electoral support of the incumbent in presidential elections (2018) to be a similar marker.

The principal-agency framework is also plausible for describing the behaviour of agents, i.e., SMEs. As they possess interests of their own, agents tend to use information (informational asymmetry) to gain benefits or reduce the costs of unfavourable policy (Miller 2005). The literature on SMEs argues that excessive regulation and expectations regarding their activity are the key factors interfering with the business environment. Audit procedures are indeed excessively used in Russia as a means of monitoring and control (Paneyakh 2014), distorting agents' intentions and encouraging morally hazardous behaviour. Under the pressure of audit, and in the absence of other incentives conducive to compliance, creative compliance might be seen by agents as a plausible strategy (Tarasenko 2022).

As research demonstrates, audits and governmental monitoring partly account for the growing grey market and informal practices (Gimpelson and Kapelyushnikov 2014). For example, studies have demonstrated that SMEs tend to cut costs such as taxes or obligation to fulfil numerous regulations by hiring employees unofficially. In order to escape additional paperwork and enjoy the preferences the SME status entails, managers tend to keep the size of their business within the income limits (120 billion per year, RUB).

Growing businesses tend to create additional SMEs to secure their status (Filippova 2021). These examples demonstrate how the information about SME activity is manipulated to reduce the negative consequences of excessive regulation. We will look for similar practices to reveal the adaptation of SMEs to the crisis, taking into consideration shifts in governmental policy. Experiencing the pressure from the incentive structure, agents have several options: they can comply, not comply, or adapt to the requirements. In this study, we specifically look at the adaptation in response to the experienced incentive structure.

Methodology of Empirical Analysis

Variable Selection

The research methodology used here is related to the determination of which factors contribute to the activity of small- and medium-sized businesses in the regional context of the Russian Federation. The selection of variables in this study is based on the results of previous studies on the importance of financial support for entrepreneurship in times of crisis, as well as innovation in the SME sector. The research model builds on a linear relationship between entrepreneurial survival and influencing factors, including levels of credit, unemployment, investment, innovation, and political factors (regional and presidential elections of 2018–2020). In addition, the research model includes the age of the population in the Russian regional context because age is recognised in the academic world as one of the success factors in business activity.

Since the main unit of the analysis is a region of the Russian Federation, the sample includes 83 regions.[1] All data collection is based on secondary data taken from official sources of information and national websites for the period from 2019 to 2020 to cover statistics before the 2020 pandemic and the COVID-19 period in 2020.

Data Collection and Measurement

The main source of information collection is the Rosstat website, from which the data of the dependent variable were partially taken: (1) business turnover for 2020 (*SME turnover*) and (2) the number of able-bodied workers employed in SMEs (*SME employment*) for both 2020 and 2019 to compare (3) the difference between SME activity (*SME employment difference*) before and during the COVID-19 pandemic. *SMEs per capita* were calculated to measure their entrepreneurial activity in a given region. This dependent variable is more accurate. In contrast to the number of SMEs, which can be a signal of the business environment favourable for registering a company, SMEs per capita as a proportion shows the scope of SMEs, regardless of the size of a given region.

Independent variables include (4) the unemployment rate in 2020 (*Unemployment*), (5) the number of loans issued to small businesses at the end of 2020 (*Loans*), (6) the total amount of private investment, which does not include government support or subsidies for business development (*Investment excluding budget*), (7) the share of SMEs in the total number that worked in the field of innovative technologies (IT) observed during the pre-pandemic year of 2019 (*Innovation*), and (8) money allocated for innovation that were invested by the entrepreneurs themselves (*Spending on innovation*) in 2019. For analysis, statistics were taken on (9) the number of high-tech jobs in the Russian regions observed during the pre-pandemic year of 2019 (*High-tech workplaces*). (10) The average age of the population in the Russian regions (*Age*) in 2020 was also collected from Rosstat.

The Russian Federal Tax Service (FNS) is another source of data to measure the response variable: (11) the number of SMEs in the regional context of Russia that were registered by the end of 2020 (*SME*). To analyse (12) the dynamics of business activity among the Russian regions (*SME difference*), data on the number of registered units of SMEs in 2019 were collected from the FNS website. All the data on SMEs were taken from the Unified Register of Small and Medium Business Entities, divided by region.

Data on (13) regional elections held in 2020 (*Regional elections*) as well as (14) the 2018 presidential election (*Presidential elections*) were taken from the Central Election Commission of the Russian Federation. Twenty-five Russian regions held subnational elections in 2020 during the pandemic, including elections of governors and regional deputies. We used the percentage of votes for the incumbent in each region in presidential elections in 2018 and binary variables for regional elections. Thus, regional and presidential elections indicate an activation of distribution of financial transfers which could influence the increase of potential supportive measures for SMEs.

All the variables are represented as descriptive statistics exhibited in Appendix 1. The equation of multiple linear regression models is available in Appendix 2. To explore the impact of regional specifics on entrepreneurial activity, the response variable is measured in five different ways: the number of registered units of SMEs in a region, the difference of SMEs number of 2019–2020 in a region, the number of people employed in SMEs in a region, and the difference of employed people between 2019 and 2020 in a region, as well as the turnover of SMEs in the COVID-19 period in a region.

These ways of measuring entrepreneurship in a regional context are limited by two factors. First, measuring entrepreneurship as a share of those wishing to become entrepreneurs or attitudes towards entrepreneurship, in general, is not suitable for this study, since the purpose of this analysis is not to predict the nature of the development of the business environment in the regions but to determine the survival of an existing entrepreneurial activity. The second factor is the lack of irrelevance of data on the share of SMEs in the country's GDP since there is no official data from Rosstat for 2020–2021.

We believe that the measurement of entrepreneurship in five different ways suggested above enables to produce reliable regression analysis.

Data Analysis

Since this study assumes that business survival depends on a group of factors, the hypotheses are tested using seven separate multiple linear regression models, where different measures of business survival are used as the dependent variables. The set of independent variables consists of nine indicators, covering regional socio-economic and political peculiarities. Since the dependent variable is measured in the different ways described above, its level of dependence on the independent factors varies from model to model. Although the eight linear regressions were built to compare the dependence of the response variable on regional features, the article focused on three main regressions selected by the Akaike information criterion (AIC) value as a best-fit model criterion (see Table 6.1).

Each model assumes a linear dependence of entrepreneurial activity on a set of influencing features in the following sequence: there are positive relationships between the share of high-tech workplaces as well as the total sum of loans granted to SMEs and for SME activity. We assume a positive impact of unemployment on business adaptation in 2020, as well as an average age of the population in a given region. The model where SMEs per capita is the dependent variable is taken as the main. All other models are compared with this main model. Although entrepreneurial dependency has been tested with eight different models, the results of regressions with *SMEs per capita*, *SME employment*, and *SME turnover* (Table 6.1) are the most reliable.

The Impact of the Pandemic Crisis on SMEs in Russian Regions in 2020

SMEs are traditionally involved in service provision, including beauty services, care and nursing, the leisure sector, trade in non-food products, the hospitality sector, food, and catering. Due to the limitations on population

Table 6.1 AIC Value Comparison in All Regressions

Regression model	*AIC value*
SMEs per capita	69.7*
SME employment	8.8*
SME turnover	28.6*
SMEs	76.3
SME employment difference	222.3
SME difference	330.8
Active SMEs	154.6
Dying SMEs	121.0

*Lower AIC value.

mobility (full or partial lockdown) introduced by regional and local authorities, these spheres of the economy suffered the most (Chernova and Neklyudova 2021).

Table 6.2 highlights that the dynamics of *SME employment* are positive in 2020 compared with the previous year because the measurement of the dependent variable as a number of employed in 2019 is less than in 2020. Interestingly, the number of SMEs shrunk by 96,684 in 2020 compared to 2019, whereas the number of employees increased by approximately four times. The main explanation for this difference is that in 2020, SMEs registered all workers officially to receive state subsidies. According to the employment support loan as one of the legislative measures for SMEs in Russia (Appendix 3), the loan does not need to be paid back if 90% of employees are retained by Russian companies. We argue that during the COVID-19 pandemic, SMEs formalised their employees for interest-free loans, accounting for the increased level of employment.

In addition to the Moscow region, the top five regions as 'the most successful' include the Sverdlovsk region, the Krasnodar region, the Republic of Tatarstan, and the Novosibirsk region. Meanwhile, those which failed to cope with this external shock include the Chechen Republic, the Republic of Kalmykia, Tyva, and Ingushetia (Figure 6.1).

The analysis of governmental regulations and support measures helps to reveal their role in SME survival and adaptation, especially in terms of informal practices. There was a set of supportive measures addressing SMEs in crisis introduced by the federal and regional governments (Appendix 3). In addition to tax incentives, financial support (loans and subsidies), moratoriums on penalties for government contracts, tax penalties for non-submission of documents, on-site inspections, and bankruptcy were introduced. The latter could have been especially important from the point of measuring actual SME activity and dynamics during a pandemic crisis.

This excessive regulation has influenced supportive measures in the following ways. In addition to Rospotrebnadzor and the Ministry of Emergency Situations, the Federal Agency on Labour Relations is the third most likely

Table 6.2 SME Dynamics Measured as Number of SMEs, Employed People, and SME Turnover

	Number of SMEs		*Number of SME employment (thousands)*		*SME turnover (Bln rub)*	
	2019	*2020*	*2019*	*2020*	*2020*	*2021*
Total	1,823,760	1,727,076	9,264	34,471	7,368.3	86,662.2
Average	21,973	20,808	111.6	415.3	88.77	104.41

government organisation to undertake regulatory and control actions (monitoring of agents by the principal), according to the societal organisation for SMEs 'OPORA Rossii' (OPORA, 2020). In particular, altogether there were up to 200,000 actions initiated in 2019 by this agency. The number of casual, unscheduled regulatory checks was equal to 129,000 in 2019. Planned actions accounted for 17,100 actions in 2019. Therefore, the moratorium on scheduled inspections introduced by the federal government in 2020 is not expected to significantly relieve SMEs from the pressure of extensive regulation. It also signals that the monitoring tools of the principal to control agents remained unchanged.

The national government adopted a list of economic sectors which are eligible for state support to help relieve the effects of the pandemic. These sectors include transport, culture and leisure activities, education, tourism, hotels, public nutrition, consumer services, health care, and retail business. Small businesses operating in these areas became eligible for direct financial support. The subsidy that compensated for the costs of COVID-19 prevention was intended for 500,000 SMEs in the field of hospitality, personal services, catering, sports, and additional education. Insurance payments for covering pension contributions and medical insurance were halved for small businesses, going from 30% to 15%. This reduction of insurance payments was available until the end of 2020. Direct payments for small businesses operating in areas of the economy which were harmed the most were provided. In addition to that, bank loans with zero interest rates that could only be used to pay salaries were introduced.

We consider that loans encouraged SMEs to formalise their employees and reduce the number of unofficially employed workers. As a result, the increase in the number of people employed in SMEs during the pandemic can be exampled by the decrease of grey employment relationships which become formalised. If this consideration is correct, it means that in regions with a high level of unemployment and a low level of innovative SMEs, businesses were indeed motivated by loans to legalise previously unofficially employed people, which partially led to an increase in the number of SMEs. As Filippova (2021) demonstrated, to continue enjoying preferential treatment from the government, managers tend to keep the size of their business within the income limits (120 billion per year, RUB). The legalisation of employment could result in the registration of additional companies to secure SME status. This demonstrates how SMEs acting as agents employed informational asymmetry to deceive the principal and benefit from unfavourable circumstances.

To sum up, despite figures suggesting the improvement in SME scope and numbers employed in these enterprises, the interpretation suggested above clearly demonstrates that we hardly witnessed the actual growth of these enterprises during the pandemic. Instead, the adaptation of SMEs to the circumstances is obvious.

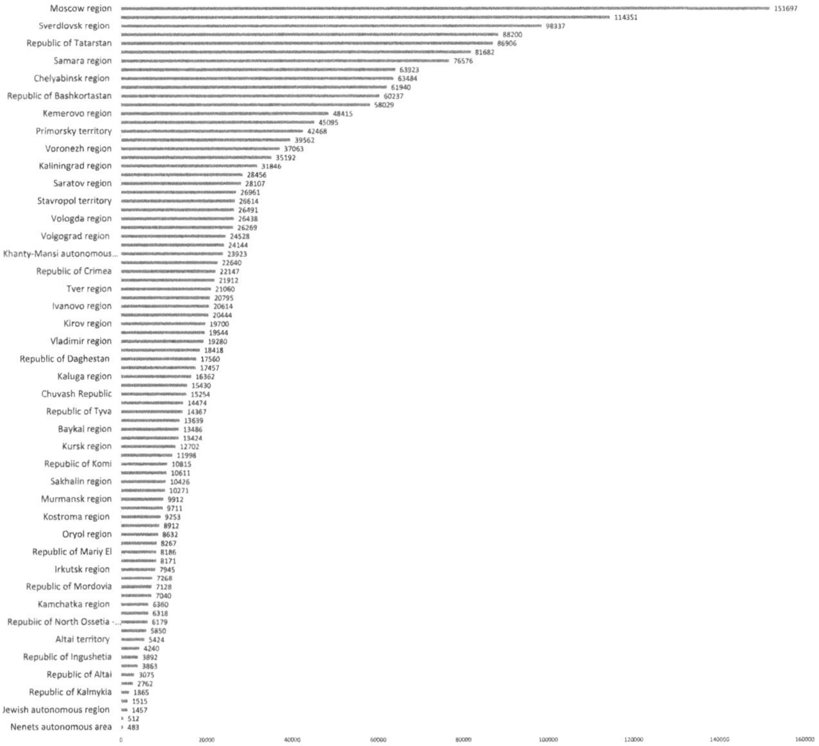

Figure 6.1 The number of SMEs in Russian regions in 2020.

Incentives Created by the Principal and Informational Asymmetry Employed by Agents

The main findings of the regression analysis are summarised in Figure 6.2. The explanatory models present the results of the level of entrepreneurial activity in the regions of Russia during the COVID-19 pandemic and its dependence on socio-economic features. Below are the results of the analysis in which entrepreneurial activity was measured in different ways. The conclusions are quite ambiguous since different social and economic measures become influential factors for different measurements. But even with conflicting explanatory variables, we see a strong relationship between the number of loans in 2020 and the level of entrepreneurship, as well as a positive relationship between the average age of the population in the region and entrepreneurial activity.

We consider SMEs per capita as the most reliable dependent variable, which mitigates the effect of the legalisation of unofficially employed. The explanatory models for the number of SMEs and the scope of their workforce are identical and include the same financial, economic, and social

Model 1

Dep. Variable	**SME per capita**	R2	0.588
Model:	OLS	Adj. R2	0.572
Method:	Least Squares	F-Statistic:	37.55
No.Observations:	83	Prob (F-statistic):	3.47e-15
Df Residuals:	79	Log-Likelihood:	-30.853
Df Model:	3	AIC:	69.71
Covariance Type:	nonrobust	BIC:	79.38

	coef	std err	t	P>|t|	[0.025	0.975]
const	4.7748	2.260	2.113	0.038*	0.277	9.273
Unemployment	-0.3957	0.112	-3.537	0.001**	-0.618	-0.173
Age	0.0650	0.016	3.960	**0.000*** **	0.032	0.098
Presidential elections	-2.5583	0.480	-5.330	**0.000*** **	-3.514	-1.603

Model 2

Dep. Variable	**SME employment**	R2	0.960
Model:	OLS	Adj. R2	0.958
Method:	Least Squares	F-Statistic:	471.6
No.Observations:	83	Prob (F-statistic):	8.70e-54
Df Residuals:	78	Log-Likelihood:	0.59708
Df Model:	4	AIC:	8.806
Covariance Type:	nonrobust	BIC:	20.90

	coef	std err	t	P>|t|	[0.025	0.975]
const	-6.7728	0.577	-11.746	**0.000*** **	-7.921	-5.625
Unemployment	0.3119	0.095	3.274	0.002**	0.122	0.502
Age	0.0661	0.013	5.219	**0.000*** **	0.041	0.091
Loans	0.4198	0.057	7.345	**0.000*** **	0.306	0.534
HiTech Wplaces	0.5814	0.072	8.069	**0.000*** **	0.438	0.725

Model 3

Dep. Variable	**SME Turnover**	R2	0.957
Model:	OLS	Adj. R2	0.954
Method:	Least Squares	F-Statistic:	342.4
No.Observations:	83	Prob (F-statistic):	4.51e-51
Df Residuals:	77	Log-Likelihood:	-8.2769
Df Model:	5	AIC:	28.55
Covariance Type:	nonrobust	BIC:	43.07

	coef	std err	t	P>|t|	[0.025	0.975]
const	-8.5634	1.330	-6.439	**0.000*** **	-11.212	-5.915
Unemployment	0.2370	0.107	2.217	0.030*	0.024	0.450
Age	0.0358	0.015	2.325	0.023*	0.005	0.066
Loans	0.6942	0.068	10.146	**0.000*** **	0.558	0.830
Investment	0.1323	0.059	2.250	0.027*	0.015	0.249
HiTech Wplaces	0.2248	0.224	1.888	0.063*	-0.012	0.462

*** p-value significance at 1%,** - 5%, * - 10%

Figure 6.2 Results of analysis.

factors. Almost all of the explanatory models exhibit a strong positive presence of three variables: (1) governmental loans in 2020, (2) high-productive workplaces in a given region, the share of SMEs in the total number that worked in the field of innovative technologies (IT), and (3) the average age of the population. The fourth significant variable is the positive effect of the unemployment rate in all models apart from the one with SMEs per capita as the dependent variable. This model includes the negative role of presidential elections and the absence of any effect of high-tech workplaces. We follow the formulated hypotheses as well as qualitative data and studies to interpret these statistical results.

First, **loans** appear to be relevant in all models with various dependent variable measurements, apart from one – SMEs per capita. When loans granted to SMEs increased by 1 million, the number of people employed in SMEs increased by 42 in Model 2, and SME turnover grew by approximately 70 million in Model 3 (Figure 6.2). The correlation is positive: the greater number of SMEs in a given region, the larger the workforce. This then correlates to a larger turnover and hence, more loans are provided. We see these loans as a part of the incentive structure created by the principal. They were aimed at reducing risks caused by COVID-19 and restrictive regulations.

Second, starting conditions such as the number of **high-productive workplaces** (data analysts, IT specialists, etc.) in a given region appeared to be a significant factor for SME turnover. Several regions prominently differed in terms of the number of high-tech workplaces, considering that the mean equals 119.5. These regions include such advanced economies as Moscow region (924.1), Tuymen region (753.3), Republic of Tatarstan (506.1), Chelyabinsk (397.6), Novosibirsk (349.1), Rostov (346.3), and Samara (376.6). The significance of the number of overall high-productive workplaces registered in the non-public sector of the economy in 2019 might show the role of innovative potential as a starting condition that helped more equipped regions survive during the pandemic. Provided that SMEs often deliver various services, this finding can be interpreted as demonstrating generally higher levels of consumption which triggered the development of SMEs. As a result, we witnessed an increase in SME turnover in regions with higher high-productive workplaces. The effect of the pandemic on these structural conditions seems to be limited.

Third, surprisingly, the relatively developed age of a population is positively associated with SME survival if it is measured in numbers and workforce. The **average age** of the population appeared to be a significant predictor with a positive correlation: if the average age of the population is higher, the number of SMEs is larger as well. This dynamic can be explained by higher demand for services provided by SMEs, such as nursing for elderly and online purchase and delivery, in regions where elderly population dominates. The average age could also indicate more restrictions in a given region, provided that COVID-19 was considered to be of disproportionate danger to the elderly and regional authorities took this into consideration when issuing restrictions.

Fourth, the negative effect of **the percentage of votes for the incumbent in presidential elections** is only present in the model with SMEs per capita as the dependent variable. It might be explained by the role of political machines that are effectively mobilised in regions with industrial economies (Panov and Ross 2013). Their presence in regions such as Bryansk, Lipetsk, and others is associated with the activity of smaller scope of SMEs during the COVID-19 pandemic. There are also relatively poor ethnic republics that are known for effective mobilisation in presidential elections (including the Republic of Daghestan, Ingushetia, Kabardian-Balkarskaya, and

Karachaevo-Cherkesskaya). In this sense, a more loyal and effectively mobilised electorate is associated with a worse performance of SMEs during the pandemic.

In the Model 1, the effect of **unemployment** became negative: the fewer unemployed people, the more SMEs per capita. We link the role of unemployment to governmental measures that were introduced (1) to motivate companies to maintain the same level of employment and (2) a simplified status registration procedure as well as an increased payment of unemployment benefits. These two measures have potentially contradicting effects: the first measure discourages unemployment while the second may encourage job loss. But as the literature above demonstrated, both measures were aimed at maintaining the purchasing power of the population.

The minimum unemployment benefit was increased from 8,000 roubles (90 euros) to 12,130 roubles (135 euros), which was available for three months regardless of employment experience and qualifications. Natalia Zubarevich and Sergei Safronov suggest that while this was only a modest increase in unemployment benefits, the new policy still encouraged people to apply for unemployment support more actively than before (Zubarevich and Safronov 2020). The Ministry of Labour and Social Protection calculated that 450,000 unemployed people received this increased minimum unemployment benefit in April–May 2020. However, these measures were temporary and terminated on 1 October 2020 (Governmental Decree #844, adopted 10 June 2020). As a result of this short-lived policy measure, the number of people turning to public employment agencies for obtaining the minimum unemployment benefits increased by 250% in June 2020 in comparison to February 2020. The unemployment rate increased from 4.6% (3.5 million people) to 6% (45 million) compared with early 2019 (Zubarevich and Safronov 2020). It is hard to evaluate the impact of employee decisions on SME activity. Nevertheless, this finding supports assumptions about the significance of employment policy during the pandemic. This also emphasises the volatility of such policy and its direct effect on the behaviour of ordinary people and SMEs.

The effect of regional elections appeared to be a mediating factor for the unemployment rate (Figure 6.3). Additionally, in those regions where there were no regional elections in September 2020, the SME turnover is significantly smaller. Following the hypothesis about the redistributive effect of elections, we treat regional elections as a proxy for additional social benefits and financial support available for a given region during the peak events of an electoral cycle.

Conclusion

The COVID-19 pandemic challenged the activity and survival of SMEs in Russia. In contrast to other external shocks, analysis of SMEs' survival and activity brings several additional dilemmas into focus. The federal government

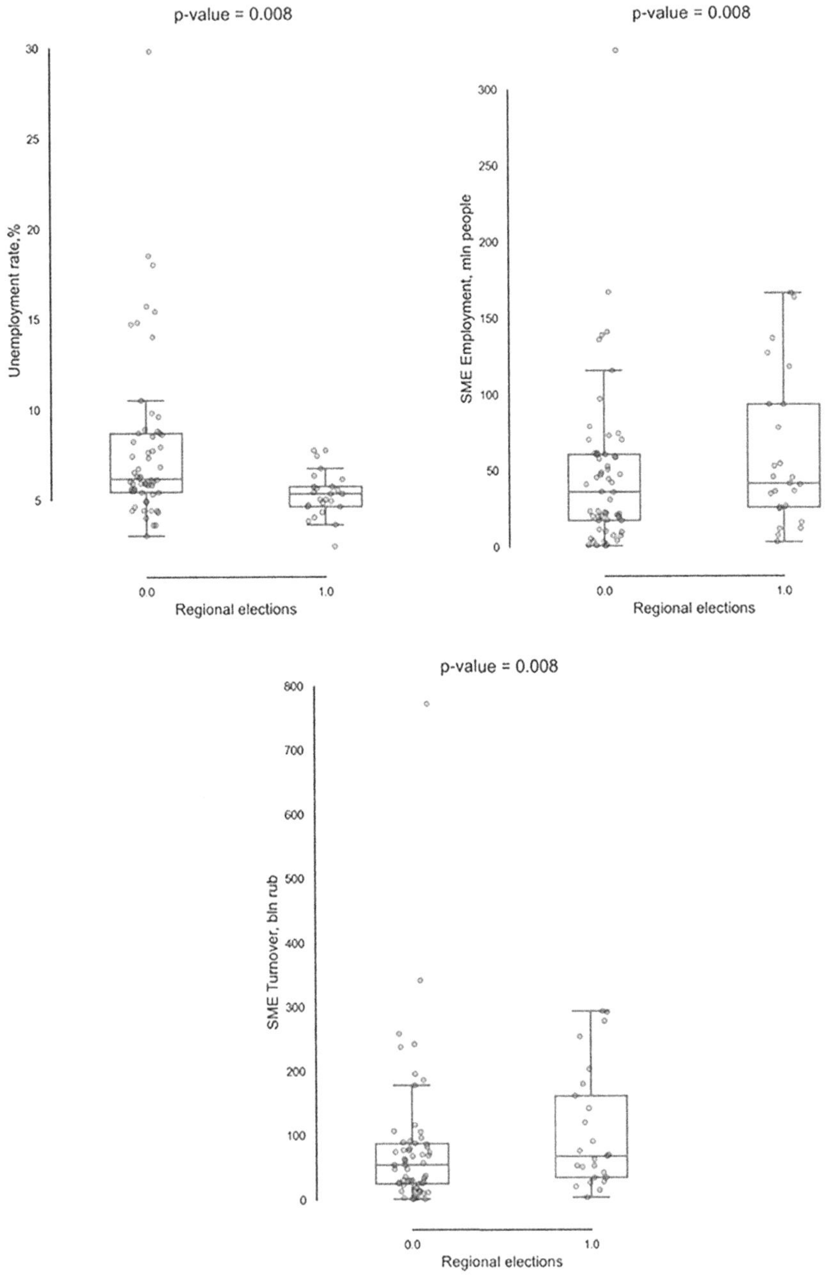

Figure 6.3 The comparison of unemployment rate, SME employment, and SME turnover distribution by regional elections held.

Source: Authors.

faced a choice: either to support businesses, which in turn would take care of employees, or to support citizens directly. The Russian government pursued both policy measures: issuing loans for SMEs and increasing the unemployment rate, though also lifting bureaucratic barriers for registering as unemployed. The pandemic forced businesses to fire employees, and the Russian government entered the employment market to regulate this process, offering compensations for businesses, on the one hand, and increasing unemployment benefits, on the other. Data on SMEs in 2019 and 2020 demonstrate the immediate effect of cost-reduction tools employed by the principal. In particular, public loans aimed at supporting businesses that did not fire employees in the face of reduced income. This brought about a change in businesses' strategies concerning employment in SMEs. In particular, the benefits loans offered caused SMEs to reduce the number of unofficially employed workers. This governmental regulation brought about immediate but ambiguous consequences. This finding contributes to the scientific literature on SMEs by reconsidering the influence of the principal-agent relations on SME activity. The principal-agent framework suggests that the principal engages both positive incentives (benefits) and negative sanctions to ensure certain behaviour of agents. This analysis demonstrates how sanctions and information asymmetry interfered with the activity of SMEs. These findings can be interpreted in line with previous research demonstrating how agents manipulated information to manoeuvre within the incentive structure and benefit from the circumstances. This opportunistic nature of agents acting in the Russian context seems to be one of the key aspects of the principal-agent relations during COVID-19.

Unfolding the composition of the incentive structure created by the principal, this chapter showed that the national government has not only focused on financial assistance for SMEs but also lifted some bureaucratic barriers and relaxed fiscal regulations. Since these policies were applied to all Russian regions and data were not available to test their effects separately, the analysis is limited to studying the impact of loans in addition to other social-economic and political factors. In addition to that, the analysis shows that some lifted barriers were not substantial to limit the monitoring of SMEs. As a result, the principal secured outcome-based incentives for evaluation of performance of agents during COVID-19.

It is hard to estimate how effective lockdowns and other restrictive measures were in Russia. Examples of societal discontent in the North Caucasus demonstrated that to secure their business, people did not follow the restrictions. This might be an important explanatory factor that requires further exploration. It should be taken into consideration that social-economic factors such as gross-regional product per capita were not found to be significant in explaining SMEs' survival.

Interestingly, the electoral cycle does not appear to be a significant regional factor itself. At the same time, it served as an intermediate factor explaining the increase in SME turnover and the level of employment in regions where regional elections were held in 2020. The hypothesis about the relevance of elections was formulated in line with the policy cycle argumentation. The role of previous electoral mobilisation during the presidential elections in 2018 proved to predict the performance of SMEs, measured as SMEs per capita. The presence of an active political machine in the past was associated with lower likelihoods of SMEs surviving the pandemic.

Note

1 Moscow and St. Petersburg are excluded from the sample because these two federal cities may bias the results of the analysis due to their status and, hence, economic characteristics as well as political significance.

References

Barinova, Vera, Zemtsov Stepan, and Tsareva Yulia. 2018. "Entrepreneurship and Institutions: Does the relationship exist at the regional level in Russia (in Russian)." Predprinimatelstvo i Instituty: Est li Svyaz na Regionalnom urovne v Rossii, *Voprosy Ekonomiki* 6: 92–116.

Batley, Richard. 2004. "The politics of service delivery reform." *Development and Change* 35, no. 1: 31–56.

Busygina, Irina, and Filippov Mikhail. 2020. "Russian Federalism: Informal Elite Games Against Formal Democratic Institutions." *PONARS Eurasia Policy Memo*, June 22, 2020. https://www.ponarseurasia.org/russian-federalism-informal-elite-games-against-formal-democratic-institutions/.

Chernova, Christina, and Neklyudova Natalia. 2021. "The Impact of the Coronavirus Pandemic on Small and Medium-sized Enterprises in Russian Federation." *SHS Web of Conferences* 135, 01005 (2022) ECCW 2021. https://doi.org/10.1051/shsconf/202213501005.

Chunikhin, Sergey. 2020. "Modelling the development dynamics of small and medium-sized enterprises in Russia." *Amazonia Investiga* 9, no. 27: 116–128.

Filippova, Evgenia. 2021. "Number of Small and Medium-sized Companies in Russia Might Increase Steeply." *Parlamentskaia Gazeta*. August 19, 2021 (in Russian). https://www.pnp.ru/economics/chislo-malykh-i-srednikh-predpriyatiy-v-rossii-mozhet-rezko-vyrasti.html.

Gel'man, Vladimir, and Zavadskaya Margarita. 2021. "Exploring varieties of governance in Russia: In search of theoretical frameworks." *Europe-Asia Studies* 73, no. 6: 971–988.

Gilev, Aleksei, and Dimke Daria. 2021. "'No time for quality': Mechanisms of local governance in Russia." *Europe-Asia Studies* 73, no. 6: 1060–1079.

Gimpelson, Vladimir, and Rostislav Kapelyushnikov. 2014. "Between Light and Shadow: Informality in the Russian Labour Market. Institute for the Study of Labor (IZA)." *Discussion Paper* No. 8279, June 2014.

Gimpelson, Vladimir, Kapelyushnikov Rostislav, and Lukyanova Anna. 2010. "Employment protection legislation in Russia: Regional enforcement and labor market outcomes." *Comparative Economic Studies* 52: 611–636.

Gourinchas, Pierre-Olivier, Şebnem Kalemli-Özcan, Veronika Penciakova, and Nick Sander. 2020. "Covid-19 and SME failures." *National Bureau of Economic Research. Working paper* No. 27877.Hud, Martin, and Katrin Hussinger. 2015. "The impact of R&D subsidies during the crisis." *Research Policy* 44, no. 10: 1844–1855.

Huskey, Eugene. 2010. "Elite recruitment and state-society relations in technocratic authoritarian regimes: The Russian case." *Communist and Post-Communist Studies* 43: 363–372.

Juergensen, Jill, José Guimón, and Rajneesh Narula. 2020. "European SMEs amidst the COVID-19 crisis: Assessing impact and policy responses." *Journal of Industrial and Business Economics* 47, no. 3: 499–510.

Kaneva, Maria, and Galina Untura. 2019. "The impact of R&D and knowledge spillovers on the economic growth of Russian regions." *Growth and Change* 50, no. 1: 301–334.

Knight, John, and Shi Li. 1999. "Fiscal decentralization: Incentives, redistribution and reform in China." *Oxford Development Studies* 27, no. 1: 5–32.

Kuzmin, Evgeny, Marina Vinogradova, and Valentina Guseva. 2019. "Projection of enterprise survival rate in dynamics of regional economic sustainability: case study of Russia and the EU." *Entrepreneurship and Sustainability Issues* 6, no. 4: 1602–1617.

Miller, Gary. 2005. "The political evolution of principal-agent models." *Annual Review of Political Science* 8: 203–225.

Naudé, Wim. 2020. "Entrepreneurial recovery from COVID-19: Decentralization, democratization, demand, distribution, and demography." *IZA Discussion Papers*, No. 13436, Institute of Labor Economics (IZA), Bonn.

OPORA. 2020. "Analiz Kontrolno-nadzornoi Deyatel'nosti Organov Gosudarstvennoi Vlasti." *OPORA Rossii* (Analysis of Monitoring Activity of State Authorities), in Russian. https://opora.ru/upload/iblock/86a/86a6807fa453230466d7f48436aca10e.pdf.

Orttung, Robert. 2004. "Business and politics in the Russian regions." *Problems of Post-Communism* 51, no. 2: 48–60.

Paneyakh, Ella. 2014. "Faking performance together: Systems of performance evaluation in Russian enforcement agencies and production of bias and privilege." *Post-Soviet Affairs* 30, nos. 2–3: 115–136.

Panov, Petr, and Ross Cameron. 2013. "Sub-National elections in Russia: Variations in United Russia's domination of regional assemblies." *Europe-Asia Studies* 65, no. 4: 737–752.

Pedraza, Jorge Morales. 2021. "The micro, small, and medium-sized enterprises and its role in the economic development of a country." *Business and Management Research* 10, no. 1: 33–44.

Power, Michael. 2000. "The audit society - second thoughts." *International Journal of Auditing* 4, no. 1: 111–119.

Razumovskaia, Elena, Yuzvovich Larisa, Kniazeva Elena, Klimenko Mikhail, and Valeriy Shelyakin. 2020. "The effectiveness of Russian government policy to support SMEs in the COVID-19 pandemic." *Journal of Open Innovation: Technology, Market, and Complexity* 6, no. 4: 160.

Sharafutdinova, Gulnaz. 2010. "Subnational governance in Russia: How Putin changed the contract with his agents and the problems it created for Medvedev." *Publius: The Journal of Federalism* 40, no. 4: 672–696.

Sharafutdinova, Gulnaz, and Turovsky Rostitslav. 2017. "The politics of federal transfers in Putin's Russia: Regional competition, lobbying and federal priorities." *Post-Soviet Affairs* 33, no. 2: 161–175.

Starodubtsev, Andrey. 2014. "Agency matters. The failure of Russian regional policy reforms." *Demokratizatsiya: The Journal of Post-Soviet Democratization* 22, no. 4: 553–574.

Tarasenko, Anna. 2022. "Outsourcing elderly care to private companies in Russia: (Non) Compliance and creative compliance as responses to the principal-agent problem." *East European Politics*. Published online, DOI: 10.1080/21599165.2022.2139683.

Vargo, John, and Seville Erica. 2011. "Crisis strategic planning for SMEs: Finding the silver lining." *International Journal of Production Research* 49, no. 18: 5619–5635.

Zubarevich, Natalia, and Safronov Sergei. 2020. "Regions of Russia in the acute phase of the COVID crisis: Differences from previous economic crises of the 2000s." N.V. January

Appendix 1

Descriptive Statistics

Variable (year)	*SME (2020)*	*SME employment (2020)*	*SME turnover (2020)*	*SME difference (2020–2019)*	*SME employment difference (2020–2019)*	*Loans (2020)*	*Unemployment (2020)*	*Innovation (2019)*	*Cost on innovation (2019)*	*Investment excluding public (2017)*	*High-tech workplaces (2019)*	*Regional elections (2020)*	*Presidential elections (2018)*	*Age (2020)*
Measurement	*Units*	*Mln people*	*Bln rub*	*Units*	*Mln people*	*Mln rub*	*% people*	*Share of SMEs in IT*	*Mln rub*	*Thousands rub*	*Thousands places*	*1 – held, 0 – no*	*% Votes*	*Year*
Mean	20808	415.3	88.77	942	24189	41416	7.087	8.25	16005.59	168411826	164.61	0.3	76.5	39.54
Minimum	401	5	0.90	–231	3	245	2.400	0.20	1.88	58212227	5.4	0.0	64.4	28.940
Median	13713	276.4	57.10	804	748	25311	5.900	7.80	5156.06	89600261	119.5	0.0	76	38.525
Maximum	127956	2907	771.90	7472	140621	259071	29.800	21.2	155191.23	2251696929	924.1	1.0	93.4	43.65
Standard deviation	22074	473.7	110	3081	36917	47244	4.094	4.27	27691.66	292411574	163.5	0.462	6.621	2.904

Appendix 2
Equation for MLR Models

(Models 1 – 8) $SMEj$, $ASMEj$, $SMEEj$, $SMEDifj$, $SMETj$, $SMEDj$, $SMEPCj$, $DSMEj = b0j + b1Lj + b2Uj + b3Ij + b4Cj + b5IEBj + b6HTWPj + b7REj + b8PEj + b9Aj + ej$,

SMEj is the activity of small- and medium-sized enterprises (SMEs) in Russian regions measured as the number of registered units in 2020. *ASMEj* is the number of working SMEs at the end of 2020. *SMEEj* is the number of people employed in SMEs in 2020. *SMEDifj* is the difference in the total number of SMEs between 2019 and 2020. *SMETj* is the total amount of regional revenue of all SMEs in 2020. *SMEDej* is the difference in the number of people employed in small firms between 2019 and 2020. *SMEPCej* is the share of SMEs per person in the Russian regions. *DSMEej* is the number of non-surviving SMEs of 2020. *Lj* is the total amount of loans granted to SMEs in 2020. *Uj* is the regional unemployment rate. *Ij* is the regional share of IT SMEs. *Cj* is the total regional business expenditures on IT. *IEBj* is investment for SMEs. *HTWPj* is the total workplaces in IT sphere. *REj* is the number of elections held at the regional level (this is the binary variable where 1 – if a region held election in 2020, 0 – otherwise). *PEj* is the percentage of votes for V.V. Putin in the 2018 presidential election. *Aj* is the average age of the regional inhabitants. *b1*, *b2*, *b3*, *b4*, *b5*, *b6*, *b7*, *b8*, and *b9* are the slopes, and the coefficients for influence of explanatory variables to study the relationship between these factors and response variables are traced. *ej* is a random error.

Appendix 3
The List of Supportive Anti-COVID-19 Legislative Measures for SMEs in Russia

Legislative measure[a]	*Description*
Suspension of penalties	For SMEs from affected industries, no collection measures will be applied for already formed tax arrears.
Reduced requirements for government contracts	The initial (maximum) contract price is increased from 1 to 5 million roubles, after which SMEs must provide security for bids from procurement participants.
Remote account opening for individual entrepreneurs and SMEs	SMEs can open a bank account without the personal presence of the person opening the account or his/her representative.
Renewal of licences and permits	Several licences and permits are automatically renewed, including production, turnover, and retail.
Tax exemption for SMEs and NPOs	SMEs from the industries most affected by the coronavirus epidemic are exempt from taxes, fees, and insurance premiums for the second quarter of 2020.
Tax exemption for SME subsidies	The possibility for SMEs not to consider subsidies received from the federal budget in the structure of income for the purposes of corporate income tax in connection with the unfavourable situation created by coronavirus.
Tax holidays (*industries impacted*)	SMEs in the affected industries may receive a deferral or instalment plan for taxes (advance payments), including insurance premiums, with due dates in 2020, except for VAT, MET, excise taxes, and tax on additional income from hydrocarbon production. Planned to be extended from three months to three years.
Tax reporting deadline	For all taxpayers, the deadlines for submitting reports to the Federal Tax Service are extended by up to three months from 2 April 2020.
Reduced insurance premiums	For SMEs, the aggregate rate of insurance premiums is reduced from 30 to 15% for the part of salaries that exceed the minimum wage during the month (12,130 roubles). The rate of insurance premiums for compulsory pension insurance will be 10%, for compulsory health insurance – 5%. Insurance contributions for compulsory social insurance in case of temporary incapacity for work and in connection with maternity are not paid.

(*Continued*)

(Continued)

Legislative measure[a]	*Description*
Lease deferral	Rent arrears for the grace period for SMEs are paid during 2021–2022, in equal monthly amounts. If the lessor refuses to comply with these requirements, the lessee has the right to go to court.
Moratorium on penalties for government contracts	Writing off the amounts of penalties accrued and unpaid under the state contract as a result of non-fulfilment of obligations under the state contract in connection with the spread of a new coronavirus infection.
Moratorium on tax sanctions for non-submission of documents	A moratorium on the application of tax sanctions for non-submission of documents, the deadline for submission of which falls on the period from 1 March 2020 to 30 June 2020.
Moratorium on on-site inspections	All on-site inspections are suspended, including tax and customs.
Moratorium on bankruptcy	The acceptance of bankruptcy petitions of the debtor by creditors is suspended. From the moment the moratorium is imposed, the debtor is not charged a penalty and sanctions for late payments.
Simplified requirements for SMEs to receive microloans and guarantees	The presence of overdue debts in taxes and fees is not a reason for refusing support. The term for existing microloans has been increased to five years. The conditions for providing support for the introduction of an emergency are as follows: commission – 0.5% per annum; the amount of security under the agreement will be 80%; newly issued microloans are granted for two years.
Credit vacation	Small- and medium-sized businesses from the affected sectors of the economy have the right, upon request, to receive a six-month grace period for any loan agreements concluded before 3 April.
Interest-free payday loans	Lending to SMEs from affected industries to pay salaries to employees. For the first six months, the rate on loans is 0%, and for the next six months, the rate is determined as the key rate of the Bank of Russia, reduced by 2 percentage points (currently – 3.5%).
Employment support loans	Enterprises from impacted industries can get a loan according to the formula: number of employees × minimum wage (12,130 roubles) × six months. The final rate for consumers will be 2%. The loan matures on 1 April 2021. Companies that retain at least 90% of their employees will not have to pay the loan along with interest.
Concessional lending	The conditions for granting loans at the final rate of 8.5% are softened. SMEs will be able to take advantage of the following options: interest 'holidays'; deferral of repayment of the principal; loan restructuring for three to ten months; a moratorium on the payment of interest and principal for a period of up to six months.
COVID-19 prevention subsidies	A subsidy that compensates for the costs of COVID-19 prevention is intended for 500,000 SMEs in the field of hospitality, personal services, catering, sports, and additional education. The size will be 15,000 roubles for initial expenses and another 6,5 thousand roubles for each employee in terms of headcount as of May 2020.

a Russian government (2020). Measures of the Russian government to combat coronavirus infection and support the economy, available online: http://government.ru/support_measures

7 Protest as an Appeal

How and Why Russians Struggled with Vaccinations in 2021

Aleksandra Rumiantseva, Alexandra Arkhipova, Irina Kozlova and Boris Peigin

Introduction

'*What Alexei Navalny*[1] *failed to do in Russia, people with syringes and illiterate medical propaganda did*', said a 45-year-old participant in protests against mandatory vaccinations and QR codes, which in the fall of 2021 affected at least 122 cities. In the fall of 2021, the Russian government (amid a spike in COVID-19 infections) decided to intensify the vaccination campaign and bring back restrictive measures, under which only those vaccinated or with a negative PCR test within the last three days could visit shopping centres, museums, and restaurants. To achieve this, the Russian government sent to the State Duma two bills: according to the first, mandatory QR codes should be introduced in public places (except for grocery stores and pharmacies), while the second established the procedure for using QR codes on planes and trains.

The huge protests appeared to be a response to these restrictions on rights and to government-mandated vaccinations. However, after the protests consideration of both bills was postponed[2] and subsequent policies did not improve the COVID-19 situation in Russia. New measures resulted in anger from ordinary citizens. These protests reflected an important idea for many Russians: the need to refuse or gently reject vaccination. According to polls conducted from February to July of 2021, 55–65%[3] of respondents said that they were not going to be vaccinated despite the fact that Russia was the first country to develop a vaccine (Sputnik V) against COVID-19 and that in autumn 2021, the daily death and infection rates were at their highest rate since the beginning of the pandemic.

So, the main aim of this chapter is to discover the real causes of this failure. Why were Russians dissatisfied with vaccines and how did Russians protest against obligatory vaccinations?

Design, Methods, and Materials of the Research

To uncover protesters' motivation and their perspectives on vaccination, we used a combination of quantitative and qualitative anthropological and sociological methods.

DOI: 10.4324/9781003364870-8

First of all, we collected several semi-structured interviews with people who participated in protests or were in activists' chats. Since the most prominent of the official (registered) political forces that supported the movement were from left-wing Russian political parties, we talked with members of the Communist Party of the Russian Federation (CPRF) and its youth sector – the Leninist Communist Youth Union (LCYU), to research their intentions to mobilise people against QR codes and vaccinations. Moreover, we talked with representatives from other non-systemic left-wing political forces such as the Russian Socialist Movement (RSD), Marxist Tendency (MT), Class Policy, and the New Reds. These groups all expressed their intentions to be vaccinated but with a bit more scepticism towards QR codes. Still, they did not join the protest against immunisation.

Second, we took several interviews with activists without party affiliations that protested against obligatory vaccination. To obtain a complete picture, we spoke with respondents from both sides, i.e., those who were against vaccination and those who kept a neutral position on COVID-19 restrictions and medical treatment. The interviews were collected from December 2021 to June 2022. In sum, we collected 16 interviews with people from Arkhangelskaya and Tumenskaya regions, as well as the federal cities Moscow and Saint Petersburg. More information about respondents can be found in the Appendix.

Finally, to gain a general picture of protests against QR codes and vaccination, we collected original data about protest events in Russia in 2021. Our data includes parameters such as date, geography, type of event, number of protesters, and persecution that followed the protest if any. We also collected information about the leaders of every action. In sum, we collected 287 unique events. As a source, we used social networks (both ones common for Russians like VKontakte, and more limited, like Facebook and YouTube) and regional social media. Our data covers 65 regions (out of 85, including Crimea and Sevastopol, which are under Russian annexation). Also, to analyse patterns of public protests, as additional material we transcribed texts from protesters' appeals on YouTube and other social platforms from November to December 2021.

This chapter proceeds as follows: First, we explain the reasons why the Russian vaccination campaign largely failed. Then, in section two, we describe our data on protest actions and show the main characteristics of dissent against QR codes. Finally, we explore the main actors of mobilisation.

The Failure of Vaccination in Russia, Past and Present

The lack of trust in vaccinations is not a new phenomenon in Russia. Doctors in the Soviet medical system interacted with parents like a parent with a stupid child. Children received part of mandated vaccine regimes initially in maternity hospitals and then partially in schools: vaccination sometimes took place in the medical offices of the state-run schools. It was not easy for parents to refuse vaccination: a doctor needed to be convinced by parents that vaccination was dangerous. The harsh, uncompromising nature of Soviet medicine and the almost complete deprivation of parents' agency in this matter led to an eventual backlash. Parents began to struggle against such pressure and attempted to regain agency as well as the right to decide for their children. Referencing stories about the dangers of vaccines – that they cause infertility – was just one strategy to rationalise not getting vaccinated. As a result, many parents from families of the Soviet intelligentsia (including families of doctors) quietly and imperceptibly tried to refuse vaccinations. Refusing vaccines has become a disguised privilege.

This form of 'medical dissent' was close to and sometimes combined with political dissent. In 2012, folklorist Andrea Kitta (2012) examined why so many educated people resist vaccination in Canada (even before vaccine-resistance became mainstream). She studied the attitudes of educated middle-class Canadians towards vaccinations. The conclusion she came to may seem surprising, but it explains a lot. In modern life, children are the highest value, and prosperous Canadians are anxious to become the right 'parents' from the moment of conception (and sometimes even earlier). In particular, anxious parents (who are not committed anti-vaccinators) try to study (mainly on the internet, of course) the arguments for and against vaccinations. They accumulate a large number of questions to potentially raise with healthcare providers in the process of discussing future vaccinations. As a rule, medical workers do not have the time and desire to explain why it is necessary to vaccinate a child here and now, so they start to intimidate parents. As a consequence, parents start to resist vaccines, half out of spite and half out of concern that there is an agenda. This case, described by Andrea Kitta, explains well Soviet and post-Soviet resistance to vaccines. The COVID-19 vaccine policy in Russia was very similar to such a strategy. It was inconsistent and lacked transparency. The obligatory form of vaccination only worsened societal trust in the Russian vaccine Sputnik V.

It is important to understand that the level of distrust in vaccines was high in Russia and the post-Soviet space well before 2020, a consequence of the abandonment of the Soviet legacy. Six months before the Sputnik vaccine appeared and vaccination began in Russia, two comparative surveys on the readiness to vaccinate were conducted in June 2020 (Lazarus et al. 2021). The first survey reveals that of the 20 countries surveyed, Russians gave the highest proportion (41%) of negative responses to the question of their future readiness to vaccinate. In November 2021, this number was still very high: 45% still didn't want to be vaccinated. This vaccine hesitancy is not only for COVID vaccines – it turns out that in Russia, only 48% of the population believe that *any* vaccines are safe, despite how almost 100% of the population is vaccinated against tuberculosis, diphtheria, and measles. This scepticism is characteristic of the entire post-communist world, albeit less so in the former Warsaw Pact countries than in the post-Soviet countries.

Since the beginning of the pandemic in Russia, there have been numerous infections, even accounting for the manipulations in open real-time data presented by official sources on the website 'StopCoronavirus.rf'.[4] The introduction of policies on self-isolation, mandated vacation days, and the first advent of a COVID-19 vaccine in the world did not help stop the spread of COVID-19 in Russia. The vaccination campaign began in Moscow in December 2020, followed by a nationwide campaign in January 2021. Nevertheless, it was unsuccessful, and by the beginning of Summer 2021, only about 11% of the population was vaccinated, while the government's target was from 20 to 60%. By October 2021, officials were forced to admit their failure. To increase the number of vaccinated citizens in the country, officials began an obligatory vaccination campaign.

The early problem with vaccines was the lack of accessibility. On one hand, foreign vaccines were not allowed to be used in Russia; on the other hand, Russian vaccines were not consistently available in all Russian regions. As a result, even if a person was ready to get vaccinated, it was sometimes impossible for him or her to do so. For those who wanted to get vaccinated only with a foreign vaccine, they would need to travel abroad, which was costly and almost impossible in the time of COVID-19. Furthermore, Russian officials have not approved foreign vaccines. The illegality of foreign vaccines created barriers to having a choice in vaccination and caused further dissatisfaction. For example, as one of our informants, a 39-year-old journalist Ivan reasoned:

> I think it is not right that we had problems with access to get vaccinated. I don't know how it is going now, but in spring, we definitely had a small deficit; there were lines at vaccine stations. At the same time, the state actively exported vaccines abroad, as we engaged in diplomacy, yes? They slowed down internal vaccination to show, 'we are cool; we can export our vaccine to a variety of other countries!' But from my point of view, it is not the right place for geopolitical considerations. I think people should have a choice, and vaccines should be from different manufacturers. – Respondent 5.

Nevertheless, what proved more critical was how the vaccine campaign in Russia was marked by inconsistent policy and a lack of clear information about the virus from the government. Altogether, it created ideal conditions for protest moods, scepticism, and rumours about COVID-19 and vaccination against it. Below we discuss the two most significant causes of the failure of the government's COVID-19 vaccination policy: lack of trust (*transparency*) and absence of choice (*obligation*).

Lack of Trust and Transparency

Russia registered three different vaccines, of which Sputnik V (Gam-COVID-Vac) was considered the most popular.[5] However, Sputnik did not receive official approval from international organisations and was not registered in most European countries and North America. Because of its lack of acceptance in international markets and a low level of trust in vaccines in general, Sputnik V did not gain widespread popularity among Russians.

The lack of trust was both in the vaccines and, critically, in the government pushing people to use them. Polls by the Levada Center showed a relationship between those who did not want to become vaccinated and those who did not trust the president.[6] People who shared this point of view believed that 'the Russian government cannot do anything well', 'they constantly deceive us, why should I believe them', and so on. Representatives of this group ('those who are afraid of Sputnik specifically') were often annoyed by the lack of vaccine alternatives ('why won't we be offered imported vaccines?'). Using experimental surveys, Boris Sokolov and Margarita Zavadskaya empirically showed the positive connection between COVID-19 scepticism and lack of trust in the government, medical system, and national institutes (Sokolov and Zavadskaya 2021). This point of view was expressed by Respondent 12:

I: If you are not vaccinated, for what reason?
R: *In short, it is out of distrust of products made in the Russian Federation (…) The vaccine is a difficult product to manufacture. I can't believe that it can be properly and in large quantities produced here, where there is no decent aspirin of its own.*
I: Are there other reasons for non-vaccination, besides mistrust of the authorities?
R: *Distrust of all the products here. There is no other reason. There is no question of 'power'. This is beyond the question of trust* […].
I: Are there any of your friends/relatives who will not be vaccinated? How do they explain this?
R: *Yes. The reasons are the same. The irritation from propaganda is so annoying.*
I: Would you be vaccinated with Pfizer?
R: *Yes. Pfizer, when it is for themselves, they will not cut corners but make sure it's good quality.*

The opinion ('you can trust Pfizer because that vaccine was made by people who are responsible for what they have done') is no coincidence. It arises from the perception of Russian society as initially corrupt. In October 2021, Russian sociologists from the 'GXPnews' company published the results of a study comparing attitudes towards vaccinations in different countries. According to this report, several factors influence attitudes towards vaccination: the number of cases (how scared the respondent was), the perception of society as corrupt (if the respondent thinks that everyone is stealing), and post-materialistic values (civil rights, including the rights of ethnic and social minorities, gender equality, the fight for the environment). If a person does not see sick people around him, he is not afraid of the disease. If he believes that everyone around is stealing and cheating, then he will not trust the vaccination process (because theft and corruption will occur there). And if in a society the struggle for civil rights is not very popular, then people in this society will think less about saving others and making decisions to be vaccinated. In Russia, there is a very low index of post-materialistic values (compared to the six other Western countries in the survey) and a very high index of perception of corruption (second only to Tajikistan), which leads to a high rate of refusal to vaccinate.[7]

Besides the generally low level of trust in government decisions, people constantly receive ambiguous information from state television and other sources of information. For example, Russian state media outlets often changed their positions regarding COVID-19 restrictions and vaccine safety. Russia Today (a state-controlled media in Russia broadcasting in different languages) published materials supporting vaccination in the Russian language and then opposite information for their broadcasts in other countries.

> First, our enemies were those, who supported the WHO, then our enemies were those who did not support them. They introduced restrictions inconsistently. They introduced restrictions but simultaneously held public events. People were nonplussed, and when people became completely freaked out (still interacted with each other and continued to infect each other at an alarming rate), further in aim to correct their own mistakes, they began to enter these QR codes [special restrictions]. But that was like flogging a dead horse. – Respondent 7.

Inconsistent policies on vaccinations were a continuation of uncertainty with general restrictions during the early days of COVID-19. In 2020, the state did not impose a formal lockdown or offer significant additional support for businesses and ordinary Russians. Instead of a lockdown, Russia declared non-working days, which were eventually cancelled because of the state's inability to continue to support paid holidays. At the same time, although the law officially banned all public events, pro-government events were held without special restrictions. In July 2020, a referendum was held on changes to the Constitution, even though the number of infections had not changed significantly.

> I'm rather annoyed because of the necessity to wear masks, although last year there were no serious sanitary norms. At least, the state did not actively enforce it. I mean, we had a lockdown last year, but rather not-at-all lockdown' in spring 2020. Then they hastily cancelled it, provided a referendum [on constitutional changes], and underestimated data on sickness and disease. They merely introduced inconsistent policies, which invoked such a distrust of vaccination. – Respondent 5.

Being inconsistent, Russian officials who were expected to prove vaccine safety only continued this vicious circle. From the beginning of the campaign, many famous and influential people in Russia showed their willingness to get vaccinated. For example, in March 2021, President Putin said he got vaccinated but did not specify by which vaccine. Moreover, this information was published in Russian sources without video materials, which led to scepticism about the reality of the event.

Finally, Russian propaganda also showed its aggressiveness towards citizens, which pushed people away from vaccination. For example, Saint Petersburg citizens complained about the billboards with pro-vaccination slogans. Billboards announced, 'How many people should die to get you vaccinated?' or 'vaccination saves our lives. Not taking care of yourselves, nearest and dearest, is madness!' People blamed the state for manipulation and use of guilt. These contradictive channels only decreased Russian citizens' willingness to participate in vaccination campaigns.

Obligatory Form

In November 2021, the government recognised the failure of the vaccination campaign and announced a resonant project that could have finally made COVID-19 vaccination compulsory. The first region that applied an obligatory vaccination was the city Moscow, followed immediately by the entire Moscow region (Moskovskaya Oblast). The central state's apparatus delegated authority to the regions to decide if they wanted to introduce new regulations or not. By November 2021, every Russian region published a Decree from its Chiefs Sanitary Doctor or its Office of Rospotrebnadzor (the federal consumer rights and well-being watchdog) except for Chukotka Autonomous Okrug.[8] As the documents stated, non-vaccinated people were prohibited from working in several industries, and all people without vaccines could not utilise public places. The *obligation* was that the list of jobs covered by the Decrees included almost all professions. For example, the list included people working in education, medicine, transport, entertainment, sport, and many others. In turn, enforcement was outsourced to the employers, who now had to ensure their worker's vaccination status within a certain period. If employees were not vaccinated on time, the company or the director had to pay a fine.

One of our respondents, Sergei, a 40-year-old worker from a railway station, blamed such a tactic for no transparency:

> For what reasons do sanitary doctors have such power? In the Decree, [the sanitary doctor] included transportation workers. Can you imagine how all these [rules] are blurred? And the energy sector. So, no real professions, nothing else, but transport and energy sectors – it is so easy [for them] to write anything. 'All workers should be vaccinated.' But *what* workers? You are a worker, you, you and you, that's all, please. There is no risk of mass infection, don't have contact with strangers. That's all. But in terms of this Decree, all without exceptions must be vaccinated. – Respondent 4.

To check that a person is vaccinated, the state introduced special codes – QR codes meant to be sent out within two weeks after vaccination. This instrument was widely used to control people and was received negatively by citizens with both pro and anti-vaccine positions. The code confirmed a person's vaccination status and allowed him or her to work and visit public spaces. Without the code, a person could be kicked out of these places. As a result, even pro-vaccine people were dissatisfied with vaccination and became more sceptical. One of the problems that was not considered before the QR codes' introduction was the lack of access to this electronic form among elderly people.

> I have heard about the case in Kazan and have read several articles and investigations about what happened there. There were large protests against QR codes because they merely could not solve the problem of public transport usage. People said, their elderly people used the transport. What are the QR codes there? They have no smartphones to use these codes! – Respondent 6.

Our respondents shared different perceptions of political engagement, but the main problem with the QR codes was their obligatory nature. While these respondents were not necessarily against vaccines, they needed to be free to make choices that were connected to their bodies.

> To be clear, I just don't want to live under the laws of a bandit state. I don't want to carry out requirements. I am not an anti-vaccine person and so on. – Respondent 2.

In some more extreme cases, respondents said they were not against the vaccine in general, but that they wanted to be more informed and did not want to be treated as if they were part of an experiment. For example, they wondered why the Russian vaccine did not pass formal tests from the WHO. They asked for equity and complained that other people ridiculed their fears and refusal to vaccinate. They say they are in the minority and should be protected like anyone else in Russia.

The obligatory forms of vaccination, in connection with a lack of trust, created a base for the anti-vaccine protest movement in Russia, in relatively new forms and with relatively new participants. These people were not politicised nor did they have activist experience: they protested because of a direct attack from the state on their bodies and lifestyle. The form and narratives of these protests are discussed below. Because of the protests, the bill that could make vaccination against COVID-19 obligatory stalled and ultimately has not been introduced. From January 2022, all regions gradually cancelled their obligatory vaccinations due to decreased COVID-19 cases.

Protest as an Appeal

Vernacular Risks of Protesting in Russia

In this section, we will talk about a very specific form that anti-vaxxist protest has taken in Russia; this form we call *protest as an appeal*. For a realistic assessment of the Russian protest activity, it is necessary to understand that the 'price of protest' in Russia has grown increasingly higher in the last 10 years. The infringement of the right to freedom of assembly began in the 2000s, when it became necessary to obtain the consent of local authorities in order to hold rallies and marches. Since 2012, the punishment for participating in an unsanctioned protest has steadily increased. Along with heavy fines, there have been numerous precedents since the so-called Bolotnaya case (2012) in which protesters faced criminal charges and prison sentences. In addition, the widespread introduction of video surveillance systems equipped with facial recognition technology in major Russian cities (primarily in Moscow and Saint Petersburg) has played a major role in the mass punishment of protesters. However, administrative and even criminal punishments are not the only means of influence on political activists in Russia: numerous cases are known of various threats made to them, such as the deprivation of parental rights, dismissal from work, etc. There are also known cases when political activists have been subjected to such 'pseudo-legal measures' as public apologies on video: as a rule, such videos are recorded at police stations to be rebroadcast on local TV news channels (Smirnova and Shedov 2020).

Gradually, this led to a perception that participation in any protest (political, social, environmental, feminist) was a kind of action which put both the marcher and his family at great risk. 'Why don't you come out to protest?' – 'Because I have children' is a typical excuse for not taking part in rallies that we have often heard in interviews recently.

The state media has gone to great lengths to shape negative attitudes towards protesters. They are portrayed in the federal channels as a small group of people who are always disgruntled, receive money from the West, and engage in suspicious activities. This attitude towards the protest has led to a perception of the protester as a freak, a marginalised person who is a threat to public tranquillity.

People who wanted to protest against QR codes and COVID-19 vaccinations had little or no experience with protest at all. Moreover, many of these protesters presented themselves in interviews as quite loyal people, and in order to reduce risks and avoid marginalisation, they invented a very specific way of public exposure. We call it a protest *as an appeal*.

The Geography of Anti-vaccination Protests

As we mentioned above in *Design and Methods*, we collected original data (287 unique protest events). The most protests appeared in the Sverdlovsk

Region (Ural Federal District), Moscow (Central Federal District), and Novosibirsk Region (Siberian Federal District). We detected more than ten protest events (45, 57, and 48, respectively) in these regions. These districts usually present a high level of dissent during protest movements, such as the campaigns in support of Alexey Navalny in 2017–2021, struggles against pension reform, or actions on local problems. Also, these regions (except Chelyabinsk) always show their protest potential during elections. In conjunction with the developed mobilisation networks, it is not surprising to see these regions at the top of the list with regard to COVID-19 vaccine actions.

To show their dissent, protesters usually chose official buildings (*local administrations*) or symbolic memorial places (monuments) for protests. We did not find any information about protest actions[9] during the first months of 2021. The first notable actions began in the summer of 2021 and peaked in November 2021 when the new law about QR codes was published. The most significant number of protests occurred between November and December when officials announced obligatory vaccinations. The median number of protesters is 20, but with time, the number of people disgruntled with the restrictions increased. In October and November 2021, most of the events attracted, on average, 30 people and, in some cases, even more than 100.

The Semi-digital Protest

People performed dissent both in traditional forms of protest such as meetings and pickets, as well as in new digital forms. Analysing the data, we identify pickets, meetings, and signature collection as traditional forms of protesting. In a variety of 'performances' (for example, religious ceremonies), we refer to a 'performative form'. Finally, we call a rather new type of protest that occurred partially on the internet *semi-digital protest* (Arkhipova et al. 2018). With the traditional forms of protest, the last one also became popular (see Figure 7.1).

A *semi-digital protest* is a form of protest in which people gather together, record video with their protest appeal and after that post pictures or videos of their demands on the Internet. Sometimes, a protester can take a selfie with the protest sign even at home and post it on his social networks with a comment.

This form of protest has become popular in Russia over the past five years, and became visible to observers in 2018–2019, when an environmental protest erupted in the Russian North (around a place called Shies). In Shies, local authorities decided to place a large toxic waste dump, and local residents began to actively protest against the construction of the landfill. Their main instrument of expression was somehow a semi-digital protest, formally made as an appeal from the villagers to the local authorities or to Putin.

This form of protest is popular for two reasons. First, there are fewer risks for protesters, and second, protesters do not need to spend extensive resources to participate (time, travel costs, etc.). Someone may launch a flash

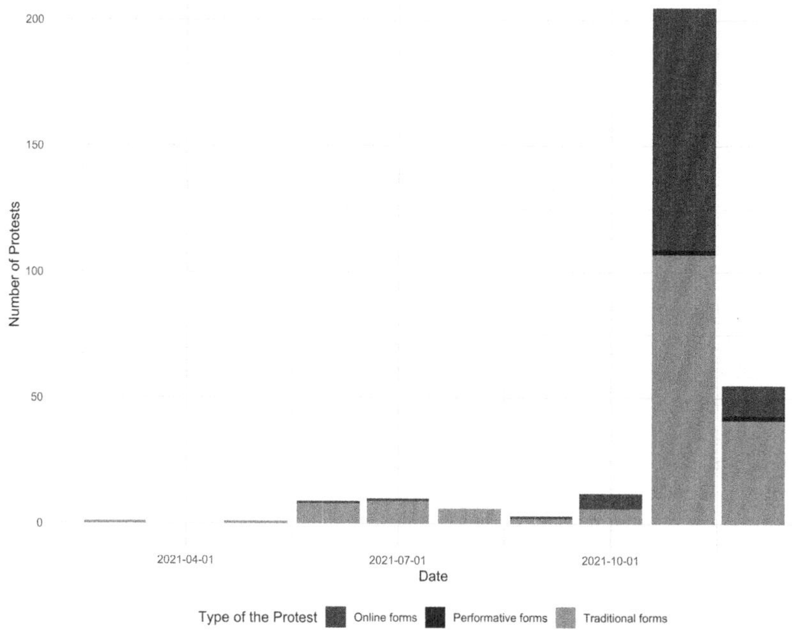

Figure 7.1 Protest format dynamics in 2021.

mob on the internet or record a special message and post it on YouTube or another popular social platform.

Protest and Appeal

The most frequent type of anti-vaccination protest in 2021 was formally an official appeal. A group of around 30 people gathered near a special sign of their city and recorded a statement. Usually, there are three speakers accompanied by other supporters in the near vicinity. Every message is addressed to a specific *addressee*. An essential characteristic of semi-digital protests is the possibility for the message to be sent to a concrete recipient with whom the citizens want to share their dissent and ask for attention to the problem (Arkhipova et al. 2018).

For example, people addressed 'our citizens and countrymen', regional officials, and even the president. Through these messages, citizens tried to attract other people's attention to the threat that may be caused by QR codes and obligatory vaccinations. In their opinion, QR codes invoked segregation that could lead to a clash in Russian society. The second problem for them was a 'clear manipulation' of society and the advent of experimentation on people. As a document that proves their opinion, they cite the Constitution, especially Articles 17 and 21. Article 17 emphasises the importance of human rights and freedom and also states that the state must guarantee these rights to every person in the Russian Federation. In turn, Article 21 affirms that 'nobody should be subjected to violence and torture' as well as be subjected to any medical or scientific experiments.[10]

This decision to cite the Constitution and other official documents to support their position highlights that the argumentation was intended for a specific audience that these citizens appealed to for help. As a guarantor of the Russian Constitution, Vladimir Putin has been perceived as a leader who should protect citizens from other officials who abuse power. For example, protesters from one of the cities in Bashkortostan finished their appeal with the following request:

> We are citizens from Neftekamsk, and we demand from you a stop to the illegal actions of the government of the Russian Federation, regional heads, Russian Consumer Supervision (Rospotrebnadzor), and a re-establishment of rights and freedoms on the territory of the Russian Federation. We demand you to hold governors and officials accountable for their abuse of power, for the social tension created, and for peoples' segregation![11]

Since COVID-19 policy implementation was transferred from Moscow to regional governments, it was easier to blame local officials. As a result, anger and blame were directed at regional officials and the president remained trusted. For example, a 40-year-old worker from a railway station said:

> After all, we have heard, yes, the president very often likes to repeat that there should be no compulsory vaccination, everything is voluntary, and so on. You need to be able to persuade people – these are his words. And on the ground, we feel that local officials either do not hear or ignore them. – Respondent 4.

As a result, protesters blamed only regional officials but not the president, and therefore, their appeal seemed to be not a protest but a special call for attention. This made them not even protesters, but a loyal part of the population that asked their president to help them in their struggle with iniquity. The popularity of appeals to officials may point out the avoidance of a real protest. People wanted to show their dissent without using traditional forms of the term 'protest'. Instead, they wanted 'to ask' the president and other people to see their problems and not be punished because of their request. They seek to find the most unpolitical and loyal way to show their dissent. At the same time, some people showed an absence of trust in all politicians in the country. In this case, they appeal to friends or fellow citizens. Since the pension reform, the approval rating of Vladimir Putin decreased by ten points[12] and the pandemic only worsened the situation.

At the same time, a uniform attitude of politically active citizens towards video appeals was ambiguous. Some of our respondents from activist or party-based circles were highly sceptical about such formats of protest against vaccination. They said it was similar to an appeal but did not yet qualify as resistance.

> Video appeals are good, but they shouldn't send a petition to the King (Tsar'). Because all of them begin with 'Dear Vladimir Vladimirovich', help us, we are under pressure, we are forced. I don't get on those well. – Respondent 1.

Another problem with online forms of protest was the absence of proof that the addressee actually received the message. This undermines the whole idea and rationality of creating and posting appeals on the internet.

> I will say it to you another time, I am not sure the president receives these appeals. I mean, whether he really watches them. His secretary or apparatus, I don't know, how it works. – Respondent 4.

Low Level of Civil Values

What is more important, protesters who participated in anti-vaccine meetings were in most cases without activist experience and do not have a strong identity as members of civil society. To investigate this supposition, we compared the sum of donations and appeals for the help that OVD-Info publishes every month in their reports.

OVD-Info[13] is a large human rights project that helps detainees from political protests in two ways: it provides extensive information about civil rights, and it raises money for lawyers. As a rule, in the last few years the number of OVD-Info's donations has grown in parallel with the number of detentions during political rallies. This is due to the fact that there are so many people in Russia who are afraid to go to political rallies but are willing to help those who are not afraid to go (Arkhipova, Zakharov, and Kozlova 2021).

In the autumn of 2021, people began to be detained at anti-vaxxing protests, and we would expect the number of references to human rights instructions from OVD-Info to increase as well as the number of donations. But it turned out that while the number of appeals increased significantly in November 2021, the sum of donations was constant. Also, the number of people who read legal instructions was constant, whereas the number of calls on the urgent line increased significantly in November compared with other months (see Figure 7.2). In sum, we can suppose that this increase includes protesters against QR codes and vaccinations, but these people are new to the system, so they are unfamiliar with the instructions and are not ready to donate to NGOs such as OVD-Info working in this field. In other words,

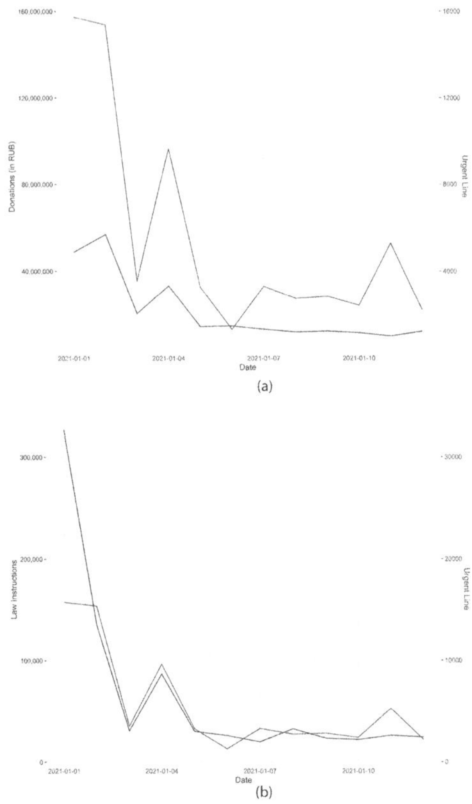

Figure 7.2 a,b Relationship between law instructions uploaded or donations and calls to the urgent line.

Source: OVD-Info[20]

when vaccination opponents were detained, they rushed for legal aid but were far less willing to engage in civil rights education and even less willing to help other detainees. This shows that they were not aware of themselves as a community.

An RSD activist commented on this new wave of protesters:

> [They] did not notice these [the rise of repressions], and it was comfortable to live with it. The regime is getting tougher, but we have some autonomy. But these long-understood and long-existing things have come to the surface in this pandemic. And people didn't like it. But, by and large, this is nothing new and, in general, with attacks on rights and freedoms and surveillance systems, it was worth discussing all these things earlier and worrying about them earlier. – Respondent 5.

For the first time, the reaction from the regime was relatively calm: we did not notice any detentions or fines before June. The increase in repressiveness against protesters began with the rise of mobilisation. The first cases of intersection between the police and citizens appeared in summer and the peak matched the peak of the protest activities in November. However, the police did not use harsh penalties for anti-vaccine protesters. We revealed only one criminal proceeding, whereas the other cases were limited to administrative deals, warnings from the police, or fines. The average number of detainees or fined people was one or two. The average fine was from 10 to 20 thousand roubles (147–294 euros), similar to all cases connected with Article 20.2. In sum, there were only 43 cases out of 287 where we found any type of punishment (fine or detention), which seems low compared to the regime's reaction to other uprisings. In contrast to the Navalny Team[14] and other political activists' situation, the regime did not seek to use coercive measures to destroy the movement against QR codes.

To sum up, *semi-digital protest* seemed to be a preferred format for those people who most likely did not have previous activist experience. They were not involved in organisational networks and did not know how to express their grievances. As a result, they see an appeal to the president as the only way to attract attention.

Incohesive Opposition

In most cases, the protests looked like popular gatherings without mobilisation processes. However, in 32% of cases (92 out of 287), the protests were organised by two main forces: political (partisan) forces or local activists and conspiracy communities. Below we describe each of the players to show why they failed to unite to increase their chances of protesting against obligatory vaccination.

Conspiracy Communities

The leading players in this group are conservative far-right forces. These movements are known for their high level of loyalty to the state and orthodox views. They created special channels in a Russian social network named Telegram where they published messages against vaccination or spread rumours about COVID-19. Anti-vaccine supporters and some influencers created different channels and chats to spread information about vaccines and COVID-19 precautions. Some of them began to promote the anti-vaccine movement on existing channels. For example, one of the far-right communities, Sorok Sorokov, changed its usual theme and started to post content with an anti-vaccine agenda. In August 2022, the median number of people on such channels was around 50,000, where the minimum was 20,000, and the maximum was 130,000. One of the private blogs where the information against vaccines was posted – Maria Shukshuna's channel – had an audience of around 330,000 people. According to Medialogia,[15] audiences for the most popular private blogs and news channels were of around 2 and 2.5 million, respectively. The most notable are 'Sorok Sorokov', 'Immune Answer', and 'All-Russia Parent Resistance'. Their audience, on average, was from 50,000 to 100,000 people. Sticking to a radical position, they constantly speak about the vaccine's threats, shifting from provocative messages to conspiracy narratives. For example, they actively developed rumours about a global conspiracy against the world population to build a new world government and diminish the population by up to 1 million people. In a situation of high uncertainty, people were ready to believe this information or at least share it. As one respondent told us:

> All this is not a vaccine that we used in the 80s and 90s when we were young. Now the situation is completely different: Extermination has already begun. And every war is cyclic; everything is severe. We have no time. – Respondent 2.

Using a very belligerent narrative, they were ready to fight against vaccinations physically. For example, one of the channels stated: 'Who will touch my kid with this vaccine will not be ready even to regret it! Sanitary doctors, think twice about this!'.[16]

At the beginning of 2022, some channels were deleted, and a few begun to support the Russian war of aggression against Ukraine. For example, Sorok Sorokov changed their name to Zorok Zorokov. Despite their loyalty to the president, all groups with pro-antivaccine positions faced oppression from the state. Their supporters were detained and prosecuted for spreading 'fakes news'. At the same time, Russian 'anti-fake laws' were seriously tightened precisely after the start of the COVID-19 epidemic. Starting from April 2020, in addition to administrative liability for the dissemination of fake news,[17] criminal liability was also introduced[18] (Arkhipova and Peygin 2021).

In sum, such forces retained a loyal position to the president, blaming only the government, Dmitriy Medvedev, or regional elites for unpopular decisions. Moreover, they pushed gratitude for Vladimir Putin between messages with aggression against the state.

Left-Wing Forces

Another essential factor in the anti-vaccine arena was left-wing forces, especially the Communist Party (CPRF). They served a more neutral position than conspiracy groups and tried to avoid a union with them. Moreover, they rejected identification with them, citing their radical position. As one of the CPRF members told us in the interview:

> If I am not mistaken, they are hard anti-vaxxers. I don't remember exactly, but there was something obscurantist. That's why I am trying to stay away from

> them. We know all of them. We also tried not to communicate with them, although they are interested in uniting with us. – Respondent 3.

As CPRF stated, they did not have a strong position against vaccination and QR codes. Instead, they tried to highlight support for protests against restrictions under constitutional liberties. Such ambiguity annoyed other left-wing forces. One respondent from a left-wing activist circle told us:

> What is interesting is their position was tricky: they have never told they were against vaccinations on the whole or on the level of the organization. They said they were against obligatory vaccinations. But from ordinary people's point of view, it was like 'if I can be not vaccinated, I would prefer not to do this.'. – Respondent 8.

Lacking a strict position about vaccinations, members of the party should individually decide whether to be vaccinated or not. Some of our respondents told us they simultaneously were vaccinated and mobilised people against vaccination. Explaining their position, they addressed sympathy for people whose decision has been considered unpopular. Another tactic to substantiate their protest was obtaining the support of this new electorate. That was a primary cause that other left-wing forces cited for why they were not ready to unite with CPRF and blame them for the populism.

> In fact, if we take CPRF and other leftist groups, they decided to hype up this obscurantism of several backward segments of the population. Instead of educating or explaining why vaccination is the right choice, they merely participated in protest actions against obligatory vaccination. – Respondent 8.

Continuing their success after the State Duma elections, CPRF pretended to reflect the interest of the broad masses without sharing a clear position. They had no central agenda for vaccination policy. All questions connected with protest events, sharing information against QR codes, or signature collection were resolved locally. To show loyalty to the ruling party, the leader of the CPRF, Gennadii Zyuganov, was vaccinated, but at the same time, did not restrict mobilisation against vaccinations inside the party.

> The party is not as centralised as someone could want, and it shares different population segments. Anti-vaccine supporters were a large group. That's why some politicians, including those from Moscow, decided to express this position and organise events for them. So, they gained their support. You may be surprised, but we have a relatively pluralistic vision in the party. In the borders of this pluralism, different situations are permissible. I will say it like this… The central committee did not pass protest actions; this is very local. But we have this local activity. – Respondent 9.

Moreover, to save their position of loyalty, Communist Party members sought to play by the rules. They followed COVID-19 restrictions and did not lead protest events: they merely organised 'meetings' with their voters and supporters. However, communists also faced repression from the state. This occurred not only when the level of their protest activity increased, but also earlier, at the beginning of the movement. This persecution could be connected with the pre-electoral campaign and overall campaign against communists before the elections for State Duma[19] positions. For example, some party members explained the attacks against one of the most popular CPRF deputies – Valerii Rashkin – as part of an information war against the party. To sum up, despite CPRF's caution during the development of anti-vaccine and QR code protests and their ambivalent actions and lack of a strict position, they also faced repression.

However, support for the anti-vaccination movement has helped the CPRF acquire new party members. Answering the question, 'Did the party manage to attract new supporters on the wave of these protests?' one of our respondents from CPRF commented:

> Well, yes, I believe. Those who were our supporters, they stayed, and they probably attracted more, yes. At least they come to us and we work all the time. I wouldn't say for sure if that was the reason for the growth of the ranks. Yes, they joined and we had an increase, but I can't say it was specifically due to distant regime and COVID-19, we also have other protests. – Respondent 10.

Support for anti-vaccination protesters, despite the fact that it caused an information war against the party and a repressive response from the regime, was also one of the reasons the party was successfully represented in the elections.

> Well, of course, our position played on the party's reputation. Because one of the litmus tests of the organization was the elections in September 2021. In which we received more support than in the previous elections. And we think that our activity on this topic also had an impact on the result. Not only that, but it was one of them. – Respondent 11.

Despite the common goals in the fight against vaccinations, both actors (conspiracy communities and left-wing forces) shared very different values. This led to the inability to combine efforts in mobilisation against mandatory vaccination.

Conclusion

In this text, we traced how vaccination policies were implemented in Russia and identified why they could not be defined as successful. The main reasons we identified were post-Soviet Russia's social and political struggle with the overall value of vaccines, a lack of open information about vaccines, the inaccessibility of timely and equally vaccine supplies across Russia, and the fluctuation of government policies between optional and required vaccinations. The latter reason caused a surge of discontent among Russian citizens and led to a wave of anti-vaccination protests.

Most of the protests involved people who were not politically active until 2021 – before COVID-19 and the introduction of compulsory vaccinations. We attribute this to the fact that the introduction of restrictions first affected people physically, placing restrictions on their ability to travel or work. Such restrictions proved to be most tangible in daily life and caused anger.

A lack of experience with activism influenced the form of protest. Protest, in addition to traditional forms such as assemblies, included numerous appeals. Through appeals published on social networks, people asked decision-makers to address their concerns and reassess the mandatory vaccination policy. On the one hand, the authorities' rejection of rallies and marches is explained by the fact that at the time of the protest wave, there were still restrictions on freedom of assembly, which were complemented by the general repressiveness of the regime. On the other hand, people who participated in these vaccine protests sought not so much to protest violently as to draw public and political attention to certain problems. As a result, the protest looked more like an *appeal* than an explosion of discontent.

At the organisational level, these protests were supported by various forces, including non-opposition ones. Among the leaders were various far-right channels as well as representatives of leftist forces. Extreme right-wing forces, known for their conservative values and extreme loyalty to the authorities, acted aggressively, refusing forced vaccinations. In turn, the left-wing forces, mainly representatives of the Communist Party, protested with restraint, offering alternatives to the official government policy. Even though the Communist Party never clearly articulated an official position against required vaccinations at their leadership level, opposition against compulsory vaccinations became an unofficial part of their agenda. Despite their common goals, the overly different views of these two coordinating forces led to fragmented protests. Those fighting against compulsory vaccination fought among themselves and were not ready to unite.

Although these protests can be considered successful, since the law on compulsory vaccination never came into force, it was unsuccessful from a long-term perspective. First, the protest did not leave behind any new organisational networks or protest experience despite the involvement of citizens who had not previously participated in activism. Second, protests were characterised by a high loyalty to the president, who was not the target of growing discontent. This was largely because protests were made against regional officials and chief doctors. Finally, the law on compulsory vaccinations was defeated mainly because of a new agenda: the outbreak of a full-scale Russian invasion of Ukraine, which diverted attention from the regime's internal problems to external threats.

Funding

Aleksandra Rumiantseva acknowledges funding by the U.S. Russia Foundation, Hans Koschnik Special Scholarship.

Notes

1 Alexey Navalny is a well-known Russian politician. In 2013, he ran second in the Moscow mayoral elections. In 2018, he was nominated for president of the Russian Federation, but was not approved as a candidate. The rejection of Navalny's candidacy and his famous film 'He is Not a Demon to You' ('On vam ne Dimon') sparked massive street protests in Moscow, Saint Petersburg, and other major Russian cities. In January 2021, Navalny was arrested and on 2 February was sentenced to prison for two years and eight months. Navalny's arrest sparked new mass street protests. In 2022, new charges were brought against Navalny, and on 22 March, he was sentenced to nine years in prison in a strict regime colony (taking into account the time already served).
2 The bills were sent to the State Duma on 12 November 2021, and their consideration was postponed until 14 January 2022.
3 Vaccination, Levada Center. Link to the source: https://www.levada.ru/2021/08/09/vaktsinatsiya/.
4 Operational Data, StopCoronovirus.rf. Link to the source: https://xn--80aesfpebagmfblc0a.xn--p1ai/.
5 Produced by Gamalei Institution in Russia.
6 Coronavirus, vaccinations and mandatory vaccinations, Levada Center. Link to the source: https://www.levada.ru/2021/07/05/koronavirus-privivki-i-obyazatelnaya-vaktsinatsiya/.
7 "Trust in authority or informed choice? What Really Affects Vaccination Rates", GXP-News. Link to the source: https://gxpnews.net/2021/10/doverie-k-vlasti-ili-soznatelnost-naseleniya-chto-na-samom-dele-vliyaet-na-tempy-vakczinaczii/.
8 Chukotka is a Russian region located in the Far East. Officials did not provide the official documents because of the low number of cases correspondingly arising from the low number of people living there.
9 We searched protest actions in social networks and also used Mediology sources to find the data.
10 Russian Constitution, Chapter 2: Human and Civil Rights and Freedoms.
11 The video message was removed from YouTube for violating community rules.
12 Government approval, Levada Center. Link to the source: https://www.levada.ru/indikatory/odobrenie-organov-vlasti/.
13 https://en.ovdinfo.org/.
14 During the protests against Navalny's arrest in January–February 2021 were arrested around 11,000 people, more than 9,000 cases of administrative offenses were initiated, and 90 criminal cases were opened. Source: 'Crackdown on peaceful protests in January–February 2021 in Russia'. OVD-Info. Link to the source: https://english.ovdinfo.org/winter-2021-supression-en.
15 Telegram-Channels: July 2022, Mediologia. Link to the source: https://www.mlg.ru/ratings/socmedia/telegram/11361/.
16 Message from the channel Zorok Zorokov Movement: https://t.me/sorok40russia.
17 Article 13.15 of the Code of Administrative Offenses.
18 Article 207.1 of the Criminal Code.
19 State Duma elections were held in Russia on 17–19 September 2021.

20 We took the data from monthly reports that OVD-Info mails to their donators. These reports include information about the donations amount and the size of work that had been done by the organisation during the given month.

References

Arkhipova, Alexandra S., and B. S. Peygin. 2021. "Ministry of truth: How the Russian state fights fake news during the COVID-19 pandemic." *Steps* 7, no. 4: 124–150.

Arkhipova, Alexandra S., Daria A. Radchenko, Alexey S. Titkov, Irina V. Kozlova, Elena F. Yugai, Sergey V. Belyanin, and Maria V. Gavrilova. 2018. "«Rally rebuild»: Internet in protest and protest on the internet." *Monitoring of Public Opinion: Economic and Social Changes* 1: 12–35.

Arkhipova, Alexandra S., Alexey. V. Zakharov, and Irina V. Kozlova. 2021. "The ethnography of protest: Who participated – and why – in the rallies of 2021." *Monitoring of Public Opinion: Economic and Social Changes* 5: 289–323. https://doi.org/10.14515/monitoring.2021.5.2032.

Kitta, Andrea. 2012. *Vaccinations and Public Concern in History: Legend, Rumor, and Risk Perception*. London: Routledge.

Lazarus, Jeffrey V., Scott C. Ratzan, Adam Palayew, Lawrence O. Gostin, Heidi J. Larson, Kenneth Rabin, Spencer Kimball, and Ayman El-Mohandes. 2021. "A global survey of potential acceptance of a COVID-19 vaccine." *Nature Medicine* 27, no. 2: 225–228.

Smirnova, Nastya., and Denis Shedov. 2020. "Suppression of Peaceful Assembly in Russia from 2015 to 2020: From a Coalition of Human Rights Organizations, Report for the United Nations Human Rights Committee." OVD-Info. https://en.ovdinfo.org/suppression-peaceful-assembly-russia-2015-2020#6.

Sokolov, Boris O., and Margarita A. Zavadskaya. 2021. "Socio-demographic profiles, personality traits, values, and attitudes of COVID-skeptics in Russia." *Monitoring of Public Opinion: Economic and Social Changes* no. 6: 410–435. https://doi.org/10.14515/monitoring.2021.6.1938.

Appendix

Information about Respondents

Respondent 1: Ilya, 18 years old. He is receiving a bachelor's degree (1 course) and lives in Arkhangelsk. Having no party affiliation, he actively protested against QR codes in his city.

Respondent 2: Viktor, 35 years old. He works in the Internet as a freelancer (not IT sector) and has primary education (he finished nine school classes). He lives in Arkhangelsk. He has no party affiliation. Having a very strong position against vaccination, he did not actively protest against QR codes and vaccination.

Respondent 3: Vladislav, 24 years old. He received a master's degree in Political Science at Saint Petersburg State University. He lives in Saint Petersburg and is a member of Communist Party of the Russian Federation (CPRF) and Leninist Communist Youth Union (LCYU).

Respondent 4: Sergey, 40 years old. He works on the railroad and had training in radio technics. He lives in Kotlas (Arkhangelskaya Region) and is a member of CPRF.

Respondent 5: Ivan, 39 years old. He works as a journalist and received a master's degree in History. He lives in Saint Petersburg and an activist in Russian Socialist Movement (RSD).

Respondent 6: Valeria, 39 years old. She works as an accountant and received a master's degree in Pedagogy. She lives in Saint Petersburg and is an activist in RSD.

Respondent 7: Igor, 33 years old. He works as a researcher and received a master's degree in Philology. He lives in Saint Petersburg and is an RSD activist.

Respondent 8: Maria, 32 years old. He works as a researcher and received a master's degree in Biology. He lives in Saint Petersburg and is a Marxist Tendency activist.

Respondent 9: Stepan, 33 years old. He works in construction and received a master's degree in Education. He lives in Saint Petersburg and is a Marxist activist (movement 'Class Politics').

Respondent 10: Tatiana, 56 years old. She lives in Tumen and is an assistant deputy. She received a master's degree in Engineering and has a CPRF membership.

Respondent 11: Dmitriy, 22 years old. He lives in Saint Petersburg and is receiving a master's degree. He has an affiliation with CPRF and LCSM.

Respondent 12: Alexander, 58 years old, is an artist and lives in Moscow.

8 The State Failing People's Expectations

Resentment at the Pandemic Policy in Belarus and Kazakhstan

Kristiina Silvan and Shugyla Kilybayeva[1]

Introduction

In spring 2020, the world watched with dismay as Aleksandr Lukashenka, Belarus's authoritarian president, dismissed the threat posed by COVID-19, praised home remedies from vodka to saunas, and stubbornly refused to shut down his country. On the other side of the post-Soviet space, Kazakhstan, headed by Kassym-Jomart Tokayev, reacted as early as January 2020 by imposing national measures in response to the COVID-19 pandemic. These ranged from border closures to severe social distancing measures. Unlike in Belarus, the spread of the disease was effectively halted in Kazakhstan (Jones and King 2021). Yet, the success was both controversial and temporary. Policy not only generated an economic and social crisis that the government struggled to manage, but also failed to prevent a peak in COVID-19 cases once restrictions were lifted in May 2020.

This chapter asks what changes – if any – took place in state-society relations during the first year of the COVID-19 pandemic in the post-Soviet region. It applies a comparative framework to examine government responses and citizen reactions to them in Belarus and Kazakhstan, two post-Soviet states with consolidated authoritarian regimes, from January 2020 until January 2021. The comparative approach is particularly suitable given a puzzle that emerged during data collection. Despite polar opposite COVID-19 policies adopted by Belarusian and Kazakhstani policymakers, citizens in both states were equally dissatisfied with the response of their respective governments – namely, the seemingly insufficient support to those in need. Addressing this key puzzle, the chapter argues that in both Belarus and Kazakhstan, this dissatisfaction was exacerbated by the dissonance between the COVID-19 policy response and the governments' pre-existing legitimisation narratives that dubbed Belarus as a 'socially oriented' and Kazakhstan as a 'listening' state that was also supportive of small- and medium-sized enterprises (SMEs). In the shifting political opportunity structures, mounting popular grievances accelerated citizens' involvement in new forms of grassroots activism as people self-organised in order to prevent the spread of the virus.

DOI: 10.4324/9781003364870-9

However, the political aftermath of the pandemic crisis was different in Belarus and Kazakhstan. While the perceived COVID-19 policy failure of the government and the emergence of a newly energised civil society paved the way for a political crisis in Belarus during the unpredictably competitive presidential election of August 8 (Charnysh 2020), Kazakhstan's uncontested Majilis election of January 2021 was marked by widespread apathy, typical for parliamentary elections organised in closed authoritarian settings (Bohr 2021). However, it could be argued that popular discontent regarding the management of the COVID-19 pandemic as well as a more general disappointment with President Tokayev's leadership contributed to the emergence of a subsequent political crisis in January 2022.

A comparative analysis of Belarusian and Kazakhstani COVID-19 responses and citizen reactions enables us to examine the transformation of state-society relations in the authoritarian political context during the first year of the pandemic. Data for this analysis were collected through semi-structured expert interviews, systematically collected media accounts, and survey data. The chapter then relies on a general pandemic periodisation, dividing the analysis into three temporal sections: spring, summer, and autumn 2020. In the spring of 2020, Kazakhstan imposed a strict lockdown, while Belarus did the exact opposite. Neither policy met the expectations of the people. In Kazakhstan, this was due to the limited social policy response during the lockdown (Greer et al. 2021) and popular dissatisfaction with the state crisis management in the summer of 2020. In Belarus, it was the contrast to other states' approaches that raised concern. Civil society actors and members of the political opposition were able to capitalise on popular grievances, and thus, the political opportunity structures of each country – understood in the framework of this chapter as the 'aspects of the political system that affect the possibilities that challenging groups have to mobilise effectively' (Giugni 2011, 271) – shifted against the government.

The empowerment of regime challengers was faster and more pronounced in Belarus than in Kazakhstan. This could be explained by the fact that the Kazakh regime entered a somewhat less repressive – and less welfare-oriented – phase after the mid-2010s. In the summer of 2020, public resentment that had been mounting in Belarus over the years found a political outlet in the upcoming presidential election. In Kazakhstan, in contrast, the failure of state management during the peak of COVID-19 cases (Ybrayev 2020) prompted an analogous grassroots mobilisation that Belarus experienced already in the spring. Like in Belarus, civil society did not appear out of nowhere but had roots in the political and social activation of previous years. Finally, in the autumn, Belarusians took to the streets to challenge the results of the rigged election. The popular uprising was crushed by the government's campaign of mass repression and torture, in which newly introduced COVID-19 regulations were instrumentalised.

In Kazakhstan, some health policy measures were reintroduced to curb the spread of a new wave in the autumn of 2020. In the run-up to the January

2021 parliamentary and local elections, state authorities managed to turn the political opportunity structure in their favour by postponing political reforms and limiting room for independent electoral observation. In this setting, the low voter turnout in the January 2021 parliamentary election (63.3%, the lowest since 1999 (Hewitt 2021)) is explained by the lack of genuine political competition. The OSCE assessed that 'while five parties participated in the electoral process, and their candidates were able to campaign freely, limits imposed on the exercise of constitutionally guaranteed fundamental freedoms restrict the political space' (OSCE 2021). What is more, President Tokayev succeeded in retaining the legitimacy narrative that portrayed him as the constructor of a new 'listening' state, while shifting the blame for pandemic mismanagement on the former minister of health and regional governors. Taken in combination, the first year of COVID-19 highlighted failures in political accountability in both Belarus and Kazakhstan, which in turn contributed to the governments' legitimacy further eroding.

COVID-19 as a Challenge to Performance-Based Legitimation Narratives in Belarus and Kazakhstan

Now that the initial global shock of the COVID-19 pandemic has arguably passed, it is possible to study the political implications of the first phase of the pandemic, which lasted from the emergence of the virus in December 2019 until the beginning of the mass vaccination campaign in the spring of 2021. Given that the virus administered a shock to every political system in the world, it is not surprising that the pandemic led to the emergence of an entirely new subfield in Social Sciences (Greer et al. 2021; Laruelle et al. 2021). In the introduction to this book, the pandemic is conceptualised as an exogenous shock that reshaped political opportunity structures. It is hypothesised that the pandemic increasingly shifted control of political, media, economic, and administrative resources to the state, thus strengthening authoritarian tendencies. However, as this chapter suggests, in both Belarus and Kazakhstan, it was the challengers of the authoritarian governments – pro-democracy political experts, activists, and ordinary citizens – that were able to improve their access to political resources. The process was facilitated by the challengers' ability to capitalise on an increasingly omnipresent social media and – especially in the case of Belarus – economic resources generated in the private sector, particularly the booming IT industry. We argue that a shifting of resources against the government in both Belarus and Kazakhstan was rooted in each governments' inability to live up to their legitimation narratives. People's dissatisfaction with the respective governments' inability to live up to their promises generated resentment, which the governments' challengers in turn managed to reframe to their advantage.

In order to ensure the survival of their regime, contemporary authoritarian rulers do not rely solely on co-optation and repression, but also seek to justify their hold on power by employing a variety of legitimation narratives

(Omelicheva 2016; Gerschewski 2018; Nathan 2020). Von Soest and Grauvogel (2017) argue that performance-based legitimation strategies, i.e. narrating purported success as a means of proving the state's role in providing material welfare and security to its citizens, are most prominent in non-democratic societies that cannot tap into free and fair popular elections as a source of political power. However, given that especially the most successful legitimation strategies are dynamic and ever-changing, there is an active debate on how, to what extent, and with what effects non-democratic rulers legitimise their rule (Dukalskis and Gerschewski 2017, 252). This chapter applies the definition of du Boulay and Isaacs who define legitimation 'as a series of claims by the regime regarding their appropriateness to rule which are then transformed through social action which then produces legitimacy' (du Boulay and Isaacs 2019, 17). Having a successful legitimation strategy is one of the components of a political opportunity structure that favours authoritarian incumbents rather than their challengers.

Like many other authoritarian leaders, both Alyaksandr Lukashenka in Belarus and Kassym-Jomart Tokayev in Kazakhstan employed various social welfare-related narratives to legitimise their rule in the pre-COVID-19 era. In Belarus, Lukashenka promised to preserve the Soviet model of a socialist welfare state once he came to power in 1994 and used the trope of a 'socially oriented state' as a legitimation narrative ever since. For example, in one press conference in 2006, he elaborated:

> We have a socially oriented state; and we support people in various ways, beginning with building houses for the young. [...] In our country, World War II veterans and heroes receive full financial support from the state. [...] We are taking care of disabled people and children. [...] I am absolutely opposed to the indiscriminate removal of benefits that will later require the allocation of three times as much money from the state budget. [...] We will support education, and health care will also be primarily state funded in our country. We will never abandon that system.
>
> (Lukashenko 2006, 15, 20)

In Kazakhstan, the social welfare-related narrative was linked with a promise of economic growth that every citizen could enjoy. Since gaining independence in 1991, the transition from central planning to the adoption of a liberal and informal welfare model led to a sharp decrease in public spending on health care and pensions (Cook 2011, 193–238). According to Laruelle (2019, 2), 'economically, Kazakhstan has grown since the terrible years of the early 1990s, when the collapse of the Soviet system saw its GDP cut in half, and now belongs to the group of states with an upper-middle income; its GDP per capita has risen sixfold since 2002, while the incidence of poverty has fallen sharply'. However, Kazakhstan has experienced economic difficulties since 2014 because of falling oil prices and sanctions against Russia.

Although a rise in oil prices allowed for GDP to again grow by spring 2020, socio-economic conditions have remained harsh. The impact of the 2015 currency devaluation remained observable in real wages, fuelling a rising number of labour and civil protests in the latter half of the 2010s (Mallinson, in Bohr et al. 2019, 18).

Kazakhstan's former President Nursultan Nazarbayev's performance-based forms of legitimation were projected through a series of development strategies during his 30-year presidency (du Boulay and Isaacs 2019, 33). Kazakhstan 2050 Strategy, adopted in 2012, was a development programme that was perceived as 'an ideal to be followed in order to be happy'. In that case, Nazarbayev promised that by 2050, Kazakhstan would become one of the 30 most advanced economies in the world and that the economy would transform into a diversified one (Official Site of the President of the Republic of Kazakhstan 2012). Omelicheva (2016, 488) finds that Nazarbayev legitimised his rule by arguing that his government would be able to satisfy citizens' needs in both socio-economic and political terms. 'Nazarbayev's "economy first, then politics" slogan meant that political reforms lagged under his presidency' (Mallinson 2019, 10).

During Nazarbayev's rule, citizens rarely had a chance to influence the political decisions of the country. During the last decade, internet and social media played a significant role in increasing people's political awareness in Kazakhstan (Kilybayeva and Nurshanov 2020). Since 2011, social media and social network users have grown in Kazakhstan. According to data from World Bank (2020), 32% of citizens in Kazakhstan used the internet in 2009, doubling in 2013 to 63%, and increasing to 86% by 2020. Thanks to the internet, the number of citizens who believed the rhetoric of the state-run TV channels about the success of Nazarbayev's leadership decreased. On the Internet, it was often possible to find videos and materials that were not shown through state channels. Later social networks became a platform for citizens to discuss, exchange thoughts, and start alliances with like-minded people. More than half of the population (55.4%) in 2020 answered that thanks to the internet and social networks, he/she became more involved in politics (Kilybayeva 2020). With the expansion of citizens' access to the internet and the decrease in their level of trust in government, in both societies there has been a growing understanding that citizens themselves can influence the political decisions of their government.

Kassym-Jomart Tokayev ascended to power in 2019 as Nazarbayev's hand-picked successor. From early on, he sought to increase his popular support by enacting legitimation narratives that were linked to performance. In his inaugural State of the Nation Address in September 2019, he introduced the concept of the 'listening state', which would respond to all 'constructive citizen requests' quickly and efficiently (Starr 2019). The wording signalled awareness of problems to be addressed as well as the parameters of acceptable criticism towards the ruling elite (cf. the notion of 'compliant' activism by Libman and Kozlov 2017). Kassym-Jomart Tokayev had a positive reputation as a Kazakh diplomat and politician, who served as a Prime Minister (1999–2002) and as Director General of the UN Office in Geneva (2011–2013). Because of this, people remained hopeful that a change was about to come, even if he had not implemented any substantial reforms improving the social welfare of Kazakh citizens before the COVID-19 pandemic. One survey conducted after Tokayev's election revealed that 50% of respondents expected the situation in the country would improve, while 33% were hoping for 'substantial reforms' (Demoscope 2019). However, the OSCE (2019) outlined in their *Statement of Preliminary Findings and Conclusions* from the 2019 presidential election that 'significant irregularities were observed on election day, including cases of ballot box stuffing, and a disregard of counting procedures meant that an honest count could not be guaranteed'. Moreover, they mentioned that there were 'widespread detentions of peaceful protesters on election day in major cities' (OSCE 2019).

This chapter analyses the Belarusian and Kazakhstani governments' response to the COVID-19 pandemic and people's reactions to it against the backdrop of the legitimisation narratives of a 'socially oriented', 'listening', and 'pro-business' state. The analysis is based on a triangulated set of data. To track government responses (or lack thereof) and their justification, we utilised the Integrum database to gather a set of articles mentioning the words 'COVID-19' (Rus. *koronavirus*) and the country in question from one major independent news outlet in both countries – *Belapan* in Belarus and *Vlast* in Kazakhstan[2] (no the use of Integrum, see Kopotev et al. 2021). While it was rather easy to track the governments' health policy intervention and the accompanying social policy measures (Greer et al. 2021), it was methodologically challenging to track people's assessment and reactions to these measures. We sought to address this challenge in three ways. First, we chose to analyse the reports of independent rather than state-owned news outlets, which not only report on government decisions, but also on public reactions such as petitions, protests, and relevant survey results. Second, we studied the findings of the few publicly available public opinion polls as well as the results of a survey, which was conducted by one of the authors in Kazakhstan in June–July 2020 (Kilybayeva 2020). Third, we conducted semi-structured interviews with local experts (five in Belarus and five in Kazakhstan). The experts, sampled by snowballing method, were political and social analysts as well as civic and political activists who followed the situation closely and could share their evaluation of evolving state-society relations during the period of analysis[3].

Spring 2020: Lockdown or no Lockdown?

COVID-19 was recognised as an emerging public health threat in China's Wuhan province in late 2019. A few months later, the spread of the virus forced governments around the world to respond. In the absence of vaccines, the debate revolved around the introduction of non-pharmaceutical interventions (NPIs), the construction of test-trace-isolate-support (TTIS) systems

(Greer et al. 2021, 4–5), and accompanying social policy measures. As this section demonstrates, the Belarusian and Kazakhstani governments adopted polar opposite policies in the spheres of NPIs and TTIS, but had an equally limited social policy response, which had a corrosive effect on the regimes' legitimation narratives.

Kazakhstan

At the beginning of the pandemic, the Kazakh government was among the first to act. In February, it implemented national measures in response to the looming health crisis. First, the government introduced a TTIS system for all those arriving from China and other foreign countries, regardless of if they had been in contact with people who tested positive for COVID-19 (Vaal' 2020e, Vlast 2020f). In the sphere of NPIs, the government issued travel restrictions, social distancing orders, mask mandates, and a compulsory shift to distant work and study. Although Kazakhstan's TTIS system was not as meticulously implemented as in other parts of the world, given that not everyone with COVID-like symptoms was tested, the early measures succeeded in halting the spread of the virus (Jones and King 2021). Even though official statistics showed only a few cases of COVID-19 infections, Tokayev announced a state of emergency. From March 15 onwards, a severe quarantine with a stay-at-home order began, first for one month, and then until the middle of May (Vlast 2020k). This was the first time Tokayev declared a nationwide state of emergency (Vlast 2020a). Previously, Nazarbayev introduced a state of emergency in Zhanaozen from December 17, 2011, to January 31, 2012, when the city was rocked by mass protests (Radio Azattyq 2011). This state of emergency was probably intended to prevent any possible disturbances before the upcoming parliamentary elections scheduled for January 15, 2012.

All experts interviewed for this study agreed that the government's decision to introduce a lockdown was viewed favourably by Kazakhstani citizens. We argue that this was because the act was in accord with the government's legitimacy narrative that portrayed it as a guarantor of people's welfare. Zharas, a PhD in International Relations, explained that there was a generally positive attitude towards the initial measures taken by the Kazakhstani government in addressing the pandemic from January to March 2020. Oraz, a media expert were proud that the government was taking clear measures against the spread of the coronavirus like in many 'civilised' democratic countries. Inara told in her interview that people were satisfied that President Tokayev together with the nation was going through difficult times and was doing everything necessary to stop the spread of the virus. Anastassiya, an expert in public policy, highlighted that the government hid the real statistics of coronavirus cases, which were much more in Kazakhstan and had not closed the country's borders for too long, which led to the penetration of the coronavirus from abroad. At the beginning of the state of emergency, there were eight cases of coronavirus infection in Kazakhstan (Vlast 2020j), which led some groups of people in Kazakhstan to doubt the existence of COVID-19. The amount of misinformation and conspiracy theories circulating on social media increased significantly during the first lockdown. Besides different COVID-19 conspiracy theories in Kazakhstan, some people also were convinced that the Kazakh authorities instrumentalised COVID-19 as a pretext for 'closing' people into their homes so that they would not go out to protest rallies (Zharas interview 2022).

The lockdown carried a high cost for Kazakhstan's SMEs, which challenged the legitimation narrative of the government as a supporter of private business. According to the results of a survey conducted by the National Chamber of Entrepreneurs in Kazakhstan, more than 800,000 enterprises suffered from the lockdowns. Ten percent of Kazakhstan's 1.3 million companies were on the verge of bankruptcy (Vaal' 2020l). KPMG research (2020, 8) found that COVID-19 affected most of the revenue of companies in the sectors of aviation, fitness, hospitality, and non-grocery retail. What is more, it was not only the welfare of SMEs but also average citizens that suffered, which in turn challenged the legitimation narrative of the 'listening state' caring for its citizens. Many employers were forced to either close their companies, transfer staff to reduced working hours, begin remote working policies, or even downsize staff. A large proportion of employees, both of formal and informal economies, faced a shortage of income or even lost their jobs (the majority were self-employed people), being left without sufficient means to live. According to one of the authors' survey results, due to the state of emergency and strict lockdown, 60% of Kazakhstan families' incomes decreased significantly, 30.4% of families' incomes remained the same, and 9.7% of Kazakhstani families was left with almost no means of subsistence (Kilybayeva 2020). One-fifth of the population temporarily lost their jobs or main source of income and 11.7% of the population lost their job or main source of income permanently. 27.2% of citizens' finance were not affected by quarantine measures since they continued to work remotely. However, 15.5% of the overall population's finances shrunk significantly (Kilybayeva 2020).

Tokayev sought to meet expectations set by his legitimation strategy and resolve the issue of the crisis of SMEs by creating a headquarters to help entrepreneurs (Vlast 2020d) and asking businesses to switch to remote work (Vaal' 2020m). In addition, the president gave an order to the National Bank and the national Financial Market Regulatory Agency to allocate 600 billion tenge (for one year at a rate of 8%) to support businesses affected by the coronavirus situation (Vlast 2020h). However, in April–May 2020 self-employed and many of the owners of SMEs turned to Tokayev with a request to ease quarantine measures (Inara, Anastassiya interviews 2022). Since the loss from stagnation of SMEs was enormous for the country, the government was forced to ease quarantine measures in May 2020 and tried to restore the economy after the stagnation during the state of emergency and lockdown

(Vaal' 2020f). As the next section demonstrates, the decision had a detrimental impact on public health.

During the state of emergency, the government did introduce some social policy measures, characterised by the scholars of COVID-19 politics as 'necessary to address the social and economic costs of the stringent health policy measures' (Jones and King 2021, 202). In April, the state began disbursing a single payment of 42,500 tenge (about 100 USD), available to all those who had suffered from a loss of income. Here, the Kazakhs faced a problem that challenged the government's 'socially oriented state' legitimacy narrative. The e-governing websites *Egov.kz, 42500.enbek.kz,* and Telegram bots, where applications for social support had to be submitted, could not withstand the subsequent internet traffic, thus generating public confusion and resentment (Anastassiya interview 2022). In the end, about 4.5 million people – one-fourth of the population – did end up receiving social assistance. Allegedly some took social assistance twice. Since May 11, when the state of emergency ended, the acceptance of applications for 42,500 was suspended.

From January to March, Tokayev's government allocated 23.5 billion tenge from its reserve to strengthen the healthcare system: to purchase medicines, medical devices, and laboratory equipment (Vaal' 2020l), as well as to financially supported doctors who fought coronavirus (Vlast 2020b; Vaal' 2020h). This decision was in line with the legitimacy narrative about a listening state, but just like with the single social payment, its implementation was flawed. According to Kairgali Koneyev, an Almaty doctor, candidate of medical sciences, and activist, (Radio Azattyq 2020) Tokayev promised at the beginning of the pandemic that each health worker who caught COVID-19 at work would be paid two million tenge, and 10 million if he/she died. On behalf of doctors, Koneyev asked: 'Why in the questionnaire, when you take a test for coronavirus infection, it is necessary to indicate whether you are a health worker or not? What is this for? It would seem that the last name, first name, and contact details are enough. If you are a health worker, this result will be given to you not from the position of 'whether you are sick or not', but from a political position, hinting that this was done in order not to pay promised money to sick health workers.

Belarus

In Belarus, the response to the pandemic threat was infamously limited. Although the health sector's preparedness level was reportedly elevated at the end of January and a number of measures aimed at halting the spread of the virus were introduced early on, President Lukashenka insisted that the response should be 'effective, but not over the top' (Lukashenka, quoted in Belapan 2020a). He claimed that the Belarusian public health system was fully capable of dealing with the pandemic and refused to impose a lockdown in the country and shut its borders. The WHO representative in Belarus, Batyr

Berdyklychev, initially endorsed Lukashenka's limited pandemic response. On 17 March, he issued a statement praising the government:

> [In Belarus,] significant health system efforts and resources have been devoted to early detection of COVID-19 cases via laboratory diagnostics, isolation, patient care and contact tracing. These are key measures recommended by the WHO to stop transmission and prevent the spread of coronavirus infection. [...] The WHO believes that imposing restrictions on the movement of people and goods during periods of health emergency is not effective in most cases and can divert resources from other activities.

The alleged strength of the Belarusian health sector was linked to Lukashenka's legitimation narrative of a 'socially oriented state'. He argued that it was thanks to the decision 'not to destroy the healthcare system in the post-Soviet years [that] enabled [Belarus] to withstand the spread of the virus' (Lukashenka, quoted in Oreshko 2020). Although Lukashenka repeatedly called anxiety over COVID-19 a 'psychosis' that was 'the cause of all other illnesses' (Lukashenka, quoted in Turchina 2020b), he also portrayed himself as the supporter of the weakest members of the society for whom COVID-19 could be detrimental. This can also be interpreted as an attempt to live up to the image associated with being the leader of a 'socially oriented state'. 'We must fight for every person, especially the elderly' – he claimed – 'because unfortunately the virus affects first and foremost the old and those with a weak immunity system' (Lukashenka, quoted in Korovenkova 2020b). However, experts participating in this study spoke in unison about Lukashenka's failure to live up to public expectations. They argued that Belarusians were in shock not just about the president's *inability* to provide care as prescribed by the narrative of a socially oriented state (due to the dire economic situation) but about his *unwillingness* to do so, as exemplified by the derogatory remarks about those who fell ill and died (Alyaksei, Maksim, Polina, Lena interviews 2022).

Unlike President Vladimir Putin in Russia who just ignored the COVID-19 agenda, Lukashenka took some responsibility for pandemic management. However, he also sought to shift the blame not only to 'irresponsible' citizens and incompetent health officials, but also to political opposition and even state officials in its union state ally Russia. His statements suggest that he was the one making decisions on COVID-19 measures – for example, on April 19 he lamented that '[i]t is hard to swim against the global current. But I still decided that we should not shut down the country, we should work' (Lukashenka, quoted in Belapan 2020b). At the same time, he maintained that 'people must learn to take responsibility for themselves and their close ones', complaining about those who travelled abroad and became stranded (Lukashenka, quoted in Korovenkova 2020a), thus echoing the remarks of Moscow mayor Sobyanin who blamed reckless shashlik lovers and tourists for the spread of COVID-19 in the Russian capital. What is more, Lukashenka also criticised Russia for its decision to close the border to Belarus, for spreading misinformation about the situation with the pandemic in Belarus, and for its unwillingness to evacuate Belarusians from Thailand (Korovenkova 2020a). He also accused his political challengers of 'turning COVID-19 into politics' (Lukashenka, quoted in Nosova 2020).

While the Lukashenka government insisted that the situation was under control and COVID-related deaths were reportedly caused by health issues unrelated to the virus, a part of the Belarusian society demanded a far-reaching response. In early April, 150,000 people signed an online petition addressed to the WHO requesting that a quarantine be imposed in the country (Korovenkova 2020b). Lukashenka refused, arguing that 'The talk around here is about quarantine, curfew and so on... It is simple, we can do it within a day, but what are we going to eat then?' (Lukashenka, quoted in Korovenkova 2020b). The WHO's representative, however, was now much more critical of Lukashenka's policy and called for a stronger response against the spread of the pandemic (Turchina 2020c). At the same time, the experts interviewed for this study argued that the majority of Belarusians would have preferred some 'soft' COVID-19 restrictions as opposed to 'business as usual', which was Lukashenka's policy. Thus, Lukashenka was criticised both by those who wanted a full lockdown and those who wanted at least some restrictions.

While Lukashenka's government refused to take action, civil society mobilised. Civil society actors challenged official rhetoric about the strength of the Belarusian health sector and asserted that hospitals were suffering from overcrowding and the lack of necessary supplies (Astapova et al. 2022, 20–22). Alyaksei, a Belarusian civic activist involved in the organisation of pandemic relief, explained that while Lukashenka was blinded by his 'dissidence' and the Ministry of Health preferred to keep silent, chief doctors in hospitals understood that something should be done. Hospital department heads were the ones reaching out to civil society actors to request supplies. According to Tatsiana, the wife of an IT sector worker turned civic activist, doctors specifically requested supplies rather than money, arguing that any funds would not go to their genuine needs. Polina, an entrepreneur turned political activist, noted that doctors had to receive the supplies illegally, but they did so because the need was so great and 'the state had left us [Belarusians] to deal with the disease on our own' (Alyaksei interview 2022). Both private enterprises (especially the booming IT industry) and NGOs took on the task of crowdfunding and delivering supplies to medical personnel. As Lena, a political analyst, explained, it was 'a lot quicker and easier to deal directly with hospitals'. It became clear that while Lukashenka's Belarus was not a socially oriented state, it did have a socially oriented (civil) society (Astapova et al. 2022).

Discussions about the necessity of a lockdown became especially heated in the lead-up to the traditional Victory Day Parade of May 9. Following international recommendations aimed at halting the spread of COVID-19, the Belarusian opposition cancelled its main event of the year, Freedom Day, to be held on March 25. An online petition filed on March 21 demanded the cancellation of the Victory Day Parade. Those who signed the petition argued that the funds that were saved by cancelling the parade could be used to buy medicines and other essentials for the elderly, especially for war veterans. Money could also be used to purchase medical materials and emergency supplies for hospitals fighting COVID-19, to develop green spaces in Minsk 'to normalise the environmental situation and reduce the risk of developing various diseases among the population', as well as to repair roads and bridges of the city instead of 'current repairs after the passage of military equipment' (quoted in Shcherbakov 2020). The petition was a continuation of earlier debates criticising the costs of the Victory Day Parade, but COVID-19 added a new item to the list of desired spending targets.

Intermediary Conclusions

In the spring of 2020, Tokayev's Kazakhstan opted for a proactive health policy aimed at limiting the spread of the virus in accordance with global norms. Lukashenka's Belarus was characterised in headlines as a 'COVID-19 dissident'. Social policy measures, however, were limited in both countries. This provided regime challengers with an argument that authorities were failing to live up to their legitimation narratives. Another feature that the Belarusian and Kazakhstani cases have in common is the low level of public trust in the COVID-19 figures provided by their respective governments, evident from the very beginning. For example, as early as February, the Belarusian health minister explicitly claimed that his agency was 'working in a fully transparent manner', maintaining that they had 'no interest nor possibility to hide anything' (Karaik, quoted in Turchina 2020a). The statement can only be interpreted as a desperate attempt to counter widespread allegations of statistical forgery.

Indeed, excess mortality calculations (showing the number of deaths in a given period in comparison to the number of deaths on average in that same period) suggest that official reporting both in Belarus and Kazakhstan suffered either from underreporting and/or misreporting (Greer et al. 2021). The excess mortality rate in Belarus peaked at 9.1% in June 2020 and 17.6% in December 2020, whereas in Kazakhstan, a *decline* in average mortality rates in spring 2020 was followed by an excess mortality rate of 19.7% in July and 2.8% in December. These figures are in stark contrast with the official data (The Economist 2022). What is more, in the absence of an official diagnosis of COVID-19 (which was not provided due to political sensitivity and the lack of testing equipment), both countries would underreport COVID-19 as a cause of death, citing instead alternative complications like pneumonia or heart attack.

Summer 2020: Political and Social Mobilisation Amidst the Pandemic

At the beginning of the summer of 2020, Belarus and Kazakhstan were in different stages of the pandemic. In Belarus, the first wave was coming to an end, whereas in Kazakhstan, it was only about to start. As this section highlights, the shifting political opportunity structure paved the way for COVID-19 to emerge as a major theme for *political* mobilisation in Belarus and *social* mobilisation in Kazakhstan.

Belarus

None of the Belarusian experts interviewed for the study argued that the mass political mobilisation against Lukashenka's regime was only generated during the COVID-19 pandemic. They referred both to the declining level of repression and the emergence of new forms of political and civic activism from the mid-2010s onwards. During this time, Lukashenka's authoritarian regime experienced a 'thaw' that was sparked by the Russian annexation of Crimea in 2014 and Russia's subsequent war against Ukraine in Donbas. A pivotal element of the period was the increase in civic activism, especially in the cultural and social spheres (Astapova et al. 2022). According to Maksim, the result of the thaw was a newfound sense of increasing freedom in society coupled with a perception that it was possible 'to build a reality of one's own'. Although Lukashenka's government sought to endorse some forms of collaboration with 'apolitical' civic activists, interviewees argued that interactions between a nascent civil society and the government were limited. All five of them referred to Belarus as a country split in half, arguing that two 'parallel worlds' existed in the country (Alyaksei interview 2022). On the one hand, they recalled, there was the government, 'minding its own business', while on the other hand, there were the people who 'lived their own lives' and 'did not care about politics' (Tatsiana interview 2022).

Belarusians were not thoroughly apolitical though, as three major political milestones took place in the latter half of the 2010s. According to the interviewees, these milestones paved the way for the unprecedented political mobilisation in the summer of 2020. In 2017, challengers of the regime successfully mobilised thousands of people around the country against the introduction of the so-called 'Parasite Law'. According to Maksim, Lukashenka's decision to back down on the introduction of the law as well as his unwillingness to repress protests, allegedly because of their 'apolitical' socio-economic agenda, was important as it generated a sense of empowerment among the activists. The law was also a considerable blow to Lukashenka's legitimacy narrative of a socially oriented state, given that it threatened the unemployed with punishment rather than state support. Another moment of learning came in December 2019, when the regime permitted political protests triggered by the decision to further integrate with Russia (Maksim interview

2022). Finally, during the parliamentary elections in the autumn of 2019, new groups and new faces, for example a novel political student movement, emerged in the political arena, even while elections continued to be manipulated (Lena interview 2022). These events took place against the backdrop of the development and flourishing of independent media like *Tut.by* (Maksim interview 2022).

The new grassroots groups learned to master crowdfunding through sites like MolaMola. It is perhaps no coincidence that Andrei Strizhak, the activist who coordinated #ByCovid19, the biggest grassroots initiative to facilitate civil society support during the COVID-19 pandemic, had experience in this field. He previously coordinated humanitarian support for Donbas Ukrainians in the zone of conflict from 2014 onwards and in Belarus to those who suffered during the protests against the 'Parasite Law' (Maksim interview 2022; Reform.by 2020). These insights suggest that the Belarusian civil society, if not necessarily a political opposition, gained new resources already before the COVID-19 pandemic both in terms of human capital and popular grievances vis-à-vis the Lukashenka government. These findings echo the arguments presented in recent studies by Krawatzek and Langbein (2022) and Astapova et al. (2022), according to which the political mobilisation of summer 2020 had its roots in the activation of civil society and gradual mass disappointment with Lukashenka's rule in the latter half of the 2010s.

In Belarus, the transition from civic to political mobilisation was facilitated by the launch of the presidential campaign. According to Lena, who followed the presidential campaign closely, people were expecting the elections to be announced for some time before they were on May 8. It was on this day that Valerii Tsapkala, Belarus's former ambassador to the USA and Mexico, as well as the founder of the Minsk High Technology Park, and Siarhei Tsihanouski, a popular video blogger, announced their intention to run for political office. The third alternative candidate, a banker and philanthropist Viktar Babarika, declared his participation on May 12. According to both Lena and Maksim, the date of the election –August 9 – was selected because Lukashenka was expecting an 'easy win' in a 'quiet summer', calculating that people would self-isolate and thus not show up to polling stations and vote.

However, the opposite took place. Polina was one of the hundreds of Belarusians who became involved in political activism for the first time in their lives. Once she found out that Tsepkala, whose professional work she had been following for some time, was running, she decided to join his initiative group. It was not that the government mismanagement of the COVID-19 pandemic had sparked her interest in politics, but rather the pandemic had resulted in 'less [paid] work and thus more free time' (Polina interview 2022). According to her, the activists in Tsepkala's team were made up of both those who had been involved in politics for a long time and newcomers, especially from the newly booming IT sector. Lena, in turn, noted the involvement of 'active, young, and experienced' campaigners who were driven by 'a spirit of entrepreneurialism' as they came up with creative solutions on their own initiative (Lena interview 2022). According to her and Maksim, the newfound possibility to fundraise was one of the biggest shifts empowering the political opposition, as COVID-19-related social fundraising was 'fluently transferred' into a political effort. Reflecting on the shift from civic to political activism, Maksim noted that it was as if the 'extraordinary time' of the global pandemic was followed by the 'extraordinary time' of political awakening, during which 'there was euphoria, but there was also fear'. According to Alyaksei, the shift happened only towards the end of July, which is when the number of COVID-19 infections fell, and civic activists entered the sphere of politics.

All of the interviewees agreed that the COVID-19 pandemic 'faded into the background' (Polina interview 2022) as the country prepared for the upcoming election. The three political newcomers – Babarika, Tsepkala, and Tsikhanouskaya – sparked unprecedented interest in Belarusian society as they started collecting the required 100,000 signatures needed to be registered as a presidential candidate. Enormous queues of people willing to offer their signatures made news headlines around the world (Astapova et al. 2022). Activists involved in collecting signatures were careful to follow COVID-19 regulations that the government introduced in late spring by providing masks, gloves, and hand sanitisers. Yet, the behaviour was not informed by the need to ensure public safety, but rather to avoid government backlash (Polina interview 2022).

On July 14, the Central Electoral Committee announced its decision to disqualify Babarika's and Tsepkala's candidacy, allegedly due to forged signatures. Siarhei Tsihanouski also failed to be formally registered as a candidate because he had been arbitrarily arrested and given 'administrative detention'. His wife, Sviatlana Tsihanouskaya, was allowed to register instead, arguably due to Lukashenka's underestimation of the threat she could pose to him. Both Babarika and Tsepkala shifted their support to Tsikhanouskaya (Tolkacheva 2021). In the upcoming weeks, the three female leaders of the unified opposition – Tsikhanouskaya, Tsepkala's wife Veronika Tsepkala, and Babarika's campaign manager Mariya Kalesnikova – toured the country, attracting thousands of people to their pre-election rallies. According to Maksim, it would have been absurd if someone refused to attend the rallies due to COVID-19. According to Polina, there was simply 'no time to think' about the pandemic in the midst of the political turbulence.[3]

Based on our analysis of media accounts and expert interviews, Belarus' 2020 presidential election was not dominated by a debate about (mis)management of the COVID-19 pandemic, unlike one would perhaps have expected. Maksim compared the pandemic to Europe's experience of the Spanish flu during the First World War, while Polina noted that she did not remember any citizens questioning COVID-19 during the collection of signatures. Tatsiana recalls that mismanagement of the pandemic was a topic for debate, especially in the countryside, but she too agrees that it was perceived as an *additional* rather than a major grievance people had towards Lukashenka's rule.

Kazakhstan

In Kazakhstan, the summer months passed with both the government and the citizens trying to cope with the COVID-19 pandemic. On May 11, 2020, a state of emergency was ended, and quarantine measures were relaxed (Korastyleva 2020a). However, not all restrictions were curbed as the organisation of protest rallies continued to be outlawed (Vaal' 2020b). The Prosecutor General's Office warned Kazakhstanis that rallies under quarantine were illegal (EADaily 2020). The same was stated by the chief sanitary doctors of Almaty and Astana. Minister of Health Elzhan Birtanov urged Kazakhstanis not to violate the law and restrictions set by the country's chief sanitary doctor. Birtanov also asked to 'postpone' holding rallies, as this could lead to another outbreak of coronavirus infection (Vaal' 2020c). The places of the alleged rallies were cordoned off in advance, disinfection was carried out, and numerous police squads were on duty (EADaily 2020). The government, therefore, utilised COVID-19 regulations to uphold a favourable political opportunity structure.

Opposition forces resisted the restrictions that they viewed as pretexts for limiting their activism. On June 6, two unrelated political organisations – the Democratic Party headed by Zhanbolat Mamay and the Democratic Choice of Kazakhstan (*Demokraticheskiy vybor Kazakhstana,* abbreviated DVK) – announced their intention to protest. DVK, run by one-time government insider Mukhtar Ablyazov, was ruled as 'extremist' by a court in 2018 and banned in Kazakhstan, (Moldabekov 2020a). The Democratic Party put forward as political demands during their rally the cancellation of credit debts of Kazakhstanis, the fundamental refusal to sell land to foreigners, and the release of all political prisoners. The leader of the DVK party Ablyazov, who is in exile in France, wrote a post on his Facebook on June 3, in which he demanded the payment of '50 thousand tenge to each citizen of Kazakhstan, including 4-month-old babies' and the payment of interest on loans to individuals and legal entities for 4 months (Moldabekov 2020a). These demands reflected awareness about both socio-economic and political grievances present in society, stemming from the government's inability to live up to the narrative of a 'listening state' and unwillingness to introduce political reforms.

On the day of the protests, the police blocked rally locations and all activists were imprisoned in paddy wagons. The reason for the detentions was that *akimat*, the local administration, did not receive notifications about the organisation of peaceful rallies. The law 'On the procedure for organising and holding peaceful assemblies in the Republic of Kazakhstan' (Zakon.kz

2020), which came into force on May 25, 2020, required submitting a notification to *akimat* five days before the day of rallies holding. Thus, the new law, which allegedly softened the conditions for holding rallies, did not save the protesters from bans and detentions (EADaily 2020). On June 19, there was a trial of political activist Alnur Ilyashev (Moldabekov 2020b) for criticising government measures to combat COVID-19 (Amnesty International 2020). Again, the government utilised COVID-19 restrictions to resist shifts in the political opportunity structure.

However, limiting the opportunity to voice dissatisfaction was not a remedy for dissatisfaction *per se*. Two of the interviewees viewed political mobilisation in the summer of 2020 as a continuation of the mobilisation that had commenced a year before, upon Nazarbayev's resignation in March 2019 (Inara, Zharas interviews 2022). The leader and 'father' of the nation, Nursultan Nazarbayev, left office voluntarily, arguably as he felt that the Kazakhs were tired of his promises. The resignation immediately shifted the political opportunity structure towards the regime's challengers and marked the beginning of new political mobilisation in Kazakhstan. People widely felt a new political responsibility for the future and felt that they were able to influence political decisions in their country. It was demonstrated by the growth of citizens' political participation and self-organised initiatives. Some of the loudest voices were from Kazakhstan's young people who started to show unprecedented activism. People could no longer be silent and began to fight for real political change.

On the evening of March 19, 2019, Nazarbayev announced his decision to resign right before the Nauryz spring holiday and introduced his handpicked successor, a career diplomat Kassym-Jomart Tokayev. This sparked hope for democratic change in the country. However, hope was replaced by disappointment the next day when Tokayev renamed the capital Astana to Nur-Sultan in honour of Nazarbayev. Even if it was indeed Nazarbayev who had transformed Tselinograd from a steppe town into Astana, a million-strong city, many citizens widely expressed their disagreement with the renaming of the capital Astana, refusing to call it Nur-Sultan. It was still a surprise when Tokayev proposed renaming the capital back to Astana in September 2022.

During the Almaty marathon in April 2019, young activists put up a banner with a sign saying 'you will not run away from the truth' (Rus. 'ot pravdy ne ubezhish'), which quickly spread on social media with the hashtags 'you will not run away from the truth', 'I have a choice' (Rus. #отправдынеубежишь, #уменяестьвыбор). A new youth movement also invited Kazakh society to see the shortcomings of the regime and peacefully protest by saying 'Wake up, Kazakhstan' (Kaz. 'Oyan, Qazaqstan!'). The activists adopted the popular saying 'Wake up, Kazakh' (Kaz. 'Oyan, Qazaq')[4] used by 19th-century Alash orda[5] intelligentsia and pleaded for people to take responsibility for the development of the government.

During March and April 2019, several thousand active citizens were arrested, and journalists beaten (Starr 2019). Shortcomings in the presidential elections in June 2019 prompted massive rallies in many cities of Kazakhstan, which the police suppressed by force. However, Tokayev also expressed awareness of people's political grievances, announcing that the old formula of 'economy first, politics second' was no longer valid and he began to use narratives about being 'with the people'. In the aftermath of the unprecedented street protests against the unfair electoral process in June 2019, Tokayev signed new legislation on assemblies that required rally organisers to provide advanced warning of their protest intentions, rather than requesting permission. However, the government could still cancel or refuse permission for planned or impromptu assemblies.

The struggle between Tokayev's government and its political opponents took place against the backdrop of a worsening health crisis. In June–July, Kazakhstan experienced a dramatic rise in COVID-19 cases accompanied by a tragic death toll (Vaal' 2020j, 2020q). The media reported on hospitals in crisis, shortage of medical personnel and equipment, ambulances with people in critical condition having to wait outside the hospital or return them home, and the general struggles of COVID-19. Kazakhstan's healthcare infrastructure appeared to be chronically weak, and this revelation threatened the success of Tokayev's legitimacy as a ruler.

During the nationwide online forum *Biz Birgemiz* (*We are together*) on June 23, 2020, President Kassym-Jomart Tokayev sought to convince Kazakhstani citizens that he was, after all, living up to the expectations of his 'pro-business' and 'listening state' legitimacy narratives. He noted that all countries of the world, including Kazakhstan, were confronting the coronavirus pandemic. He elaborated:

> Significant funds have been allocated from the budget to combat coronavirus. Food was distributed to low-income families. A number of benefits are provided for small and medium-sized businesses. At the initiative of *Elbasy* [Nursultan Nazarbayev], significant funds have been allocated from the Birgemiz ('We are together') Foundation and real assistance is being provided to those in need. This work is actively carried out by the Nur Otan party. All this testifies to the inviolability of our unity.
>
> (Official Site of the President of the Republic of Kazakhstan 2020)

However, the summer of 2020 became tragic for people in Kazakhstan. COVID-19 spread rapidly after the lessening of quarantine measures in the middle of May 2020, which caused thousands of deaths. According to Violetta, an expert in public policy, there was a lot of criticism from people towards the government. 'They [government] could not contain the situation with the coronavirus and could not stabilise the situation. There was a complete lack of competent leadership, it was obvious that the person who was supposed to lead this process [Minister of Health, Yelzhan Birtanov] did not cope with his role'. Another interviewee, Inara, explained that the infection rate reached a peak in the summer 2020, hospitals were overcrowded, and there were no medicines in pharmacies: 'It was a time when all citizens actively back to medicines in pharmacies, where there were even no paracetamols and other required medications'.

All Kazakhstan experts interviewed for the study agreed that citizens were disappointed with how COVID-19 was managed by the government in the summer of 2020. Seeing government inaction, civil society stepped in – much like in Belarus in the spring. Ordinary citizens made their own initiatives to send medicines to different regions and cities of the country by post to those who needed them urgently but could not access them. Violetta noted there were many initiatives from civil society to close the 'holes' that formed in Kazakhstan because of the lack of competence on the part of the government to address the situation with the pandemic. People created websites for the exchange of help between citizens who needed medicines. For example, in the capital city, active citizens organised material aid and psychological support for medical workers who worked long hours 'on the front', providing them with hot food and essential medical supplies.

Unlike Lukashenka, Tokayev was able to limit the space for political opposition and to live up to its narrative of a 'listening state' – or, at the very least, convince the people that it was attempting to construct one. Anastassiya and Violetta both pointed out that the Tokayev government tried to assure people that the situation was under control and persuade them that they were working to solve problems, for instance, to increase the number of hospital beds and import medicines into the country. There was a clear message from the government to the people that they were controlling the process. If people would wait a little and be patient, everything would be fine.

Tokayev was also involved in shifting the blame for mismanagement of the pandemic to state officials. On June 29, during a meeting in Akorda, he stated that the tasks that he set to counter the COVID-19 pandemic 'had not been fulfilled or were far from being fully completed'. Tokayev accused *akims* (regional governors) and ministers of shutting themselves off from the people and ceasing to respond to citizens' appeals. He instructed them to organise information work, conduct regular online briefings, and organise online consultations with doctors on the broadcast of republican TV channels (Vaal' 2020a). These calls are fully coordinated with the legitimacy narrative of a 'listening state'.

The peak of the general outrage and anger of Kazakhstanis was the grandiose fireworks in honour of the birthday of Nazarbayev on July 6, organised against the backdrop of people dying from COVID-19 (Zharas interview 2022). As a result of people's indignation, on June 9, Tokayev signed an order declaring July 13 a day of national mourning in memory of citizens who suffered from COVID-19 (Vlast 2020g). On that day, former president Nazarbayev expressed condolences to the families and friends of the victims of the coronavirus pandemic (Vlast 2020c). On July 19, Tokayev threatened the government with its dissolution (Vaal' 2020p). During an extended meeting of the government, Tokayev announced the creation of a special commission that would investigate mistakes and omissions made:

> The former leadership of the Ministry of Health was not properly prepared to deal with the coronavirus pandemic, and in general, the frequent change of methods and approaches is questionable among the population. [...] The Ministry of Health made a number of mistakes in managing the situation. The majority of *akims* did not carry out their work at the proper level. The government also did not control.
>
> (Vaal' 2020o)

The experts interviewed for this study did not unanimously blame Kazakhstan's pandemic mismanagement on the president. According to Zharas, an expert international relations, 'Tokayev tried to make the situation better but was surrounded by corrupt people from Nazarbayev's era suffering from bad management skills'. Inara was also convinced that the power transition from Nazarbayev to Tokayev had not yet been completed. According to her, Tokayev was genuinely interested in managing the country effectively, but the 'old' system did not allow it. She added that 'Tokayev is insistently changing the country and creating his team of like-minded people to strive for his vision of the country's development'. Journalist Yelbol Karimov (2021), for his part, blamed Kazakhstan's COVID-19 policy failure on the unsatisfactory work of *akims* and the Interdepartmental Commission on the Non-proliferation of COVID-19, systemic errors of the Ministry of Health, as well as an underestimation of the scale of the disease. This was paralleled by the poor foresight of the Minister of Health Birtanov, who in early March 2020 predicted that the 'maximum' number of coronavirus cases in the country would be 3,000–3,500 people (Karimov 2021).

Intermediary Conclusions

Both Belarus and Kazakhstan witnessed a new wave of activism in the summer of 2020. For Belarus, the approaching presidential election provided the challengers of the regime with a window of opportunity to confront Lukashenka at the polls. The gradual increase in their resource base and the decline in state repression from the mid-2010s onwards, combined with Lukashenka's decision to allow Tsikhanouskaya to run, enabled the emergence of mass protests. COVID-19 faded away from public consciousness. In Kazakhstan, in contrast, the pandemic dominated public debates and contributed to the activation of civil society organisations that had been paused in spring. However, unlike in Belarus, citizens of Kazakhstan refrained from participating in large-scale political demonstrations due to the lingering shock stemming from the significant death toll observed during the summer of 2020 at the peak of the pandemic. (Astapova et al. 2022). Instead, unlike Lukashenka, Tokayev was still able to shift the blame for pandemic mismanagement to others.

Autumn 2020: Repression and Apathy

After a politically turbulent summer, both the Belarusian and Kazakhstani authorities started to push back against their challengers. While in Belarus, crude repression became the only tool available for Lukashenka to achieve his objectives, Tokayev relied on his earlier legitimacy narrative of a 'listening state' and succeeded in overseeing a parliamentary election where the political mobilisation of his challengers was limited.

Belarus

After August 9, 2020, the political opportunity structure in Belarus changed again. On the day of the presidential election, Lukashenka's challengers appeared stronger than ever. Thousands of people throughout the country were queueing in order to cast their ballots on the main day of elections as instructed by the opposition. Hundreds decided to stay in the vicinity of the voting premises in anticipation of the preliminary results. Tsikhanouskaya's supporters took photos of their ballots and submitted them to Golos, the opposition's vote calculation initiative (Tolkacheva 2021). According to Polina, this was one of the most important initiatives of the new political opposition, as it got people involved in the political process with the means of new technology. Although no official election results were yet announced, people gathered on the streets protesting against (potential) fraud. Security services repressed the protests violently, according to official statistics arresting 3,000 people in 33 cities (Tolkacheva 2021). On the next day, the Central Electoral Commission announces the results of vote counting: 80.23% for Lukashenka and 9.9% for Tsikhanouskaya.

The violent repression of protests continued for days, weeks, and months. The events in Belarus are already the subject of many scholarly and non-scholarly analyses (see, e.g. Way 2020; Hall 2022; United Nations High Commissioner for Human Rights 2022,). According to all the interviewees, it was in this phase that the COVID-19 pandemic became instrumentalised by the Lukashenka government as a pretext for repression. As Mitikka 2023 notes in this volume, this practice was a common feature of all autocracies in the region, including Russia. The situation was especially severe in prisons. Given the high number of detainees in the autumn of 2020, protesters were put into overcrowded cells, where COVID-19 spread quickly. Authorities refused medical assistance to those who fell ill and in general did not seek to protect detainees from catching the virus (Maksim interview 2022). Regulations introduced in order to stop the virus from spreading were used to refuse detainees the right to meet people from outside. The right to receive parcels on a daily basis was amended to only receive them once per week (Alyaksei interview 2022). Finally, detainees were forced to wash the prison cell floors with chloride, which caused pain in their skin and eyes (Polina, Alyaksei, Maksim, Tatsiana interviews 2022).

Masks that people wore to protect themselves against COVID-19 became a tool for hiding one's identity for both the protesters and members of the security apparatus. The Telegram channel *Black Book of Belarus,* which has 100,000 subscribers, was devoted to 'de-anonymising' police officers that were involved in the suppression of protests (Walker 2020). At the same time, protesters would also wear masks in order not to be identified by representatives of the security apparatus (Polina interview 2022). Later on, mask-wearing became a political marker of one's opposition to Lukashenka (Lena interview 2022). Because of repression, Lukashenka's challengers were disempowered. However, it would not be accurate to claim that the political opportunity structure shifted away from the political opposition even if the 'window of opportunity' subsequently closed. After all, Lukashenka's regime depends primarily on repression and is the target of major popular grievances after the failed revolution of 2020. In the context of economic hardship, Hall (2022, 22) concludes, it is Lukashenka's entire performance legitimacy – not just the narrative of a 'socially oriented state' – that failed outright.

When a new wave of COVID-19 swept over Belarus, civic activists were no longer there to support the state. Public health initiatives were almost completely diverted to help the victims of repression, while grassroots civic movements became one of the major targets of state repression. However, according to Alyaksei, this did not leave people in trouble, given that the availability of international COVID-19 relief meant that additional support from civil society was not as vital as in the spring. What is more, in December 2020, Belarus became one of the first countries to start vaccination programmes, given that the Belarus-based company *Belmedpreparaty* acquired the rights to produce Russia's Sputnik-V (Turchina 2020d).

Kazakhstan

In Kazakhstan, the difficult summer was followed by a natural decrease in COVID-19 cases in the autumn. Yet, the improvement of the public health situation did not yield more space for voicing criticism towards the government. Altayev Nurzhan, the chairman of the *El Tiregi* Union of Industrialists and Entrepreneurs and a member of the parliament from the ruling *Nur Otan* party, lost his position for 'discrediting the party'. Nurzhan's misstep was voicing a sharp statement criticising the government for its poor performance during the pandemic and calling for political and economic reforms (Sputnik 2020).

Meanwhile, President Tokayev sought to narrate himself as an ally of the people and a guarantor of the 'listening state'. On October 7, he spoke at a meeting discussing preparations for the second wave of coronavirus infections, reminding the government of the need to 'communicate' with society in order not to lose people's trust.

> I want to note the critical importance of communications and feedback with the citizens of our country. Practice has already shown that the success of the fight against the pandemic largely depends on the degree of people's confidence in the measures and decisions taken. Trust, in turn, depends on the understanding and involvement of citizens in the actions of the authorities.
>
> (Tokayev, quoted in Vaal' 2020d)

Tokayev stressed that it was necessary to continue a constant dialogue with citizens, to talk about problems and risks honestly and openly, while also offering solutions. He presented that businesses and citizens should understand that the development of the situation depended on strict adherence to sanitary and preventive measures (Vaal' 2020d). This statement reflected yet another attempt to shift the blame from Tokayev's administration, this time onto irresponsible members of the citizenry and the business community.

A new wave of COVID-19 in the autumn raised questions about the need to cancel or postpone elections for the lower house of the parliament (Majilis) and local councils (Maslikhats), scheduled for 10 January 2021. However, in late October, a member of the Central Election Commission Serik Sydykov said that both elections would be held regardless of the COVID-19 situation (Vaal' 2020r).

Unlike in Belarus, elections passed amidst popular apathy. Although elections can serve as windows of opportunity, for regime challengers, this time the political opportunity structure remained favourable to the incumbent, regardless of some grievances that were present in society. Five political parties supportive of the regime participated in the elections: Nur Otan, Ak Zhol Democratic Party of Kazakhstan, Auyl People's Democratic Party, Adal Party, and People's Party of Kazakhstan. No independent or opposition party candidates were allowed to run due to Kazakhstan's electoral legislation. What is more, independent observers were not allowed to enter polling stations for various reasons, some of which were related to social distancing measures put in place to counter the spread of COVID-19. At some polling stations, surveillance cameras were covered with objects. Thus, the rights of observers were violated (Violetta interview 2022). Dozens of those who came out to protest the 'staged' and 'undemocratic' vote in 'unauthorised rallies' were detained in mass in various cities across the country. The kettling strategy was again used against some activists in Almaty. Surrounded by frost, they spent six to 10 hours outdoors (Radio Azattyq 2021). According to Inara, people were more active in the parliamentary elections of 2021 than in previous years. Overall, however, the elections were not perceived to be as meaningful as presidential elections.

Conclusions

In this chapter, we set out to explore policy introduced by the governments of Belarus and Kazakhstan vis-à-vis the COVID-19 pandemic and the evaluation of that policy by the public, from January 2020 until January 2021. We found that while the two countries witnessed polar opposite responses to the pandemic threat from the beginning, there were some notable commonalities between them. First and foremost, citizens in both countries were dissatisfied with the government's approach to COVID-19 in the long run. We have argued that this was because both governments failed to live up to the legitimacy narratives they had constructed in previous years: one that is 'socially oriented' and capable of providing security and welfare in Belarus, or efficient, pro-business, and responsive to citizens' needs in Kazakhstan. However, there are nuances. Lukashenka's legitimacy crumbled completely because it was already 'corroding' in the 2010s, especially due to attempt to introduce the infamous 'Parasite Tax' in 2017 (Moshes and Nizhnikau 2019; Krawatzek and Langbein 2022). The political opportunity structure shifted in favour of Lukashenka's challengers not only because of his resented COVID-19 'dissidence', but also by other factors that fell into place both before and during 2020. In the latter half of the 2010s, the 'softening' of the authoritarian regime generated space both for a stronger civil society and alternative political candidates, whereas the boom in the IT sector and the shift away from paternalistic values (Krawatzek and Langbein 2022) fuelled the drop in support for Lukashenka's command style politics (cf. Moshes and Nizhnikau 2019). In 2020, letting Tsikhanouskaya challenge him on the ballot was a major miscalculation (Way 2020).

In Kazakhstan, Tokayev's legitimacy narrative was dented by the meagre and chaotically distributed compensation for lost income in the spring, lack of support for SMEs, collapse of the healthcare system, and failure of local government management during the peak of the pandemic in summer 2020. Overall, Tokayev's promises for reform did not bring meaningful improvements. However, the president managed to shift the blame of pandemic mismanagement to other state actors and, in the end, convinced most Kazakhstanis of his commitment to the legitimacy narratives of a 'listening' and 'pro-business' state.

We have argued that failing to live up to one's legitimacy narrative is dangerous for an authoritarian leader because popular grievances generate political resources for the regime's challengers, thus shifting the political opportunity structure in their favour. However, grievances alone are not enough for a political crisis to erupt. In Belarus, it was the emboldened and empowered civil society that played a key role, transforming into a channel for political activism in the run-up to the August 9 presidential election (Astapova et al. 2022). Lukashenka's challengers had also another important resource: technological savviness. Already before the COVID-19 crisis, they learned to engage with citizens on social media and to raise funds, thus laying the groundwork for the new civil society – business nexus that bypassed the state in the spring of 2020. In Kazakhstan, political opposition remained marginalised even though grievances vis-à-vis the regime constructed by Nazarbayev were strengthened in the aftermath of Tokayev's ascension to power. Moreover, like many authoritarian rulers around the world, both Lukashenka and Tokayev utilised measures designed to halt the spread of COVID-19 to their advantage. In Kazakhstan, the threat posed by the virus was cited as a reason for restricting opposition activists' right to protest and refusing electoral observers the chance to be present in polling stations (Hewitt 2021). In Belarus, the measures functioned as an additional method of repression in the autumn of 2020, while not being utilised in the spring. It could be argued that Lukashenka could have easily utilised the pandemic to his advantage in both the spring and summer of 2020 – but the opposite happened. This finding points to the importance of agency in the process of authoritarian learning in the region.

According to the experts interviewed for this study, COVID-19 had a consolidating effect on Belarusian society. The government's inability to live up to the standards of a 'socially oriented state' accelerated people's alienation from the government, as 'people realised that they are on their own, that the state will not help them' (Tatsiana interview 2022). According to Polina, the pandemic forced people to learn how to self-organise with the help of social media and new technologies. She argued that it was members of the IT community, nurtured by Lukashenka since the mid-2010s, that acted as a 'catalysator' for this process. Indeed, all five interviewees pointed to President Lukashenka's role in accelerating the empowerment of the political opposition. If he had signalled that he cared for the people as his legitimacy narrative of a leader of a 'socially oriented state' entailed – by introducing some social distancing measures, for example, or showing sympathy for those who suffered – his core electorate might still have voted for him in August 2020. Experts argued that if he had blocked Tsikhanouskaya's registration, most of the people might have remained apolitical, given the lack of a suitable alternative candidate, as arguably had been the case in the presidential election of 2015.

In Kazakhstan, COVID-19 functioned as a limelight exposing underlying problems: not only in the healthcare system, public management, and communications, but also limited capabilities in central and local governments. According to the interviewees, the citizens of Kazakhstan have a very low level of trust in the government. Citizens are sure that the government does not work to improve the situation in the country, and they are only interested in profiting at the expense of taxpayers and natural resources. Moreover, people do not go to vote in parliamentary elections because they know that there are no such parties or people for whom they would like to vote. Everything there is predetermined, and the results are artificially constructed. However, Tokayev's recent ascension to power resulted in an ambiguous attitude towards his regime among the Kazakh people. Some experts believed in the sincerity of Tokayev's intentions to become a listening and hearing ruler, but they believed that the environment and the system did not allow him to achieve good results. Other experts believed that Tokayev did not differ from Nazarbayev in that Tokayev also seeks legitimisation of his power through promises and, just like Nazarbayev, shifts the blame on his subordinates and threatens to fire them. In reality, everything remains as before. All in all, Tokayev turned out to be better at playing the 'blame game' than Lukashenka for two reasons. First, it is because Lukashenka did not properly try – instead, the Belarusian president expressed pride in his decision to 'swim against the global current' (Lukashenka, quoted in Belapan 2020b). Second, Tokayev could use his otherwise unfavourable public image as a weak actor to argue that the pandemic was mismanaged because his hands were tied.

Although the human toll of COVID-19 was enormous in both Belarus and Kazakhstan, the pandemic had a surprisingly positive effect on the development of civil society. A lot of people participated in grassroots activism, showed solidarity, and developed initiatives to help those in need. Those who had started to fight for democratisation at the beginning of Kazakhstan's 2019 power transition were convinced that the state needs political reforms because COVID-19 crisis management showed a lack of independence and capability in state apparatuses. January 2022 grassroots mobilisation showed how people in Kazakhstan became tired of promises and longed for real political reforms. However, peaceful protests turned into organised riots and civilian bloodshed. Although the future of protests in Belarus looks grim given the still ongoing repression, the legacy of mobilisation is expected to be decisive for the country's future development.

Russia's war in Ukraine has shifted the political opportunity structure in both Belarus and Kazakhstan. After the launch of Russian aggression against Ukraine from Belarusian territory, thousands of people around Belarus came out to protest regardless of the extremely repressive nature of the contemporary Belarusian regime. Moreover, regime challengers in Belarus hope that if Russia is fully defeated in Ukraine and Putin's regime collapses, Lukashenka can be forced to resign and free and fair elections can finally be organised. All in all, it can be argued that Lukashenka's position has been weakened by the war, even if for the time being regime challengers have not been able to capitalise on it. In Kazakhstan, Tokayev has managed to use the war to his advantage, promoting himself as a guarantor of Kazakhstani independence and the only actor able to navigate through internationally turbulent times. In November 2022, he secured a landslide victory in the presidential elections.

Acknowledgement

Shugyla Kilybayeva's research was supported by a Marie Curie RISE scheme within the H2020 (grant acronym: SHADOW, no: 778118).

We would like to express my heartfelt gratitude to Dr. Abel Polese, the project coordinator, for his unwavering support, invaluable academic and professional mentorship throughout my time in Estonia.

We would like to express my gratitude to TalTech Law School, Tallinn University of Technology, for warmly hosting me. The environment of kindness and care provided by the faculty has made my experience truly extraordinary.

In addition, we acknowledge the input of the ten anonymous experts interviewed for this chapter. Thank you for your time and analytic insights.

Notes

1 *Vlast* is a popular independent daily online newspaper. While it is published in both Kazakh and Russian languages, we only analysed the Russian language material due to accessibility and linguistic comparability.
2 The experts argued that COVID-19 faded away and moved out of the public limelight in the summer. This is also reflected in the systematically collected newspaper data, with *Belapan* publishing no articles featuring our COVID-19 keywords between June 18 and December 23, 2020.
3 We would like to thank all of the experts for the time and the analytic insights they contributed to this research project.
4 Myrzhakyp Dulatov, a poet, writer, publicist, and educator, together with Alikhan Bokeikhanov and Akhmet Baitursynov, played a great role in the revival of the national identity of the Kazakhs in the 20th century. Dulatov is the author of the poems 'Oyan, Qazaq!' ('Wake up, Kazakh!'), which was published in 1909 and immediately sold out. It was republished in 1911. The title of the book served as a manifesto, an appeal to the Kazakh intellectuals of the early 20th century.
5 The main goal of the creation of the national liberation movement Alash in 1917 was the restoration of Kazakh statehood. The founders of the party program were political leader Alikhan Bokeikhanov, educator and linguist Akhmet Baitursynov, as well as writer and poet Myrzhakyp Dulatov.

References

Amnesty International. 2020. "Aktivist iz Kazakhstana Al'nur Ilyashev prigovoren k "ogranicheniu svobody" za kritiku pravitel'stvennyh mer po bor'be s Covid-19." June 22, 2020. https://eurasia.amnesty.org/2020/06/22/aktivist-iz-kazahstana-alnur-ilyashev-prigovoren-k-ogranicheniyu-svobody-za-kritiku-pravitelstvennyh-mer-po-borbe-s-covid-19/.

Astapova, Anastasiya, Vasil Navumau, Ryhor Nizhnikau, and Leonid Polishchuk. 2022. "Authoritarian cooptation of civil society: The case of Belarus." *Europe-Asia Studies* 74, no. 1: 1–30. https://doi.org/10.1080/09668136.2021.2009773.

Belapan. 2020a. "Lukashenko: Mery po preduprezhdeniyu zavoza koronavirusa dolzhny byt' effektivnymi, no ne izbytochnymi." February 12, 2020.

Belapan. 2020b. "Lukashenko: V Belarusi vybrali pravil'nuyu taktiku bor'by s koronavirusom." April 19, 2020.

Bohr, Annette. 2021. "Elections in Kazakhstan yield results as predicted." Chatham House Expert Comment, January 21, 2021. https://www.chathamhouse.org/2021/01/elections-kazakhstan-yield-results-predicted.

Bohr, Annette, Brauer Birgit, Gould-Davies Nigel, Kassenova Nargis, Lillis Joanna, Mallinson Kate, and Satpayev Dosym. 2019. *Kazakhstan: Tested by Transition*. London: Chatham House Royal Institute of International Affairs.

Charnysh, Volha. 2020. "The Uninteded Consequences of the Pandemic on Belarus' Presidential Elections." July 29, 2020. https://www.ispionline.it/en/pubblicazione/uninteded-consequences-pandemic-belarus-presidential-elections-27109.

Cook, Linda J. 2011. *Postcommunist Welfare States: Reform Politics in Russia and Eastern Europe*. Ithaca: Cornell University Press.

Demoscope. 2019. "Vybory prezidenta Kazakhstana." https://www.demos.kz/old/rus/index.php?poll=77.

Du Boulay, Sofya, and Rico Isaacs. 2019. "Legitimacy and Legitimation in Kazakhstan and Turkmenistan." *Theorizing Central Asian Politics: The State, Ideology and Power*, 17–41. https://doi.org/10.1007/978-3-319-97355-5_2.

Dukalskis, Alexander, and Johannes Gerschewski. 2017. "What autocracies say (and what citizens hear): Proposing four mechanisms of autocratic legitimation." *Contemporary Politics* 23, no. 3: 251–268. https://doi.org/10.1080/13569775.2017.1304320.

EurAsia Daily. 2020. "Kazakhstantsy proveli mitingi, nesmotrya na zapret sanitarnyh vrachei." June 7, 2020. https://eadaily.com/ru/news/2020/06/07/kazahstancy-proveli-mitingi-nesmotrya-na-zapret-sanitarnyh-vrachey.

Gerschewski, Johannes. 2018. "Legitimacy in autocracies: Oxymoron or essential feature?" *Perspectives on Politics* 16, no. 3: 652–665. https://doi.org/DOI:10.1017/S1537592717002183.

Giugni, Marco. 2011. "Political opportunity: Still a useful concept." In *Contention and trust in cities and states*, edited by M. Hanagan, C. Tilly, 271–283. Dordrecht: Springer Netherlands.

Greer, Scott L., Elizabeth J. King, and Elize Massard da Fonseca. 2021. "Introduction: Explaining pandemic response." *GREER*, SL et al. 3–33. http://www.jstor.org/stable/10.3998/mpub.11927713.3.

Hall, Stephen. 2022. "The end of adaptive authoritarianism in Belarus?" *Europe-Asia Studies*. 1–27.

Hewitt, Simon. 2021. "The 2021 Kazakhstan Legislative Elections: Reflections on the 'Listening State." *EIAS Op-ed*, February 9, 2021. https://eias.org/publications/op-ed/the-2021-kazakhstan-legislative-elections-reflections-on-the-listening-state/.

Jones, Pauline, and Elizabeth J. King 2021. "COVID-19 response in Central Asia: A cautionary tale." In *Coronavirus Politics*, edited by E. M. da Fonseca, S. L. Greer, E. J. King, and A. Peralta-Santos. Ann Arbor: University of Michigan Press. http://www.jstor.org/stable/10.3998/mpub.11927713.3.

Karimov, Elbol. 2021. "God s koronavirusom v Kazakhstane: chto bylo i chego zhdat' dal'she." *Liter*, March 13, 2021. https://liter.kz/odin-god-s-koronavirusom-v-kazahstane/.

Kilybayeva, Shugyla, and Nurshanov Azamat. 2020. "The impact of social media on Kazakhstani youth's political behavior." *Central Asia and the Caucasus* 20, no. 1: 62–75.

Kilybayeva, Shugyla. 2020. "Citizens and Politics". Unpublished survey conducted in Kazakhstan in May–July, 2020.

Kopotev, Mikhail, A. Mustajoki, and A. Bonch-Osmolovskaya. 2021. "Corpora in text-based Russian studies." In *The Palgrave Handbook of Digital Russia Studies*, 299–318. Cham: Palgrave Macmillan. https://doi.org/10.1007/978-3-030-42855-6_17.

Korovenkova, Tatiana. 2020a. "Lukashenko: Nado lyudei zastavit' otvechat' za sebya i tekh, kto ryadom." *Belapan*, March 20, 2020.

Korovenkova, Tatiana. 2020b. "Lukashenko: U nas segodnya 794 cheloveka gospitalizirovany, 31- na IVL." *Belapan*, April 7, 2020.

Korastyleva, Yuna. 2020a. "Glavnyi sanvrach Kazakhstana rasskazala ob etapah smyagcheniya karantinnyh mer." *Vlast*, May 12, 2020.

KPMG. 2020. "Vliyanie Covid-19 na klyuchevye sektora ekonomiki Kazakhstana. Mnenie uchastnikov rynka." May 2020. https://assets.kpmg/content/dam/kpmg/kz/pdf/2020/05/covid-rk-economy-sectors.pdf.

Krawatzek, Félix and Julia Langbein. 2022. "Attitudes towards democracy and the market in Belarus: What has changed and why it matters." *Post-Soviet Affairs* 38, nos. 1–2: 107–124.

Laruelle, Marlene, Mikhail Alexseev, Buckley Cynthia, Ralph S. Clem, J. Paul Goode, Gomza Ivan, Henry E. Hale et al. 2021. "Pandemic politics in Eurasia: Roadmap for a new research subfield." *Problems of Post-communism* 68, no. 1: 1–16. https://doi.org/10.1080/10758216.2020.1812404.

Laruelle, Marlene. 2019. "Introduction: The Nazarbayev generation: A sociological portrait." In *The Nazarbayev Generation: Youth in Kazakhstan*, edited by M. Laruelle, 1–22. Washington, DC: Rowan & Littlefield.

Libman, Alexander, and Kozlov Vladimir. 2017. "The legacy of compliant activism in autocracies: Post-communist experience." *Contemporary Politics* 23, no. 2: 195–213. https://doi.org/10.1080/13569775.2016.1206275.

Lukashenko, Aleksandr. 2006. "We are building a socially oriented state." *Russian Politics & Law* 44, no. 4: 6–22. https://doi.org/10.2753/RUP1061-1940440401.

Mallinson, K. 2019. "Governance in Kazakhstan: Tested by transition." Chatham House Report.

Moldabekov, Daniyar. 2020a. "Miting v Almaty 6 iyunya: protest na fone dezinfektsii." *Vlast*, June 6, 2020.

Moldabekov, Daniyar. 2020b. "Prokuror zaprosil tri goda lisheniya svobody dlya Al'nura Il'yasheva." *Vlast*, June 19, 2020.

Moshes, Arkady, and Ryhor Nizhnikau. 2019. "The Belarusian paradox: A country of today versus a president of the past." FIIA Briefing Paper 258.

Mitikka, Eemil. Forthcoming. "Authoritarian Responses to Protest Participation During COVID-19: The Russian Case". *The Politics of the Pandemic in Eastern Europe and Eurasia: Blame Game and Governance,* edited by M. Zavadskaya. London: Routledge.

Nathan, Andrew J. 2020. "The puzzle of authoritarian legitimacy." *Journal of Democracy* 31, no. 1: 158–168. https://doi.org/10.1353/jod.2020.0013.

Nosova, Marina. 2020. "Lukashenko o koronaviruse: Segodnya malen'kij luchik nadezhdy zabrezzhil." *Belapan*, April 17, 2020.

Official Site of the President of the Republic of Kazakhstan. 2012. "Strategy 'Kazakhstan-2050': New Political Course of the Established State." State of the National Address, December 14, 2012. https://www.akorda.kz/ru/official_documents/strategies_and_programs.

Official Site of the President of the Republic of Kazakhstan. 2020. "Glava gosudarstva prinyal uchastie v obschenatcional'nom onlain-forume 'Biz Birgemiz'." https://primeminister.kz/ru/news/glava-gosudarstva-prinyal-uchastie-v-obshchenacionalnom-onlayn-forume-biz-birgemiz-235024.

Official Site of the President of the Republic of Kazakhstan. 2022. "President Respubliki Kazahstan." https://www.akorda.kz/ru/president/president.

Omelicheva, Mariya Y. 2016. "Authoritarian legitimation: assessing discourses of legitimacy in Kazakhstan and Uzbekistan." *Central Asian Survey* 35, no. 4: 481–500. https://doi.org/10.1080/02634937.2016.1245181.

Oreshko, Alyaksei. 2020. "Lukashenko o koronaviruse: Uspokaivat'sya nel'zya, no i dlya paniki u nas net osnovanii." *Belapan*, March 12, 2020.

OSCE. 2019. "International Election Observation Missions Republic of Kazakhstan – Early Presidential Election. Statement of Preliminary Findings and Conclusions." June 9, 2019. https://www.osce.org/files/f/documents/4/2/422510.pdf.

OSCE. 2021. "International Election Observation Missions Republic of Kazakhstan – Parliamentary Election. Statement of Preliminary Findings and Conclusions." January 10, 2021. https://www.osce.org/files/f/documents/c/6/475538.pdf.

Radio Azattyq. 2011. "V Zhanaozene vvedeno chrezvychainoe polozhenie." December 17, 2011. https://rus.azattyq.org/a/zhanaozen_state_of_emergency_kazakhstan/24424972.html.

Radio Azattyq. 2020. "Kairgali Koneyev: Koronavirus v Kazakhstane byl ne pandemiei, a chistoi vody politikoi." September 8, 2020. https://rus.azattyq.org/a/kazakhstan-coronavirus-pandemic-interview-kairgali-koneyev/30825364.html.

Radio Azattyq. 2021. "Parlamentskie vybory-2021. Rezultaty exitpolla." January 11, 2021. https://rus.azattyq.org/a/with-no-opposition-on-ballot-kazakhstan-holds-parliamentary-elections/31040111.html.

Reform.by. 2020. "Koordinator #ByCovid19 Andrei Strizhak s semei vyekhal iz Belarusi". July 6, 2020. https://reform.by/145756-koordinator-bycovid19-andrej-strizhak-s-semej-vyehal-iz-belarusi.

Shcherbakov, Zakhar. 2020. "Minoborony: Ehpidemiologicheskaya obstanovka pozvolyaet provesti voennyi parad." *Belapan*, April 20, 2020.

Sputnik. 2020. "Nurzhana Al'tayeva iskluchili iz partii Nur Otan." February 1, 2020. https://ru.sputnik.kz/20201202/Nurzhan-Altaev-lishilsya-deputatskogo-mandata-posle-ukhoda-iz-partii-Nur-Otan-15627961.html.

Starr, Frederick. 2019. "First Glimpses of Tokayev's Kazakhstan: The Listening State?" *Atlantic Council Commentary*. September 17, 2019. https://www.atlanticcouncil.org/commentary/long-take/first-glimpses-of-tokayevs-kazakhstan/.

The Economist. 2022. "Coronavirus Excess Death Tracker." October 20, 2021. https://www.economist.com/graphic-detail/coronavirus-excess-deaths-tracker.

The World Bank. 2020. "Individuals using the Internet (% of population) – Kazakhstan." https://data.worldbank.org/indicator/IT.NET.USER.ZS?locations=KZ.

Turchina, Irina. 2020a. "BNTU perevodyat na individual'nuyu programmu obucheniya v svyazi s vyyavleniem u studenta koronavirusa." *Belapan*, February 28, 2020.

Turchina, Irina. 2020b. "Lukashenko o koronaviruse: Vyderzhim do pravoslavnoj Paskhi — znachit, zhit' budem." *Belapan*, March 24, 2020.

Turchina, Irina. 2020c. "Missiya VOZ: Belarus' vkhodit v novuyu fazu vspyshki COVID-19." April 11, 2020.

Turchina, Irina. 2020d. "V Belarusi nachinaetsya vaktsinatsiya ot COVID-19." *Belapan*, December 29, 2020.

United Nations High Commissioner for Human Rights. 2022. "Situation of human rights in Belarus in the run-up to the 2020 presidential election and in its aftermath." March 4. https://documents-dds-ny.un.org/doc/UNDOC/GEN/G22/276/97/PDF/G2227697.pdf?OpenElement.

Vaal', Tamara. 2020a. "Akimy i ministry v period pamdemii zakrylis'ot naroda, zayavil Tokayev." *Vlast*, June 29, 2020.

Vaal', Tamara. 2020b. "Birtanov zayavil o vtoroi volne koronavirusa v Kazakhstane." *Vlast*, June 4, 2020.

Vaal', Tamara. 2020c. "Glava Minzdrava prizval povremenit's mitingami v period karantina." *Vlast*, June 4, 2020.

Vaal', Tamara. 2020d. "Kazakhstan dolzhen izbezhat' zhestkogo karantina – Tokayev." *Vlast*, November 7, 2020.
Vaal', Tamara. 2020e. "Kazakhstan zapretit v'ezd esche iz neskolkih stran iz-za koronavirusa." *Vlast*, March 10, 2020.
Vaal', Tamara. 2020f. "Kompleksnyi plan po vosstanovleniu ekonomicheskogo rosta Kazakhstana utverdilo pravitel'stvo." *Vlast*, May 19, 2020.
Vaal', Tamara. 2020h. "Nadbavki do 850 tysyach tenge poluchat vrachi, zadeistvovannye v bor'be s koronavirusom." *Vlast*, March 30, 2020.
Vaal', Tamara. 2020j. "Oslablenie karantinnyh mer privelo k rostu zabolevaniya koronavirusom." *Vlast*, May 25, 2020.
Vaal', Tamara. 2020k. "Pochti 1 tysyach chelovek nahodyatsya na karantine v Kazakhstane." *Vlast*, March 5, 2020.
Vaal', Tamara. 2020l. "Poryadka 23.5 milliarda tenge vydelili iz rezerva na bor'bu s koronavirusom v Kazakhstane." *Vlast*, April 1, 2020.
Vaal', Tamara. 2020m. "Pravitel'stvo prosit biznes pereyti na distantsionnuyuy raboty." *Vlast*, March 16, 2020.
Vaal', Tamara. 2020o. "Spetskomissiya budet razbirat'sya v dopuschennyh oshibkah v bor'be s koronavirusom v Kazakhstane." *Vlast*, July 10, 2020.
Vaal', Tamara. 2020p. "Tokayev prigrozil pravitel'stvu rospuskom." *Vlast*, July 10, 2020.
Vaal', Tamara. 2020q. "V Kazakhstane uvelichilos chislo samoobraschenii s simptomami koronavirusa." *Vlast*, May 20, 2020.
Vaal', Tamara. 2020r. "Vybory v mazhilis sostoyatsya v srok, vne zavisimosti ot epidsituatsii." *Vlast*, October 10, 2020.
Vlast. 2020a. "Chrezvychainoe polozhenie. Onlain." March 15, 2020.
Vlast. 2020b. "Halyk bank perechislit 100 million tenge medikam, boryuschihsya s koronavirusom." March 16, 2020.
Vlast. 2020c. "Nazarbayev vyrazil soboleznovaniya rodnym i blizkim zhertvy pandemii koronavirusa." July 13, 2020.
Vlast. 2020d. "NPP sozdala operativnyi shtab dlya pomoschi predprinimatelyam." March 16, 2020.
Vlast. 2020f. "Svyshe 400 kazakhstantsev obratilis' v MID s pros'boy ob evakuacii iz Kitaya." February 5, 2020.
Vlast. 2020g. "Tokayev podpisal rasporyazhenie ob ob'yavlenii traura v Kazakhstane." July 9, 2020
Vlast. 2020h. "Tokayev poruchil vydelit' 600 milliardov tenge na kreditovanie oborotnogo kapitala MSB." March 19, 2020
Vlast. 2020j. "V Kazakhstane nachal deistvovat' rezhim chrezvychainogo polozheniya." March 16, 2020.
Vlast. 2020k. "V Kazakhstane vvedeno chrezvychainoe polozhenie iz-za koronavirusa." March 15, 2020.
von Soest, Christian, and Julia Grauvogel. 2017. "Identity, procedures and performance: How authoritarian regimes legitimize their rule." *Contemporary Politics* 23, no. 3: 287–305. https://doi.org/10.1080/13569775.2017.1304319.
Walker, Shaun. 2020. "'The only way to stop violence': Why protesters are unmasking Belarus police." *The Guardian*, September 17, 2020. https://www.theguardian.com/world/2020/sep/17/the-only-way-to-stop-violence-why-protesters-are-unmasking-belarus-police.
Way, Lucan Ahmad. 2020. "Belarus uprising: How a dictator became vulnerable." *Journal of Democracy* 31, no. 4: 17–27.

Ybrayev, Zhandos. 2020. "Covid-19 in Kazakhstan: Economic Consequences and Policy Implications." *Central Asia Program Paper, № 234*. July, 2020. https://centralasiaprogram.org/wp-content/uploads/2020/07/CAP_Paper_No.234_by_Zhandos-Ybrayev.pdf.

Zakon Respubliki Kazakhstan. 2020. "O poraydke organizatsii I provedeniya mirnyh sobranii v Respublike Kazakhstan." https://online.zakon.kz/Document/?doc_id=36271780&pos=5;-106#pos=5;-106.

Interviews

Belarus

Alyaksei, Minsk, civic activist. Interviewed by the authors on 8 June 2022 via Zoom.

Lena, Minsk oblast' / Minsk, political analyst (PhD in Political Science). Interviewed by the authors on 6 June 2022 via Zoom.

Maksim, political analyst (PhD in Cultural Studies). Interviewed by one of the authors on 7 June 2022 via Zoom.

Polina, Hrodna oblast' / Minsk, entrepreneur turned political activist. Interviewed by the authors on 16 June 2022 via Zoom.

Tatsiana, Minsk, partner of a Belarusian IT specialist turned civic activist. Interviewed by the authors on 17 June 2022 via Zoom.

Kazakhstan

Anastassiya, Almaty/Pavlodar, expert in Public Policy, Master of Sociolinguistics. Interviewed by the authors on 10 June 2022 via Zoom.

Inara, Almaty/Shymkent, PhD in Social Science. Interviewed by the authors on 15 July 2022.

Oraz, Almaty, expert in Media, lecturer. Interviewed by the authors on 3 June 2022 via Zoom.

Violetta, Almaty, expert in Public Policy. Interviewed by the authors on 17 June 2022 via Zoom.

Zharas, Nur-Sultan/ Shymkent, PhD in International Relations. Interviewed by the authors on 18 June 2022 via Zoom.

9 The COVID-19 Pandemic and the Performative State in Uzbekistan

Mirzokhid Karshiev and Kristiina Silvan

Introduction

On March 15, 2020, Mirzokhid, one of the authors of this chapter,[1] was in Qarshi, the administrative centre of the Qashqadaryo region of southern Uzbekistan, attending a local Navruz[2] celebration, when the news of the first patient with COVID-19 in the country came through. At a governmental meeting in Tashkent, harsh measures aimed at containing the spread of the virus within the country were announced. Schools, kindergartens, and universities were to be closed nationwide and all international travel was halted overnight from March 16 forward. Prime Minister Abdulla Aripov explained at the briefing that the measures were necessary to minimise social contact and prevent further dissemination of COVID-19 in the country (Kun.uz 2020a). In Qarshi, the ongoing celebrations were called off hastily and thousands of people in the park were asked to go home. The established power vertical demonstrated how fast decisions could be taken and implemented.[3]

Several days later, Mirzokhid went for a scheduled interview with the regional administration (*khokimiyat*) in Termiz, Surxondaryo region. A huge crowd of over 100 people gathered in front of the building to participate in a conference call with their superiors, still better known to locals by its Soviet name of a 'selector' meeting (Rus. '*selektornoe soveshchanie*'). The attendees were heads of local government bodies and key management personnel, some of whom travelled over 150 km to attend this two-hour gathering. It was ironic that the meeting was meant to consider the government's response to the developing COVID-19 situation, and yet was not organised fully online.[4] This was an early indication of how administrative practices were and are slow to change. Decision-making at the national level and implementation at the sub-national level may diverge.

Researchers of Central Asia have long noted the apparent duality of the state: it can be overwhelmingly present and control some spheres of community life, while at the same time fail to deliver basic public services (Heathershaw 2014). The pandemic, as with many other crises, has laid bare the various aspects of the public administration and governance system in the countries of the region. In the past three years, the way the decisions were

DOI: 10.4324/9781003364870-10

taken, communicated, implemented, (re)evaluated, changed, and if/how these processes prevented the mass dissemination of COVID-19 as well as the general state-society nexus in Central Asian countries have been a focus of numerous studies and publications (Laruelle et al. 2020; Dzhuraev 2021; Caron and Thibault 2022). This chapter contributes to this new body of literature by providing a unique ethnographic multi-level perspective of the response of Uzbekistan's public administration to the pandemic threat. It asks how the executive and especially local bureaucrats perceived their work in the context of the evolving COVID-19 pandemic and whether COVID-19 posed a threat to the government's image of public performance. To address these questions, we analyse the national and the sub-national government's response to the pandemic through the lens of a 'performative state', considering the prevalent administrative culture and practices they are embedded in.

Authoritarian Modernisation and Performance Legitimacy

In the world of global rankings and indicators, most post-Soviet countries cannot boast about their achievements in governance. According to Gel'man (2017), post-Soviet Eurasia could compete with sub-Saharan Africa for the dubious honour of representing the epitome of bad governance. There is a plethora of academic and policy-oriented scholarship that provides possible explanations for this phenomenon. Firstly, these countries all had to address a common Soviet legacy – a system based on undemocratic public administration that was designed for authoritarian rule and a command economy over the wellbeing of its citizens (Barabashev and Straussman 2007; Liebert, Condrey, and Goncharov 2013). The transition from the Soviet governance system required a triple transformation affecting nation-building (constructing a state and nation), constitution-reformulation (democratisation), as well as the 'normal politics' of allocation (market economy) (Offe and Adler 1991).

The different pace and path of administrative reforms in former post-Soviet countries led researchers to emphasise the role of national leaders (Gleason 1997; Cummings 2002), transitional contexts, institutional design (Jones Luong 2002), and the role of networks and patron-client relationships (Ledeneva 1998; 2007; 2013; Lewis 2012; Hale 2014), including those of clans (Collins 2006) and informal elite networks (Radnitz 2010).

Portraying bad governance in post-Soviet Eurasia as a primarily agency-driven rather than structure-induced phenomenon, Gel'man (2017) considers bad governance practices as a consequence of elite rent-seeking combined with weak and limited domestic and international resistance. The literature on the governance system in Uzbekistan also underlines the role of elite agents in an authoritarian context, persisting through neopatrimonial relations (Ilkhamov 2007; Laruelle 2012; Isaacs 2014), effective authoritarian legitimation techniques (Omelicheva 2016), and increasing 'social control' (Urinboyev 2014). Perlman and Gleason (2007), who conducted a comparative analysis of administrative reforms in Kazakhstan and Uzbekistan, concluded that policy choices rather than cultural values played a determining role in the administrative change in the countries reviewed. The bottom-up, ethnographic accounts of everyday life in the country referred to the dualism of state presence/absence and the state itself turning into an informal institution (Rasanayagam 2011), thus making the boundaries between the formal and informal difficult to delineate.

We argue that administrative behaviour and underlying administrative culture need to be understood in relation to the broader social environment. In the real world, states are seldom the only actors in societies and are almost never autonomous from social forces (Migdal, Kohli, and Shue 1994). Bottom-up ethnographic research has demonstrated that ordinary citizens as well as state bureaucrats encounter the state in a far more decentralised and disaggregated form (Gupta 1995). An 'analysis of the state' requires us to conceptualise a space that is constituted by the intersection of local, regional, national, and transnational phenomena.

One way of analysing the state is to look at its legitimation practices. On the one hand, the scholarship on fragile states argues that effective governance increases the legitimacy of the responsible governance actors, and higher levels of legitimacy increase their effectiveness (Schmelzle and Stollenwerk 2018). This mutually dependent and reinforcing relationship came to be known as a virtuous circle and has been popular among development policy practitioners (World Bank 2011), who have been supportive of interventions, aimed at improving state performance and effectiveness.

On the other hand, legitimacy that state performance generates is often identified as one of the three pillars of authoritarian stability (along with repression and co-optation) (Gerschewski 2013). Due to the nature of the regime that is mutually exclusive with rule-based mechanisms for handing over power and implementing policies, procedural legitimacy is difficult to obtain for authoritarian governments, which leads them to rely on identity-based legitimacy claims (foundational myth, ideology, and personalism) (von Soest and Grauvogel 2017). What is seen as performance depends on the context: it can be the provision of safety and security or the ability to provide economic growth or public services. While the idea of political decision-makers' legitimacy (i.e. the right to rule) based on performance has been used to describe communist governments in the past (White 1986), particularly in the Chinese case (Zeng 2014), authoritarian governments all across the world have embraced the potential of performance for producing legitimacy in order to maintain power. The so-called 'informational autocracies' (Guriev and Treisman 2019) and 'spin dictatorships' (Guriev and Treisman 2022) tend to adopt a rhetoric of performance and competence to boost their popularity. Guriev and Treisman (2019) argue that 'like democratic leaders, most dictators today focus on economic performance and service provision when they address the public and avoid the violent rhetoric of old-style autocrats' (Guriev and Treisman 2019, 123). Here, performance not only refers to the substantive delivery of outputs, sought after by citizens, but also to the theatrical deployment of language, symbols, and gestures to foster an impression of good governance among citizens. Currently, performative governance techniques are mostly associated with authoritarian settings, like China (Ding 2020; 2022), but researchers have highlighted that democratic and semi-democratic regimes may also include performative elements, especially by populist politicians (Moffitt 2016; Kissas 2020).

In his classic study of Soviet *nomenklatura*, Michael Voslenky (1984) described Soviet senior bureaucrats as an exploitative and parasitic class that was career oriented due to the many benefits that their work entailed. He argued that members of the administrative elite saw themselves as hard-working intellectuals but in fact they were primarily focused on the 'imitation of vigorous activity' (Rus. '*imitatsiya burnoy deyatelnosti*'), which remains a well-understood phrase of bureaucratic jargon in post-Soviet settings up to this day.

The transformation of the Soviet bureaucracy into post-Soviet ones followed a variety of different trajectories, but throughout the former Soviet Union, the process entailed the adaptation of Soviet practices to those trends in public administration that were dominant at the time, in the early 1990s. In particular, the principles of new public management (NPM) were popular among development practitioners. Indeed, NPM with its priority towards improving the *performance* of state bureaucracy – as if they were a market entity – became the leitmotif for reconstructing the system of public administration. We argue that the performative governance studied in this chapter is a rather peculiar adaptation of these two trends: Soviet-style hand-waving and NPM.

Joe Migdal's differentiation between the 'image' and 'practices' of the state (Migdal 2001, 16) is also insightful for the further analysis of a 'performative state' put forward in this chapter. According to Migdal, 'the routine performance of state actors and agencies, their practices, may reinforce the image of the state or weaken it; they may bolster the notion of the territorial and public-private boundaries or neutralise them' (Migdal 2001, 18).

In the following sections, we analyse how this rhetoric and practices of 'performance' have influenced policymaking and implementation in sub-national public administration bodies in Uzbekistan both before and during the pandemic. The analysis put forward in these sections is built on a unique set of qualitative data that consists of secondary sources (media reports, news items, analytical essays, official statistics, and legislative acts) as well as primary sources collected by Mirzokhid Karshiev while at field work in Uzbekistan in spring-summer 2020 (field notes and 12 semi-structured interviews conducted with local bureaucrats, civic activists, and ordinary people).

The interviews were multi-sited, conducted in Southern, Central, and Western parts (regions) of Uzbekistan, mainly organised in three patterns. Firstly, as Mirzokhid originally comes from Uzbekistan and has a work experience of working as a civil servant and as a consultant in local governance support projects, implemented by international organisations, he utilised the network of acquaintances and former colleagues for arranging interviews. Secondly, thanks to the relative transparency of the civil service system, Mirzokhid directly contacted the public officials in the central and local government (via social networks, through email, and phone) and requested interviews with them. Thirdly, the interviewees were asked for other potential interlocutors, who could be beneficial for the project (snowballing). We believe, this approach allowed us to go beyond the 'social bubble' problem, especially in regards snowballing, when study participants only refer researchers to those who share their beliefs and inclinations. Eighty percent of interviewees were men and 20% women, which mostly reflects the demographics structure of the public administration system in Uzbekistan. Most of the interviewees wished to remain anonymous. Given the risks involved, the authors decided to anonymise the data related to personal information of the interviewees. Two-thirds of the interviews were conducted online and via phone as the possibilities for face-to-face interviews were limited in April–May and July of 2020.

Public Administration Reforms and the Performative State on the Eve of the Pandemic

Uzbekistan, a post-Soviet state, was ruled by a former Communist party secretary-turned-president, Islam Karimov, for 25 years after the collapse of the Soviet Union and the country's independence in 1991. After Karimov's sudden death in 2016, Shavkat Mirziyoyev, the prime minister of the country since 2003, took over and among other things, launched an ambitious governance reform. The reform signalled an intention to make a transition from a closed and heavily repressive type of authoritarianism towards a softer version of authoritarianism (Lemon 2019). Some of these reforms, especially related to the eradication of forced labour, earned Uzbekistan the 'country of the year' award by The Economist (2019).

Immediately after assuming the head of state role, Mirziyoyev underlined the need for faster reactions to citizens' needs, improved service delivery mechanisms, and greater powers for local authorities. In this framework, Mirziyoyev proclaimed a new motto: 'the state should serve its citizens, not vice versa'. The Concept of Administrative Reforms, adopted by the president in September 2017 (Lex.uz 2017), indicated many problems in the public administration system, including the declarative nature of many tasks, extreme centralisation of decision-making (superiors' tendency to micromanage that public officials usually refer to as 'manual control' (Rus. '*ruchnoye upravleniye*')), and duplication of functions and powers, for example with one state body combining functions of policy implementation and oversight. Decentralisation, civil service reform, improvement of public service delivery, public-private partnership, and greater transparency and accountability of the state and its institutions were the cornerstones of the new reform agenda. Since 2016, many participatory platforms have been introduced on the national level, including ones geared toward the discussion of new legislative initiatives and for introducing petitions to the parliament.

Similar developments have taken place on the level of local governance, where the system also received a facelift. One of the most popular decisions made by President Mirziyoyev was the establishment of presidential reception houses in each region, city, and district of the country. According to the decree that established the virtual and on-site reception points, the aim was to 'organise direct dialogue with the population' and 'ensure the functioning of a new system of working with appeals of individuals and legal entities to protect their rights, freedoms and interests' (*UzDaily* 2016). People could address their grievances online, via telephone, or by attending in person. A specific unit within the presidential administration monitored all the cases and made sure that these cases were 'closed' properly. Another administrative change introduced by Mirziyoyev was the requirement for local *khokims* and other top managers to live in their respective districts/regions and spend a significant amount of their time visiting communities and solving their problems.[5]

These changes could be interpreted as a sign that 'participatory' (Owen 2020) and 'responsive' (Heurlin 2016) authoritarianism was taking hold in the Uzbek political system. Following Dimitrov (2023), the newfound responsiveness can also be seen as an institutional solution to the 'dictator's dilemma' that allowed the authorities to gather information about the elite and popular discontent more effectively and use this knowledge to prevent potential challenges, thus stabilising its rule. However, given how little *substantive* change these reforms introduced to Uzbekistan's system of public administration, we maintain that these amendments can be seen as an attempt to build an authoritarian performative rather than a performance state.

Another characteristic of Mirziyoyev's Uzbekistan in the pre-pandemic period was the newfound frequency of institutional and organisational changes. This was geared towards making an impression of a new era of performance while only introducing cosmetic changes to the system of public administration. In 2016–2020, the number of ministries in Uzbekistan went up by two-thirds (from 15 to 24). Almost all ministries and other governmental bodies faced personnel, administrative, and functional reshuffling, while numerous new state agencies, committees, associations, and other state bodies were established. Just before the COVID-19 pandemic, in September 2019, the state sanitary and epidemiology system in Uzbekistan was thoroughly restructured and the former sanitary-epidemiology oversight service of the Ministry of Public Health was divided into two separate bodies, namely the State Inspection under the Cabinet of Ministers and the Agency under the Ministry (Lex.uz 2019). The main justification for this reform was to significantly improve the epidemiological welfare of the population. Little did the decision-makers know that the state's ability to care for the health of its people was to be tested in the very near future.

The Performative State and the Outbreak of the COVID-19 Pandemic in Uzbekistan

Beginning of the Pandemic

As is well known by now, the story of the global COVID-19 pandemic started in Wuhan, Hubei province, China, in December 2019. In the initial 'information repression phase', the virus spread widely around China, whereas in the 'mobilization for containment phase', which began after mid-January 2020, the entire country was locked down in a push to halt the spread of the disease (Shih 2021). On January 25, President Xi Jinping announced the formation of the Central Leading Group on Confronting the Novel Coronavirus Pneumonia (CLGCNCP) and warned his subordinates: 'Preserving life is the highest priority [...] all will be held responsible for preventing and controlling the epidemic' (Xinhua 2020, quoted in Shih 2021, 72). In effect, the authorities mobilised to contain COVID-19 with astounding success, albeit in a way that kept society under full control of the Communist party (Shih 2021). The Chinese ability to uphold its 'zero-COVID policy' during the initial phase of the pandemic was seen as a clear case of the state's ability to strengthen its legitimacy through effective crisis management.

Similarly, Uzbekistan's initial response to the pandemic was praised by many, including international organisations and experts.[6] The Uzbek government demonstrated an early understanding of the challenges of COVID-19 as a novel virus. Already on 29 January 2020, it created a special anti-COVID-19 commission, tasked with preventing the dissemination of COVID-19 in the country (Lex.uz 2020). Its composition was almost like the Cabinet of Ministers, with the prime minister as its chair. Initially, the commission's role seemed minor, but it soon became clear that it was the one that made most decisions related to the introduction of health policy measures (lockdowns; travel, work, and other limitations), albeit without the established procedures of transparency and accountability. The decisions were made during meetings behind closed doors. While this was possible under the Uzbek legislation, a professor of law in Tashkent pointed out in his interview with Mirzokhid that the practice was 'against the spirit of the law'.[7]

It seems that the authorities' response was based on the advice from the leading state epidemiologists that argued that 'the dissemination of the virus could be stopped with early, draconian measures' (Gazeta.uz 2020). This was partially based on China's then seemingly well-handling of COVID-19 pandemic in its territory (BBC News O'zbek 2020) and the Uzbek government's invitation to Chinese medical professionals early on to share their 'zero-COVID' practices. When confronted by a journalist in March 2020 about the projections that the global COVID-19 pandemic could last for up to two years, Nurmat Atabekov, Uzbekistan's chief sanitary inspector, argued that the virus would be 'won over' in a month or two (Kun.uz 2020b). Correspondingly, we argue that the expectation of a 'sprint' rather than a 'marathon' led to many officials perceiving the outbreak of the pandemic as an opportunity to deliver quick results and demonstrate performance in the eyes of their superiors, or, in other words, enact the authoritarian performative state.

The way in which the public administration demonstrated performance followed the Chinese example. From mid-March 2020 onwards, the majority of the people were locked in their houses. Local officials blocked roads to stop people from getting around, issued penalties for not wearing a mask in public, disinfected streets with firefighting machines, and built special 'disinfection tunnels' that would protect people entering public buildings and venues from the virus.

These measures were, of course, felt among the people. As Mirzokhid was doing his fieldwork in southern Uzbekistan, gossip about an upcoming closure of intercity and interregional borders spread. He arranged a shared taxi to Tashkent because by that time, all buses, trains, and airplanes had already stopped operating. The taxi driver said that the road to Tashkent was full of police checkpoints and warned that if Mirzokhid doesn't have a temporary or permanent registered address in the capital, they might not be let through. Luckily, he did have the necessary registration in Tashkent and was let through. However, it was not only the police that followed state instructions for halting the spread of the virus. Upon entering Tashkent, Mirzokhid's taxi driver thoroughly disinfected his car with a chemical solution – both inside and outside.[8]

The novelty of the COVID-19 virus meant that the entire world was in a curious state of callowness (or ignorance?) about how the virus spread and what were the best ways to protect oneself. This uncertainty was also expressed in Uzbekistan. In an online conversation with a male member of parliament who helped build a 'disinfection tunnel' to the market in his constituency, he explained: 'Everyone coming to enter (i.e., not everyone, but those with special permission) the market would need to go through a "tunnel" where they were sprayed with a disinfectant'. His initiative was showcased on national TV as a successful method for enabling people to do their shopping while staying safe from the virus. However, in his conversation with Mirzokhid, the politician said he didn't know the contents of the chemical disinfectant, given that the local branch of the state sanitary and epidemiology agency had prepared the solution and controlled the whole process. He was not sure if the tunnel could really stop the spread of the virus.[9]

Local Governance Hyperactive Mode

The strict national lockdown did not mean that the public administration had taken a step back – quite the opposite, it was working full steam, breathing life into the performative state and entering a state of hyperactivity. A senior manager in local *khokimiyat* (body of governance) in central Uzbekistan lamented to Mirzokhid on the phone:

> Do you think I'm working from home? No, of course. Every day there's a new instruction from above. We're blocking roads, distributing food, organising

> quarantine facilities, and doing whatever comes to the mind of superiors. Maybe I'm meeting more people now than before (the pandemic). I rented a place near *khokimiyat* and am staying there. I don't want my family to get the virus from me.[10]

The deeply permeated culture of the performative state was indeed demonstrated in countless ways during the COVID-19 pandemic. One of the interviewees of Mirzokhid reflected:

> One of the pertaining features of our system is that it values quick delivery of results. I can definitely say, that in our *khokimiyat*, the guys, who can rapidly execute whatever orders from above, get better promotions compared to those who want their actions to be consistent with all the laws.[11]

Another respondent suggested:

> Most local government officials are engaged in what they call '*ochko yig'ish*' (Uz. 'ollecting points')…What it means in practice is that they're constantly following signals from superiors and trying to deliver expected outcomes as fast as they can. It's a kind of competition.[12]

Although the participants of this study were critical of the way 'working hard' was equated with efficiency and performance – regardless of whether it was purposeful or not – they viewed it as an unchangeable part of one's career in public administration. One junior civil servant lamented:

> We usually have to stay at work late into the evening, as long working hours are considered to demonstrate hard work and performance. Our superiors are used to receiving calls and instructions from the centre at eight or nine p.m., and if they don't pick up their office phones or do not deliver reports on short notice, they're labelled 'lazy' and could be penalised during the next 'selector' meeting.[13]

It would be wrong to claim that the culture of performativity had emerged recently, whether during Mirziyoyev's tenure or as a response to the outbreak of the COVID-19 pandemic. On the contrary, one of the senior-level officials, interviewed by Mirzokhid, said that he had not had a proper holiday for 15 years.[14] There is reason to believe that his state of affairs was indicative of most public servants.

Performative Spending

As the insights of the previous section highlight, the COVID-19 pandemic put Uzbekistan's public administration into a mode of hyperactivity. While the phenomenon can indeed be explained primarily by the governance system's focus on performativity *vis-à-vis* one's superiors, it seems that the unprecedented activity was also driven by financial incentives in the form of a sudden relaxation of budgetary constraints.

Like in many parts of the world, the government announced bonuses for medical personnel taking care of patients who contracted COVID-19. What was exceptional in Uzbekistan, however, was how substantial these extra payments were, amounting to around seven to ten times the average salary. A representative of the state sanitary and epidemiology agency, interviewed by Mirzokhid, complained that the considerable financial compensation created an incentive to medical workers to *over*report COVID-19 cases and falsely claim pneumonia or flu patients as COVID-19 ones. In effect, the state sanitary agency introduced the practice of a centralised *triple* check of samples in district, regional, and national laboratories, which in effect increased the cost of testing and put a strain on the testing capacity. What is more, the sudden budget increase was seen by some of the agency managers as an opportunity to make money by purchasing medical and sanitary supplies at higher, 'above market' prices (Kun.uz 2020c).

The flurry of activities aimed at halting the spread of COVID-19 was also explained by the spending spree of local officials, sometimes with their corrupt interests at play. One middle-aged local official in Surxondaryo hinted at this in his conversation with Mirzokhid:

> Some of these decisions [like street disinfection, and tunnels] seem funny from a medical side. But when you follow the money, [see] who is selling the equipment, materials, constructing the facilities and so on, you will understand not to criticise this publicly.[15]

While the economic cost of the COVID-19 pandemic is well known, it is also true that some companies and individuals benefited greatly from the outbreak of the pandemic if they were able to provide the now much needed products and services. For example, in Uzbekistan, like almost everywhere in the world, large-scale quarantine facilities were organised for those arriving from abroad. These facilities were built and equipped first in Tashkent and later in other parts of the country with millions of dollars of government funding. Given the urgency of their construction, no public tenders were held, which is why government critics voiced concerns that the large contracts could have gone to companies affiliated with high-level officials.

The representative of the state sanitary and epidemiology agency interviewed by Mirzokhid confirms that the agency's leadership and personnel were astonished by the unprecedented level of attention and funding. Regardless of the uncertainty of what was the most effective way to halt the spread of the virus, the agency was facing growing pressure to do something – *anything* – that would visibly demonstrate that they were actively fighting against the spread of the pandemic.[16]

When the pandemic had to be halted, no resources were spared. One of the social distancing measures that were introduced before the quarantine regulations had come into force was the requirement that people who arrived from abroad should stay at home and avoid contact with others. As a demonstration of state capacity and performativity, the Uzbek police force was mobilised to ensure that the rule was followed. In some cases, local police officers were patrolling in front of the homes of the arrivals, making sure there was no outside contract with these people. The story told to Mirzokhid by a man who had travelled to Andijan from one of the EU countries at the beginning of March to visit his parents is indicative both of state presence and its absence (Cf. Heathershaw 2014):

> Two weeks after my arrival, a group of local officials came to our place and said that I would have to stay at home for another two weeks. I said it didn't make sense, but they were adamant that I should follow the rules. They tested me for COVID-19 after two weeks, but the sample was lost, and I was made to wait another two weeks.[17]

Looking into government measures of spring 2020 in hindsight, it becomes clear that the drive towards performativity would commonly override common sense. While this phenomenon was by no means unique to Uzbekistan – governments around the world reacted to real or imagined popular pressure to demonstrate that they were doing all they could to halt the spread of the pandemic within their borders – the government's hasty and contradictory measures generated major confusion on the grassroots level. A 60-year-old doctor in a local health station in Chirchiq near Tashkent told Mirzokhid that her everyday trip to work was made extremely difficult due to the cancellation of all public and private transportation except for those with specific permits. Health stations remained open to the public and people like her who worked there were obviously required to show up. The problem was that due to government restrictions, she was only allowed to drive to work, which was impossible given that she had neither a car nor a driving licence. The only option was to take illegally shared taxis that zigzagged through inter-yard passages and charged exorbitant fees. Although the issue was voiced to local authorities, they had not come up with a better solution.[18]

The Performative State Faces Reality

As disorganised and performative as Uzbekistan's response to COVID-19 was, the swift and decisive health policy measures were effective in the short term. The number of COVID-19 transmissions and COVID-19-related deaths in April–May 2020 was exceptionally low, even compared to other Central Asian countries (Jones and King 2021). However, the measures were in no way sustainable in the long run. The strict limitations on people's movement took a heavy toll on people's livelihoods. Those who suffered the most were the approximately 5.5 million people working in the informal sector of the economy,[19] such as taxi drivers, market vendors, and restaurant workers. Having partially or completely lost their income, they increasingly called for either substantial financial support from the state or the relaxation of mobility restrictions. Although the government had repeatedly considered different support mechanisms (Hoshimov's Economics [Uz. *'Hoshimov Iqtisodiyoti'*] 2020) and received significant financing from the World Bank and the International Monetary Fund (IMF) to fund social welfare programmes and to stimulate its economy, most of Mirzokhid's respondents thought state social support to the population was 'too little, too late'.[20] On the other hand, however, many local officials he encountered seemed to support the government's unwillingness to provide direct cash support to people in need, arguing that such form of support could lead to corruption and laziness.[21]

On 29 April 2020, President Mirziyoyev announced that the epidemiological situation had stabilised and that the quarantine requirements would be gradually relaxed (Mirziyoyev, quoted in Gazeta.uz 2020). Although the restrictions were indeed lifted gradually and cautiously (Jones and King 2021, 200–201), the number of reported cases of COVID-19 started to increase exponentially. The government did not reinstate any new restrictions despite the visible worsening of the situation. It was only in early July 2020 that the government reinstated interregional travel restrictions and banned most large gatherings, particularly weddings (Jones and King 2021, 201). In the spirit of performativity, a new sanitary-epidemiology service was established within the Ministry of Public Health around the same time. The restrictions remained in place until mid-August and through the global 'second wave' of the pandemic in the autumn of 2020.

As one would expect, the worsening of the epidemiological situation was felt on the buzzing level of local public administration. Starting from July 2020, national news outlets started to report cases of senior public servants being hospitalised and dying of COVID-19. However, during his fieldwork, Mirzokhid found out that local officials had a particular approach to hospitalisation. According to them, the right place for senior officials to receive medical care was at the workplace, given their high social status (i.e., doctors come to them rather than the other way around) and the assumption that their presence at work was required for governance to run smoothly. Going to the hospital for treatment was seen as either a lack of commitment and/or weakness and was frowned upon. The only socially acceptable time to be hospitalised was if the official was facing criminal investigation (usually, due to allegations of corruption) and their position was in danger. In this instance, hospitalisation could work as a legal ground for avoiding detention and/or imprisonment. Needless to say, the hyperactive performativity mode combined with the incentive to turn up at work, even if suffering from COVID-19-like symptoms, only accelerated the spread of the pandemic in Uzbekistan.

Conclusion

Since his ascension to power in 2016, President Mirziyoyev sought to promote a picture of a new Uzbekistan, effective and well-governed, both to the Uzbek people and the international community. At the beginning of the COVID-19 pandemic, his government saw the crisis as an opportunity to demonstrate to the world and its citizens that it could indeed effectively deliver results and respond to the health crisis accordingly. In doing so, it could generate legitimacy created by a performance that would in turn be translated into genuine public support regardless of the continued authoritarian mode of governance. Following this logic, one of the first decisions of the government was to form a new commission aimed at drafting a coordinated state response to the public health threat posed by COVID-19. The establishment of the commission was not supposed to improve the procedural legitimacy of the government (it justifiably raised concerns given its unchecked powers), but rather generate performance legitimacy for the government by demonstrating its effectiveness in preventing the spread of the virus.

Although Uzbekistan's swift and decisive response to the pandemic was applauded initially, the grassroots perspective of the government's COVID-19 policy, provided in this chapter, suggests that both the central and local governments prioritised a theatrical, hyperactive, and superficial – a *performative* response – over a substantive (and possible less visible and more cautious) one. In this chapter, we maintain that civil servants are the central actors who act out the performative state on the ground by carrying an excessive workload with little attentiveness to performance in the genuine, efficient sense. What is more, according to one civil servant interviewed by Mirzokhid, most of the quarantine measures were taken in the belief that otherwise it will be difficult to control the people.[22]

The performative state of Uzbekistan can look harmless, but in the context of a rapidly spreading global pandemic, it had real victims. The draconian health policy measures did not consider the variety of people's needs, and when the restrictions were lifted, thousands died of COVID-19.[23] As a result, the population's trust in the state apparatus dipped to a new low, leading to the emergence of new ways of civic activism and community self-help. In contrast to the legitimacy that the authorities in mainland China arguably succeeded in generating thanks to the introduction of its 'zero-COVID-policy' in the spring of 2020, Uzbekistan failed to do so. In this chapter, we have suggested that the core of the issue is in the embedded culture of public administration that prefers a certain impression of performance rather than performance in and of itself.

Notes

1 All of the primary data presented in this chapter was collected by Mirzokhid Karshiev during a field trip to Uzbekistan in March–July 2020, which was made possible with a funding from the European Union's Horizon 2020 research and

innovation programme under the Marie Skłodowska-Curie grant agreement No 824027. Both authors were involved in analysing the data and writing the chapter, yet Kristiina Silvan's contribution to this process was considerably smaller than Mirzokhid Karshiev's.

2 A national holiday celebrating the vernal equinox, the beginning of spring, the new year, and agricultural work.
3 Diary entry on 15 March 2020 in Qarshi.
4 Diary entry on 18 March 2020 in Termiz.
5 Previously, it was a widespread practice to travel from regional centres to rural districts.
6 It is possible that the decision to take the threat posed by COVID-19 seriously was informed by President Mirziyoyev's personal background, given that his father was a doctor who had worked all his life for the prevention, diagnosis, and treatment of tuberculosis in the rural Jizzakh region of Uzbekistan. The 'personal factor' should not be overstated, though. In neighbouring Kazakhstan, anti-COVID-measures were even quicker and harsher despite no medical background of its president Qassym-Jomart Toqaev, whereas in neighbouring Turkmenistan, President Gurbanguly Berdymukhamedov – PhD in Dentistry – claimed against all evidence that the country had managed to keep the virus out completely.
7 Zoom interview on 25 April 2020 in Tashkent.
8 Diary entry on 25 March 2020 in Tashkent.
9 Zoom interview on 16 April 2020 in Tashkent.
10 A phone interview on 25 April 2020 in Tashkent.
11 Face-to-face interview on 27 June 2020 in central Uzbekistan.
12 Face-to-face interview on 12 March 2020 in central Uzbekistan.
13 Face-to-face interview on 18 March 2020 in Surkhondaryo region.
14 Face-to-face interview on 16 March 2020 in Qarshi, southern Uzbekistan.
15 Face-to-face interview on 12 June 2020 in southern Uzbekistan.
16 Online interview on 23 June 2020 in western Uzbekistan.
17 Online interview on 31 March 2020 in Andijon region.
18 Phone interview on 20 April 2020 in Tashkent.
19 The informal sector of the Uzbek economy is very large, paralleling the number of formal employed.
20 Diary entry on 25 April 2020 in Tashkent.
21 Face-to-face interview on 23 March 2020 in southern Uzbekistan, online interview on 20 April in Tashkent.
22 Online interview on 7 April 2020 in Tashkent.
23 Our calculations, based on patchy data from State Statistics Committee data, show that in the month of July to September 2020, there were in average 20,000 monthly deaths, while in the same period of 2019, the average monthly deaths were 12,000.

References

Barabashev, Alexei, and Jeffrey D. Straussman. 2007. "Public service reform in Russia, 19912006." *Public Administration Review* 67, no. 3: 373–382. https://doi.org/10.1111/j.1540-6210.2007.00721.x.

BBC News O'zbek. 2020. "Ўзбекистон, Коронавирус: Мирзиёев Хитой усулини қўлламоқчи." March 24, 2020. https://www.bbc.com/uzbek/world-52004346.

Caron, Jean-François, and Hélène Thibault (eds.). 2022. *Central Asia and the Covid-19 Pandemic*. London: Palgrave Macmillan.

Collins, Kathleen. 2006. *Clan Politics and Regime Transition in Central Asia*. Cambridge: Cambridge University Press. https://doi.org/10.1017/CBO9780511510014.

Cummings, Sally, ed. 2002. *Power and Change in Central Asia*. London: Routledge. https://www.taylorfrancis.com/books/e/9780203166918.

Dimitrov, Martin K. 2023. *Dictatorship and Information: Authoritarian Regime Resilience in Communist Europe and China*. New York: Oxford University Press.

Ding, Iza. 2020. "Performative Governance." *World Politics* 72, no. 4: 525–556. https://doi.org/10.1017/S0043887120000131.

Ding, Iza. 2022. *The Performative State: Public Scrutiny and Environmental Governance in China*. Cornell University Press. https://doi.org/10.1515/9781501760396.

Dzhuraev, Shairbek. 2021. "The Corona Pandemic in Central Asia." *Between peace and conflict in the East and the West: Studies on transformation and development in the OSCE region*, 279–285. https://library.oapen.org/bitstream/handle/20.500.12657/50420/1/978-3-030-77489-9.pdf#page=280.

Gazeta.uz. 2020. "«Принимаемые карантинные меры оправданы и своевременны» — Нурмат Атабеков." March 17, 2020. https://www.gazeta.uz/ru/2020/03/17/nurmat-atabekov/.

Gel'man, Vladimir. 2017. "Political foundations of bad governance in Post-Soviet Eurasia: Towards a research agenda." *East European Politics* 33, no. 4: 496–516. https://doi.org/10.1080/21599165.2017.1348350.

Gerschewski, Johannes. 2013. "The three pillars of stability: Legitimation, repression, and co-optation in autocratic regimes." *Democratization* 20, no. 1: 13–38. https://doi.org/10.1080/13510347.2013.738860.

Gleason, Gregory. 1997. *The Central Asian States: Discovering Independence*. Boulder, CO: Westview Press.

Gupta, Akhil. 1995. "Blurred boundaries: The discourse of corruption, the culture of politics, and the imagined state." *American Ethnologist* 22, no. 2: 375–402.

Guriev, Sergei, and Daniel Treisman. 2019. "Informational autocrats." *The Journal of Economic Perspectives* 33, no. 4: 100–127.

Guriev, Sergey, and Daniel Treisman. 2022. *Spin Dictators: The Changing Face of Tyranny in the 21st Century*. Princeton and Oxford: Princeton University Press. https://press.princeton.edu/books/hardcover/9780691211411/spin-dictators.

Hale, Henry E. 2014. *Patronal Politics: Eurasian Regime Dynamics in Comparative Perspective. Problems of International Politics*. Cambridge: Cambridge University Press. https://doi.org/10.1017/CBO9781139683524.

Heathershaw, John, 2014. "The Global Performance State: A Reconsideration of the Central Asian "Weak State"", *Ethnographies of the State in Central Asia: Performing Politics*, edited by Johan Rasanayagam, Judith Beyer, and Madeleine Reeves, 29–54. Bloomington: Indiana University Press.

Heurlin, Christopher. 2016. *Responsive Authoritarianism in China: Land, Protests, and Policy Making*. Cambridge: Cambridge University Press. https://doi.org/10.1017/CBO9781316443019.

Hoshimov's Economics («Hoshimov Iqtisodiyoti»). 2020. Jamshid Qo'chqorov va Timur Ishmetov: Pandemiyaning Iqtisodiyotga Ta'siri. https://www.youtube.com/watch?v=cwx9e9F4J40.

Ilkhamov, Alisher. 2007. "Neopatrimonialism, interest groups and patronage networks: The impasses of the governance system in Uzbekistan." *Central Asian Survey* 26, no. 1: 65–84. https://doi.org/10.1080/02634930701423491.

Isaacs, Rico. 2014. "Neopatrimonialism and beyond: Reassessing the Formal and Informal in the Study of Central Asian Politics." *Contemporary Politics* 20, no. 2: 229–245. https://doi.org/10.1080/13569775.2014.907989.

Jones Luong, Pauline. 2002. *Institutional Change and Political Continuity in Post-Soviet Central Asia: Power, Perceptions, and Pacts*. Cambridge: Cambridge University Press. https://doi.org/10.1017/CBO9780511510199.

Jones, Pauline, and Elizabeth J. King. 2021. "Covid-19 response in Central Asia: A Cautionary Tale." *Coronavirus Politics: The Comparative Politics and Policy of COVID-19*, edited by Scott L. Greer, Elizabeth J. King, Elize Massard da Fonseca, and André Peralta-Santos, 196–212. Ann Arbor: University of Michigan Press.

Kissas, Angelos. 2020. "Performative and ideological populism: The case of charismatic leaders on Twitter." *Discourse & Society* 31, no. 3: 268–284.

Kun.uz. 2020a. "Ўзбекистонда карантин чоралари: Асосий маълумотлар." March 15, 2020. https://kun.uz/news/2020/03/15/ozbekiston-karantinda-asosiy-malumotlar.

Kun.uz. 2020b. "Вирус кириб келиши, Хитойдан кутилаётган ёрдам ва карантин шароитлари. Эксперт билан суҳбат." March 19, 2020. https://kun.uz/news/2020/03/19/virus-kirib-kelishi-xitoydan-kutilayotgan-yordam-va-karantin-sharoitlari-ekspert-bilan-suhbat.

Kun.uz. 2020c. "Коронавирусга қарши курашга йўналтирилган пул маблағлари сарфи бўйича текширув ҳамда процессуал ҳаракатлар назоратга олинди - агентлик." August 28, 2020. https://kun.uz/news/2020/08/28/koronavirusga-qarshi-kurashga-yonaltirilgan-pul-mablaglari-sarfi-boyicha-tekshiruv-hamda-protsessual-harakatlar-nazoratga-olindi-agentlik.

Laruelle, Marlene. 2012. "Discussing neopatrimonialism and patronal presidentialism in the Central Asian context." *Demokratizatsiya* 20, no. 4: 301–324.

Laruelle, Marlene, et al. 2020. "Pandemic Politics in Eurasia: Roadmap for a New Research Subfield." *Problems of PostCommunism* 68, no. 1: 1–16. https://doi.org/10.1080/10758216.2020.1812404

Ledeneva, Alena V. 1998. *Russia's Economy of Favours: Blat, Networking and Informal Exchange. Cambridge Russian, Soviet and Post-Soviet Studies*. Cambridge: Cambridge University Press. https://www.cambridge.org/gb/academic/subjects/sociology/political-sociology/russias-economy-favours-blat-networking-and-informal-exchange.

Ledeneva, Alena V. 2007. *How Russia Really Works: The Informal Practices That Shaped Post-Soviet Politics and Business. Culture and Society after Socialism*. Ithaca, NY: Cornell University Press. https://www.cornellpress.cornell.edu/book/9780801473524/how-russia-really-works/.

Ledeneva, Alena V. 2013. *Can Russia Modernise?: Sistema, Power Networks and Informal Governance*. Cambridge: Cambridge University Press. https://doi.org/10.1017/CBO9780511978494.

Lemon, Edward. 2019. "Mirziyoyev's Uzbekistan: Democratization or Authoritarian Upgrading?" *Central Asia Papers*. Foreign Policy Research Institute. https://www.fpri.org/wp-content/uploads/2019/06/lemonrpe4.pdf.

Lewis, David. 2012. "Understanding the authoritarian state: Neopatrimonialism in Central Asia." *The Brown Journal of World Affairs* 19, no. 1: 115–126.

Lex.uz, 2017. "УП-5185-Сон 08.09.2017. Об Утверждении Концепции Административной Реформы в Республике Узбекистан." August 9, 2017. https://www.lex.uz/docs/3331176.

Lex.uz. 2019. "ПФ-5814-Сон 09.09.2019. Ўзбекистон Республикаси Санитария-Эпидемиология Хизмати Тизимини Тубдан Такомиллаштириш Чора-Тадбирлари Тўғрисида." September 9, 2019. https://lex.uz/uz/docs/4504360.

Lex.uz. 2020. Ф-5537-Сон 29.01.2020. Ўзбекистон Республикасига Коронавируснинг Янги Тури Кириб Келиши Ва Тарқалишининг Олдини Олиш Юзасидан

Чора-Тадбирлар Дастурини Тайёрлаш Бўйича Республика Махсус Комиссиясини Ташкил Этиш Тўғрисида. https://lex.uz/docs/4720398.

Liebert, Saltanat, Stephen E. Condrey, and Dmitriy Goncharov, eds. 2013. *Public Administration in Post-Communist Countries: Former Soviet Union, Central and Eastern Europe, and Mongolia.* Public Administration and Public Policy 170. Routledge. https://www.routledge.com/Public-Administration-in-Post-Communist-Countries-Former-Soviet-Union/Liebert-Condrey-Goncharov/p/book/9781439861370.

Migdal, Joel Samuel. 2001. *State in Society: Studying How States and Societies Transform and Constitute One Another.* Cambridge: Cambridge University Press. https://doi.org/10.1017/CBO9780511613067.

Migdal, Joel Samuel, Atul Kohli, and Vivienne Shue, eds. 1994. *State Power and Social Forces: Domination and Transformation in the Third World.* Cambridge: Cambridge University Press. https://doi.org/10.1017/CBO9781139174268.

Moffitt, Benjamin. 2016. "The performative turn in the comparative study of populism." *Political Studies* 41, no. 1: 3–23.

Offe, Claus, and Pierre Adler. 1991. "Capitalism by democratic design? Democratic theory facing the triple transition in East Central Europe." *Social Research* 58, no. 4: 865–892.

Omelicheva, Mariya Y. 2016. "Authoritarian legitimation: Assessing discourses of legitimacy in Kazakhstan and Uzbekistan." *Central Asian Survey* 35, no. 4: 481–500. https://doi.org/10.1080/02634937.2016.1245181.

Owen, Catherine. 2020. "Participatory authoritarianism: From bureaucratic transformation to civic participation in Russia and China." *Review of International Studies* 46, no. 4: 415–434. https://doi.org/10.1017/S0260210520000248.

Perlman, Bruce J., and Gregory Gleason. 2007. "Cultural determinism versus administrative logic: Asian values and administrative reform in Kazakhstan and Uzbekistan." *International Journal of Public Administration* 30, nos. 12–14: 1327–1342. https://doi.org/10.1080/01900690701229475.

Radnitz, Scott B. 2010. *Weapons of the Wealthy: Predatory Regimes and Elite-Led Protests in Central Asia.* Ithaca, NY: Cornell University Press. https://www.cornellpress.cornell.edu/book/9780801466144/weapons-of-the-wealthy/.

Rasanayagam, Johan. 2011. "Informal economy, informal state: The case of Uzbekistan." *International Journal of Sociology and Social Policy* 31, nos. 11/12: 681–696. https://doi.org/10.1108/01443331111177878.

Schmelzle, Cord, and Eric Stollenwerk. 2018. "Virtuous or vicious circle? Governance effectiveness and legitimacy in areas of limited statehood." *Journal of Intervention and Statebuilding* 12, no. 4: 449–467. https://doi.org/10.1080/17502977.2018.1531649.

Shih, Victor. 2021. "China's Leninist response to COVID-19." In *Coronavirus Politics. The Comparative Politics and Policy of Covid-19,* edited by Scott L. Greer, Elizabeth J. King, Elize Massard da Fonseca, and André Peralta-Santos, 67–85. Ann Arbor: University of Michigan Press.

Soest, Christian von, and Julia Grauvogel. 2017. "Identity, procedures and performance: How authoritarian regimes legitimize their rule." *Contemporary Politics* 23, no. 3: 287–305. https://doi.org/10.1080/13569775.2017.1304319.

The Economist. 2019. "Which Nation Improved the Most in 2019?," December 21, 2019. https://www.economist.com/leaders/2019/12/21/which-nation-improved-the-most-in-2019.

Urinboyev, Rustamjon. 2014. "Is There an Islamic Public Administration Legacy in Post-Soviet Central Asia? An ethnographic study of everyday Mahalla life in rural Ferghana, Uzbekistan." *Halduskultuur – Administrative Culture* 15, no. 2: 157–178.

UzDaily.uz. 2016. "Народные приемные Президента будут созданы в Узбекистане". *UzDaily.uz*. December 29, 2016. http://www.uzdaily.uz/ru/post/31012

Voslenky, Michael. 1984. *Nomenklatura: The Soviet Ruling Class*. New York: DoubleDay.

White, Stephen. 1986. "Economic performance and communist legitimacy." *World Politics* 38, no. 3: 462–482. https://doi.org/10.2307/2010202.

World Bank. 2011. *World Development Report 2011: Conflict, Security, and Development*. https://doi.org/10.1596/978-0-8213-8439-8.

Zeng, Jinghan. 2014. "The debate on regime legitimacy in China: Bridging the wide gulf between Western and Chinese scholarship." *Journal of Contemporary China* 23, no. 88: 612–635. https://doi.org/10.1080/10670564.2013.861141.

Index

Note: Bold page numbers refer to tables; *italic* page numbers refer to figures.

For Product Safety Concerns and Information please contact our EU
representative GPSR@taylorandfrancis.com Taylor & Francis Verlag GmbH,
Kaufingerstraße 24, 80331 München, Germany

Printed and bound by CPI Group (UK) Ltd, Croydon, CR0 4YY
14/09/2026
02216240-0002